Testimonials

As a nurse-midwife working with women experiencing medically complicated pregnancies, I try to educate women and their families, empower them, grasp onto whatever hope we can find, and navigate the complex medical world into which they have been thrust. Kelly understands, and gives women this support in the form of a comprehensive, practical, honest tome. She's got a great style. This is your sister talking to you. She doesn't mince words. She aims to help the women who have suffered through pregnancy loss and trauma and she succeeds brilliantly!

> —Carol Sudtelgte, M.S., C.N.M.
> Thomas Jefferson University Division
> of Maternal Fetal Medicine

Why Me? is a must-have guide for any woman at risk for a premature birth. Kelly Whitehead has done a brilliant job of addressing all the issues that weigh on the hearts and minds of mothers facing a high-risk pregnancy.

> —Carol Cirulli Lanham, P⊦ᴰ
> *Author, Pregnan*

This 'in-your-face' book provides t⸍   ⸍   ⸍ breaking it down into clear and hon   ⸍ ⸍s it how it is, while being very easy to comprehen⸍   ⸍ard as it can be, when in this situation, to grasp all that is going on, the magnitude of emotions, and the many questions, I truly wish I had this book during my pregnancy and during the time in which we lost our son Tanner. I felt so in the dark. Knowledge is power! Kelly has done an excellent job gathering the information and organizing it. I plan on giving one to my OB, the Labor and Delivery floor, and my Perinatologist!

> —Danah Claridge
> Founder/Creator of the Incompetent Cervix
> Support Forum (http://ic.hobh.org/forums)

DISCARD

DEC

2012

Westminster Public Library
3705 W. 112th Ave.
Westminster, CO 80031
www.westminsterlibrary.org

I LOVE this book and Kelly's 'no-nonsense' approach to dealing with a high-risk pregnancy. Why Me? echoes Sidelines' straightforward method of educating and empowering a woman with pregnancy complications to become the most important member of her medical team. A must read, physicians and midwives should be handing it out along with prenatal vitamins to women at risk!

> —Candace Hurley
> Founder/Executive Director
> Sidelines National Support Network
> (www.sidelines.org)

If a non-medical person wants to get reliable, practical, and understandable information about preterm birth, you now have a source. Kelly Whitehead's new book is a must read for all women in this situation.

> —Daniel OKeeffe, M.D., Maternal Fetal Medicine
> Specialist, Phoenix, Arizona

High-Risk Pregnancy-Why Me? is a book that every woman who is facing this difficult life scenario should have near them at all times. Kelly not only gives accurate and extremely useful information about every aspect of early labor and its' complicated medical maze, but she also gives the reader emotional support. Her voice is comforting, reassuring, and even funny at times. I highly recommend this book to all women faced with early labor and the possibility of a preterm birth.

> —Dianne I. Maroney, RN, MS, CS
> Co-author of *Your Premature Baby and Child*
> (www.premature-infant.com)

This will be one of the only books on the market that tries to address the emotional impact of high-risk pregnancies, such as those complicated by preeclampsia, often an overlooked but important component of healing and preparing for another pregnancy.

> —Eleni Z. Tsigas
> Executive Director, Preeclampsia Foundation
> (www.preeclampsia.org)

HIGH-RISK PREGNANCY–
Why Me?

*Understanding and Managing
a Potential Preterm Pregnancy*

A Medical and
Emotional Guide

by Kelly Whitehead
with Dr. Vincenzo Berghella

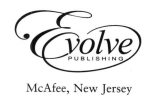

McAfee, New Jersey

Copyright ©2012 by Kelly Whitehead. Printed and bound in the United States of America. All rights reserved. No part of this book may be reproduced or transmitted in any form or by any means, electronic or mechanical, including photocopying, recording, or by an information storage and retrieval system- with the exception of a reviewer who may quote brief passages in a review to be printed in a newspaper or magazine- without written permission from the publisher. For information, contact Evolve Publishing, PO Box 276, McAfee, New Jersey 07428.

This book includes information from many sources, including research abstracts, articles, various reviews, medical texts, opinion pieces, website information, etc., as well as many quotes/commentaries based on personal experiences. It is published for general reference and is not intended to replace consultation and guidance from a medical care provider. The book is sold with the understanding that neither the author nor the publisher is engaged in rendering any medical or psychological advice. The publisher and author disclaim any personal liability, directly or indirectly, for advice or information presented within. Though the author and publisher have prepared this manuscript with utmost care and diligence, and have also made every effort to ensure the accuracy and completeness of the information presented, we assume no responsibility for errors, inaccuracies, omissions, or inconsistencies.

Library of Congress Control Number: 2011926580

ISBN: 978-0-9832647-4-3

Printed in the United States of America

ATTN: QUANTITY DISCOUNTS ARE AVAILABLE TO YOUR COMPANY, CHARITY, HOSPITAL, PRACTICE, OR EDUCATIONAL INSTITUTION for reselling, educational purposes, patient education resources, subscription incentives, gifts, or fundraising campaigns.

For more information, please contact the publisher at:

EVOLVE PUBLISHING
PO Box 276
McAfee, New Jersey 07428
orders@hrpwhyme.com

For more information and ordering visit: www.hrpwhyme.com

Dedication

To our angels who grew their wings too soon:
you will always be remembered
and live forever in our hearts.
We will treasure the memories of your short stay here
on Earth for eternity.
(Ashton John Whitehead, February 12, 2004)

For those who come too soon:
keep that "preemie fire" burning,
fight the fight.

For the families living in fear, who are scared,
anxious, or starting parenthood in the NICU...
Hang in there and keep up hope!

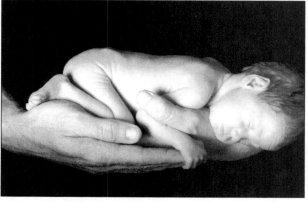

*Baby Kaiyah was born two-and-a-half months early.
She suffered a severe brain hemorrhage and wasn't
supposed to survive, yet here she is. I find this picture
to be truly inspiring, and I hope you will, too.*

Acknowledgements

To my kids for showing me a love I never thought possible, making everything to get them here well worth the struggle, stress, and tears. (Okay, so I still wish it would've been easier; I won't lie.) For my husband for dealing with me (somewhat) throughout the writing and obsessing to complete this book. I owe him for everything he had to do for me on the many, many months of bed rest and "out-of-commission time" to bake our babies. The laundry, shopping, cooking, cleaning toilets, dealing with the stress, my constant depression and an ocean full of tears, not to mention becoming a born-again virgin not once, but two times over. To my parents, family, and friends—you know who you are—for the support after the loss of my son and through the difficult times to bear my children.

Now on to the people who helped me to put together this book and gave me tips on how to write a good book. (Hey, I never wrote anything longer than a few pages before this.) To Peter Bowerman (www.wellfedwriter.com), for showing me the ropes and his hard-ass approach; I appreciate and learned more from our discussions than I ever thought possible. To my designer, Chris at DiNatale Designs (www.dinataledesign.com), for her beautiful cover and all her insights into the business. To Amy for her help on two of the most emotionally difficult chapters of this book to write. Your insights as a mom who has experienced losses made these chapters better so they could help others. Of course, a huge thanks to my Aussie editor, Geoff. All I can say is, "Couldn't have been easy dealing with a newbie like me." Thanks for all your patience. To my interior book designer, Marian, I can't thank you enough for your talent, experience, and guidance. Also, to Linda for her chart designs and her design insights. A huge thanks to Anthony Ziccardi Studios (www. aziccardi.com) for capturing memories, taking beautiful pictures of my children, and of couse, for a great cover picture. You have a way of making me look awesome. I always have fun and laughs at our 'sessions.'

There are not enough kind words for all the ladies who spilled their hearts out and shed many tears to write their stories in order to give hope to other families going down this road. (Even those that, due to space, could not be included in this book. These will be posted on the website.) Thanks to all the women who contributed to this book to make it a thousand times better with their words of hope, advice, wisdom, tips, and understanding about managing a difficult pregnancy. You guys are the best.

Finally, to Dr. Berghella, for agreeing to be part of a project by someone who was "just" a determined mom. I'm so grateful you took a chance to work with me. You've dedicated your life to helping women like us and our babies...we can't thank you enough.

Table of Contents

Foreword

Just as you are reading this line, one baby has died of being born too early. There are over 10 million babies born prematurely in the world every year. Preterm birth represents one of the leading causes of "years of life lost," because it kills babies just as they are born, preventing a whole life of 80-plus years. In terms of years of life lost, as important as or more so than, cancer or cardiac disease.

Kelly Whitehead has experienced preterm birth herself. She has educated herself on this complex topic and now is sharing her knowledge with you, from both a medical and an emotional point of view.

Often medical books, including some of the ones I have written, are too complex for the public to digest. We write them for our physician and nursing colleagues. Educating the women who actually are, or can become, pregnant and those who are at risk for, or experience, preterm birth is just as important, if not more. Kelly valiantly, with clear and frank language, goes through the main issues related to preterm birth.

I hope this text enlightens everyone—not only reproductive-age women but also their partners, health care workers, researchers, politicians, and the public at large—regarding how to best prevent preterm birth and give a healthy future to our next generations.

—Vincenzo Berghella

Introduction

Here I am, watching my daughter graduate from preschool. For me this is a lot more than just a childhood ritual. I'm on the verge of tears, hiding them from those around me. My tears are those of extreme gratefulness, thankfulness, and absolute happiness.

There are things that happen to you that forever change your life, how you view the world, and the path you take. This happened to me one terrible day in 2004, when I lost my son at 22 weeks of pregnancy. The innocence of carrying and birthing a child was then lost to me forever.

Over five years ago I wasn't sure that my baby would be born alive, never mind become a healthy, energetic, sweet, loving kid. Almost every day I'm reminded how lucky I am to be blessed with both my children. At 21 weeks I hoped every day that I would make it to 24 weeks. At 24 weeks the doctors urged me to shoot for 28 weeks. Beating the odds, there she was, born at term with the build of a football player. The biggest neck of a newborn you've ever seen. Here was the baby we thought wouldn't make it, weighing in at almost nine pounds.

Babies, who many believe have little chance of surviving, never mind making it to term or near term, defy the odds every day. This could be your baby...so **never** give up hope.

You won the lottery, only this lottery isn't the good kind. This isn't the one that allows you to live it up and let go of all your worries. This lottery is the chance of having your baby early. When considering all child-bearing women, the majority have normal pregnancies, free of all the extra worries that go along with a high-risk pregnancy. Not us.

After the loss of my son, I struggled to find answers to my questions and clarity on what to expect in any future pregnancies. When you're at risk for having your baby early, there are many, many unknowns and lots of stuff to figure out. After becoming annoyed at my inability to find information written for me, I became determined to help other women down this difficult road. I'm really just like you—nothing special, just someone who wanted to help others have better pregnancies.

The book is broken up by subject in an attempt to make it an easy reference tool to help you through this experience physically, medically, and emotionally. Provided within each chapter are years of research I've done looking at many, many studies and reviews. The goal is for you to be as knowledgeable and informed as your providers are, or as close to it as you can get.

At times this can get heavy and hard to digest. I understand this, but I feel that it's important for this information to be made available. If you want to read it—great. If you're not ready, that's okay too. Skip it! There's a lot to consider…that I know.

I've also included a large selection of quotes, tips, and stories from women on their journeys to motherhood. Some of these, too, can be difficult to read—expect a few tear-jerkers. But the take-home message is that we've made it to have healthy babies, and you can too. Making it through a difficult pregnancy isn't easy, but it can be done, and actually it is done everyday by women just like you.

Throughout the book you will notice text boxes that contain the summaries of what are called "Cochrane Reviews." A Cochrane review is the medical world's platinum standard (not even gold, but better). These reviews look at and summarize the findings of all the highest quality studies on that particular topic, i.e., randomized, controlled studies.

You'll also notice little superscript numbers. These, for those of you who aren't sure, are the reference, to the particular research article, study, website, or quote. If you look at the end of each chapter you will see the full reference should you want to look further at this topic or piece of work.

Many of the scientists, researchers, and doctors who are referenced have spent a large portion of their lives looking into the whole spectrum of stuff covered within. I thank them for all their dedication and efforts to help us to have healthier babies.

I know more often than not, as shown throughout, that the research tends to open a can full of 'unknowns.' More doors are opened, and more questions arise. The knowledge of these conditions, the human body as a whole, and especially the processes that lead to an early delivery is an evolution of understanding. Hopefully, in time, all the research will come full circle, and solid answers will be known. Currently, there's still much that is not well understood.

This book has two main goals: 1) to educate you, and 2) for you to take away the fact that there is hope and you can do this! You're not alone. What you're feeling is normal. You are going to be okay ... seriously.

There were many sections that triggered very difficult memories and feelings within me while writing this book. At times I couldn't stop my tears, and I've literally poured my heart into this with the hope that it will help someone else going through these tough times. Ladies, if I've made it here ... so can you.

My heart goes out to all of you in the midst of a difficult pregnancy, dealing with the reality of a premature baby, or grieving the loss of your precious angel. My only advice is to hang in there. Times will get better.

This book was born from the worst experience and period of my life. I hope you find it to be helpful and that it gives you the strength, courage, and hope to keep moving forward.

Even though much of this book talks about "risk" and "chance" and all that stuff, please keep this very important bit of advice close to you:

> *"Remember that statistics and risks are tricky things. Even if your risk of something is high, like 1 in 5, that still means that 4 women out of those 5 were fine and you are no more likely to be that 1 than those other 4. Doctors love risks and statistics— while they help you make important medical decisions, they don't really speak to what a specific individual will experience. And one last piece of advice: if possible, try to enjoy your pregnancy. It's so easy to get caught up in the anxiety and what-ifs, and you may even want to distance yourself from the emotions. You deserve to enjoy your pregnancy as much as anyone else."*
> ~ Liz, Massachusetts (awesome words of wisdom)

"I never thought I'd be a mother to a sleeping child, and I hate that I'm not the only one, but I'm glad I'm not alone."
~ Courtney, Ohio

For more information, resources, a glossary of terms, stories, and advice, or to order books, please visit my website at www.hrpwhyme.com. The research surrounding preterm birth, the conditions leading to early babies, treatments, etc. are constantly changing as new studies are being added to the existing literature. To stay on top of what's happening, see the website under the 'New Research' page. A portion of all profits will go to charities dedicated to helping women and babies in the fight against prematurity and related causes. If you would like to donate, this can also be done through my website.

—Kelly Whitehead

PART I

CHAPTER 1

An Early Baby Can't Happen to Me... Can It?

What is preterm birth? Why is it on the rise? And why are the causes still mostly unknown? Thirty-seven weeks of pregnancy is considered a full-term pregnancy, so a preterm birth is when your baby is born prior to this gestation. This can be confusing, because your pregnancy clock starts ticking on the presumed day of ovulation, or the release of the egg, not when you technically become pregnant (i.e., sperm meets egg).

Thirty-seven weeks wasn't always the magic cut-off to define a preterm birth. In 1950, the World Health Organization (WHO) defined prematurity as a birth weight of 2,500 g (5.5 pounds) or less, but then in 1961 changed it to mean a gestation period of less than 37 weeks.[1]

Preterm birth is a major problem for those within the field who care for pregnant women. Early birth leads to between 60 and 80 percent of all neonatal deaths.[2] Importantly, the actual survival rate of these babies depends on where you live. If you live in a poor country or region with no access to decent facilities, your baby is not going to get the care he or she needs. Is this right? No, but unfortunately this is how our world works. More money = better care.

According to *Preterm Birth: Prevention and Management*, more than $26 billion was spent in the U.S. on medical care, educational assistance, and other expenses associated with preterm birth in only one year.[3] That's a lot of money, which, being the U.S., we have more of than most other countries. However, the ability to handle preemies also varies by region, even within the U.S. A wealthy suburban area will be able to offer better care than a rural setting, where the closest hospital might be 50 miles away; think areas like Kansas or Maine.

When it became apparent that I might not make it to full term, my doctors had me aim for 32 weeks. Babies born at 32 weeks in the U.S. where I live do very well—almost as well as full-term babies—but it's not uncommon for a 32-weeker born to a mom who lives in a poor or developing country, as they are known, to have barely a chance of survival.[3] That's quite a striking difference, and very sad. Think about the poor moms who can do nothing to save their babies, when they would have been fine if only they'd lived elsewhere. It hardly seems fair, and so I guess I realize how lucky I am.

The unfortunate reality is that preterm birth is also the main cause of infant illness and death in developed countries (think the U.S., Canada, Australia, and Italy, for example). Unfortunately, this is a puzzle that has yet to be completely solved. There are numerous factors and pathways that initiate or lead to preterm birth. These can be uncontrollable things, such as your genetics or environment, or problems related to the actual development of your baby. Preterm birth can also occur as a result of your age or socioeconomic status, or through smoking or drug use.[3]

Sure, there are known ways to help reduce the chances of an early birth, and even treatments to control or keep contractions at bay, but it's by no means an exact science. Often, our doctors just don't know. They can make assumptions, tell you the facts, and provide you with the scary numbers, but really they don't, and can't, know what will happen to you with complete certainty. They don't know for sure how your body or baby will react along the way, and they don't have a crystal ball to enable them to see your future or to know when your baby will actually arrive.

Even though doctors are never absolutely sure how things will turn out, always remember, miracles happen every day. Even if you give birth prematurely, your baby *can still* have the chance of a good life.

The effectiveness of many of the treatments for prevention of early birth, like cerclages, bed rest, or tocolytics (these will all be discussed in detail later) is still largely unknown, unproven, or unclear.

Even though thousands of research studies exist on the issues surrounding preterm birth, there's still much that is unknown, and even more information that falls into hazy, gray areas. Researchers who dedicate their lives to seeking answers are, in some cases, no closer to finding the answers than they were a decade ago.

A lot of information has been discovered over recent years. For those of us who are high risk, there are many strategies and interventions to screen for and help prevent preterm birth, including: 17Alpha-Hydroxyprogesterone Caproate (17P) to reduce early birth, low-dose aspirin for preeclampsia or IUGR, ultrasound-indicated cerclage or progesterone for a short cervix, antibiotics for bacterial infections, and fetal fibronectin testing.[3] Each of these is discussed at length, and then some, later on.

According to one author, "Fetal fibronectin testing and endovaginal ultrasonography for cervical length are useful for triage." Additionally, it has been shown that "for the patient in preterm labor, only antenatal corticosteroids and delivery in a facility with a level III neonatal intensive care unit have been shown to improve outcomes consistently."[4]

I wish I could provide you with concrete answers for everything. I thought I'd easily be able to do this, until I actually read all the stuff out there in the course of educating myself, and it's extremely frustrating to realize that I can't. The thing is, if I've had a hard enough time over the past four years deciphering all the information that's available, how can the average time-crunched doc running a small local obstetrics practice figure it all out?

That's why I've written this book—to help those of you who are going through, or are about to go through, this very challenging, grueling, and anxiety-ridden marathon. It's for those of you who are trying to understand what's happening, what you're likely in for, and how to make the best decisions for both you and your baby.

What Does Being High Risk Really Mean?

You can be labeled high risk for any number of reasons. As I've said before, and I'll say again a hundred times...just because you are "high risk" doesn't necessarily mean you will deliver early. You just fall into the category of women who are more likely to develop issues and/or deliver before term. You should take some comfort from the fact that in several studies that looked at high-risk women, only around 20% actually delivered early. (These are referenced throughout the book.)

There are lots of resources out there that skim over, or even outline in detail, the many aspects of a high-risk pregnancy. These can also be great references that you may choose to explore, and some even extend beyond the scope of this book, covering topics like caring for a preemie baby or focusing solely on bed rest or nutrition. I've provided more information on my website, www.hrpwhyme.com, should you be interested in other resources.

Why Me? is different from all the other high-risk pregnancy books I have looked at, in that this book is focused solely on those conditions that commonly lead to a premature delivery. I did not attempt to cover topics like gestational diabetes, blood incompatibilities, kidney, heart, or liver diseases, and many other diseases/issues that can also lead to high-risk pregnancies. Instead, the focus of this book is quite narrow. If you've had a preemie, suffered a second-trimester loss, or think you may have a preemie, then this is the book for you. It has been written to provide coverage of thoroughly researched topics, giving you much of the same scientific and medical knowledge that your doctors are reading in their journals and then applying and using in their practices.

I wrote it because, after my 22+ week loss, I was searching for more information everywhere, specifically on an incompetent cervix (IC), and I couldn't find more than a few paragraphs that merely skimmed the surface of what I needed to know. I wasn't happy just reading that IC is a condition where the cervix is too weak to carry a baby to term, and that typically a cerclage is used to treat it. I wanted, *needed*, to know more. What is a cerclage, exactly? Is it truly effective? What are the risks of a cerclage? What are the infection rates? What are my options if a cerclage fails? Can I actually have a healthy baby?

For those of you struggling with a high-risk pregnancy and the very scary reality of maybe having a preterm and/or very sick baby, I hope to answer these questions and many more. Hang in there; it's a long, rough road, but this road can end in happiness, in the form of a healthy child. You just have to endure the ride in order to get there.

For a small percentage of you, yes, your baby will come too soon, and for some, the worst will happen, and your baby will die. For others, however, your baby may be sick but will eventually make a full recovery and thrive. Remember, the numbers are on our side. You're more likely to have a healthy baby than not.

Rates and Risk Factors

Sadly, I learned that the preterm birth rates in the U.S. are much higher than in Canada and other industrialized countries, 10.1% vs. 1.0% in 2002 according to one source.[5] Another source states that in 2005 the rate was 12.7% of all U.S. births that year, compared to a rate of only 5.9% in other developed countries.[4] The largest number of preterm births is seen in Africa and in the U.S. Yikes! What does this say? And the rate has been on the rise, too. A large increase has been observed in the U.S. over the last two and a half decades, from 9.5% to 12.7%.[3] The Centers for Disease Control and Prevention (CDC) notes that there has been a slight two-year decline in the rates for the first time in 30 years. (With a rate of 12.3% in 2008.)[6]

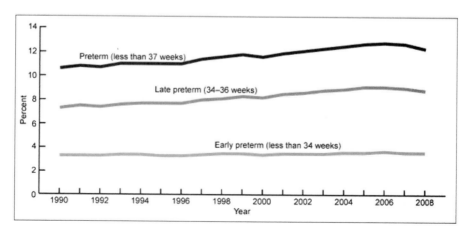

Figure 1-1. Preterm births rates: United States, final 1990–2006 and preliminary 2007 and 2008. *Source: CDC/NCHS, National Vital Statistics System.*

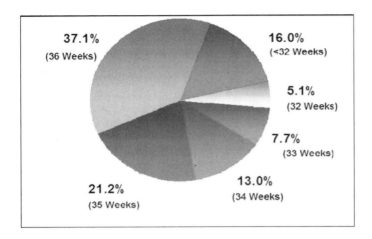

Figure 1-2. Spread of early births in the U.S.: 2003. (About 5% of all early births occur at less than 28 weeks, and about 12% occur at between 28 and 31 weeks.[3]) *Diagram Courtesy of March of Dimes.*[7]

The increase in early births in many developed countries, like the U.S., is largely due to early inductions and C-sections as a result of concern for either the mother's or the baby's welfare, known as medically indicated preterm birth or "close to term" preterm birth. This includes induction for reasons like preeclampsia/eclampsia, hemorrhage, nonreassuring fetal heart rate, or intrauterine growth restriction.[8]

The climbing rate is also caused by the increase of early births of multiples in "assisted" pregnancies, like *in-vitro* fertilization (IVF).[9] Older mommas-to-be also play a role in this increase.[3]

Could part of this phenomenon also be due, in part, to our "sue-happy" culture and our doctors' fear of being sued? I suspect the answer to that is "Yes." Doctors have been forced to become extra careful in covering their asses, including jumping in to deliver a baby just to be "safe." Nonetheless, reducing preterm birth is one of the top challenges facing obstetricians today.

It's estimated that about one-third of early births are due to early inductions/C-sections because of indications that either the mother or the baby is at risk. From 1990 to 2006, the late preterm birth rate in the U.S.—i.e., babies born between 34 and 36 weeks—rose by a whopping 20%. This means an average of 900 late preterm babies born every day. That's 900 babies with potential prematurity-related problems.[10]

As one review article concludes, "Research is needed to determine risks and benefits of induction for many commonly advocated clinical indications."[11] This raises the question of whether current practices are doing the right thing by bringing these babies into the world before they're ready.

Given the large increase in medically indicated late preterm births, one would presume that reducing this number would help to prevent many unnecessary illnesses associated with preemie babies. Maybe doctors need to be less hasty in inducing? It's a tough area, though, because even one baby saved is worth it to the family concerned. Now you can see the complexity of the issues surrounding preterm birth.

Of course, for many, there is always the cost to be considered. We all know that the cost of care for a preemie, especially a micro-preemie, is staggering. For the tiniest of babies, this cost can run into the millions for each baby. As mothers, fathers, and families, however, we couldn't care less about the cost of life-saving care for our babies. Understandably, there has been much analysis and debate in the medical and insurance communities over these costs.

In one study that looked at determining "cost-effective" strategies, they stated that, "In symptomatic women with a viable pregnancy, indomethacin [a tocolytic, which will be addressed in a later chapter] without prior testing was a potentially cost-effective strategy to prevent preterm birth occurring before 37 weeks."[12]

I have to admit that this chain of thinking scares the hell out of me. What if they find a miracle "cure" for preterm birth that happens to cost a ton of money? Will people push to have it blocked or offered only to the select few because of the cost? Is there really a price tag on the lives of our babies? I don't think so. The experiences I have had with my kids are worth more than 10 million dollars, and to take that away from even one family would be wrong.

The ethics of prematurity—not just the costs, but the actual ethical arguments of how small is too small, and what is termed "the fringes of viability," meaning the shortest gestation in which a baby can survive and still have a quality of life—is a topic of great debate and will be discussed in more detail in a later chapter.

The rate of prematurity increases dramatically with the number of babies carried: 10% of single babies are born prematurely, while for twins it is 54.9% and for triplets 93.6%.[13] Spontaneous preterm birth [caused by non-medically aided preterm labor or preterm premature rupture of membranes (PPROM)] before 34 weeks gestation occurs in only 37% of all pregnancies.[14] (Read: this is actually quite rare.)

Two-thirds of infant deaths involve babies who are born at less than 37 weeks, with only 17% of deaths actually being classified as caused by prematurity. Some believe there is actually an underreporting of prematurity-caused deaths. Based on this potential disparity, researchers looked at infant deaths in an attempt to more accurately reflect preterm birth as the cause of these deaths.

When they looked at almost 28,000 files, they found that about 34% of these deaths were actually attributed to preterm birth, i.e., double the reported amount. Ninety-five percent of those deaths were in babies born at less than 32 weeks and who weighed less than 1,500 g, or 3.3 pounds, and two-thirds of the deaths occurred within the first 24 hours.[15]

More recent data suggests that over 75% of all newborn deaths are caused by preterm birth. (The other 25% of newborn deaths are caused by infection/disease, malnutrition, etc.) Early birth causes over 50% of ALL infant and long-term illnesses/disabilities.[3]

These numbers are just staggering. Thinking about how many families suffer this terrible loss of their precious baby and are left with broken hearts and shattered dreams saddens me beyond words. Charity programs, such as March of Dimes, and various other research programs and agencies, like the World Health Organization (WHO), are hard at work every day trying to reduce this tragedy. Hopefully, one day a "cure" will be found.

It is estimated that in the U.S. alone, almost 500,000 babies are born prematurely each year. That same number of babies is born prematurely in Europe, and worldwide almost 13 million babies or nearly 10% of all babies born, arrive prematurely. Jaw-dropping numbers if you really think about it.

Most of the babies who are dying are in the poorest of countries, developing countries like India or many of the countries of Africa. The majority of babies who are born early, 85% of them, are being born to moms in Africa and Asia. This is explained simply by considering the vast number of babies being born there compared to elsewhere.[3]

So, why can't we do something to save more of our precious babies? As you will read later, there are tools and treatments that work, so why not use them? There's a simple answer—money. Many countries are unable to afford these tools or treatments to extend pregnancy in many of their undernourished mommas. Add in the need for proper training, facilities, and even just basic access to prenatal care, and you can begin to see how much is needed to solve this problem.

Certain women are at higher risk for preterm delivery, including:[3,16,17, 18, 19, 20, 21, 22, 23, 24, 25, 26, 27, 28, 29, 30, 31, 32]

+ Women with a history of pregnancy loss or preterm birth (*the* #1 risk factor)
+ Women with an incompetent cervix
+ Women with womb abnormalities
+ Women carrying multiple babies
+ Those with a family history of preterm birth (think genetics)
+ Black women (who have an even higher risk if they are underweight or overweight)
+ Obese women with a body mass index of 35 or higher
+ Very skinny ladies with a low body mass index
+ Teens
+ Heavy smokers
+ Those with diabetes mellitus
+ Those taking certain antidepressants
+ Women with periodontal disease
+ The presence of certain bacteria (*Mycoplasma genitalium* or *Ureaplasma* species)
+ Those with Crohn's disease (a gastrointestinal disease)
+ Women experiencing high stress
+ Unemployed women
+ Women with polycystic ovary syndrome (PCOS)
+ Those with a history of cervical surgeries
+ Women with a time frame between pregnancies of less than six months

✦ Those who work more than 80 hours per week or spend long
  periods standing

✦ Heavy drinkers, cocaine, or heroin users

✦ Women with bacterial vaginosis (BV), which is where the natural bacteria in the vagina are disrupted and an overgrowth
  occurs, and maybe even other genital infections like trichomoni-
  asis, chlamydia, syphilis, and gonorrhea

✦ Women whose babies are conceived via IVF

Wow…that's some list. Did you get all that? Looking at that, you
would think almost every woman is high risk. Well, not really, but as
you can see, there are a lot of factors that seem to be contributing to
preterm birth.

A Few More Specifics About Risk Factors[3]

Having already had a preterm birth is the single greatest risk factor for
having another preemie. The risk varies greatly, from around 15% to
a more than 50% chance of an early baby the next time around. Also,
the earlier your baby was born previously, or the more early babies you
have had, the higher the risk of a repeat early birth.

Almost half of all women who have had multiple preterm births
will have their next baby within one week of their previous early deliveries, and an astounding 70% will have their baby within two weeks
of that time. But it's good to know, so you can be prepared. Understand that this is not an absolute, and you can still have a healthy, full-
term baby.

Multiple spontaneous births (due to preterm labor and PPROM)
are believed to be caused by intrauterine infections. Women who suffer from conditions such as diabetes, high blood pressure or obesity are
likely to require medically assisted early deliveries in each pregnancy.
Even here, the risk is still not 100%.

Preterm birth rates in black women are high, at 16–18%, while
white women are at lower rates of 5.9%. Black women are three to
four times more likely to have their babies very early (i.e., between 20
and 24 weeks), in part because of their predisposition to infections.
(See Figure 1-3.[6])

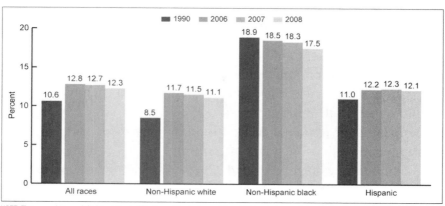

Note: The preterm birth rate is births at less than 37 completed weeks of gestation per 100 births in the specified age group. SOURCE: CDC/NCHS, National Vital Statistics System.

Figure 1-3. Preterm birth rates, by race and Hispanic origin of mother: United States, 1990 and 2006 final and 2007 and 2008 preliminary.

So, does this mean that if you're a black woman who wants a baby, you're doomed? No way. Just find a doctor who is aware of and knowledgeable about your risks, someone who will take the time to assess you and obtain a full history in order to consider your risks completely. In your case, a preventive approach is a good way to go. If I were you, I would expect some swabbing of my nether regions to make sure I didn't have any underlying BV, or other infections. Also, if I had a history of BV, I would discuss my options for preventive antibiotics (hint, hint). Make sense? I hope so.

Anywhere from 11 to 48% of women worldwide have bacterial vaginosis (BV). Genetic factors, douching, being an African-American or Afro-Caribbean, having multiple partners or a new partner, and smoking put you at a higher risk of getting BV. More than half of the women who have this show no symptoms at all. Having it has been linked to as low as a 6% risk and as high as a 49% risk of having your baby early. (This range is dependent on any other risk factors you may have.) Even considering BV as a risk factor for preterm birth, there are many who do not agree on universal screening in pregnant women.

Treatment for all women, even those with no symptoms, is not suggested, because studies have shown no reduction in preterm birth rates in women who were treated versus those who were not treated with antibiotics. Note that this was among symptom-free women. If you have symptoms, go see your doctor; you should be treated, the earlier the better.

Studies have found that treatment of periodontal disease during pregnancy did not reduce the amount of spontaneous preterm deliveries in women with this condition.[33, 34] Another study also found an increased risk of preterm birth and low birth weight babies in unintended, unwanted, or mistimed pregnancies.[35]

Interestingly, women who had polycystic ovary syndrome (PCOS) were found to be more likely to have a preemie baby. The early birth rate was 20% in women with PCOS compared to 6.9% in women without this.[31]

Many have suggested, looked at, or are researching the genetic and environmental factors that can contribute to preterm labor and birth.[4] One study looked at three genes and found that changes in one of those genes (the RLN2 gene) may lead to a genetic susceptibility to a premature baby.[36] So, now your genes and the environment are working against you as well. Will we ever win?

The genetic component of preterm birth is a hot topic and an area of study that is steadily increasing. It is now believed that preterm birth is affected by many genes, both the mama's and the baby's, along with the interactions of our genetics and the environment, including smoking. Some genes that are responsible for problems can affect our connective tissues, like in Ehlers-Danlos syndrome.

Even family genetics may play a role in preterm birth. They found that women who had sisters who had their babies early were more likely to have their babies early, too. They also found that if you have a preemie, you are more likely to have been born a preemie. This risk is far from absolute, though, and you're not doomed to a preterm birth by any stretch of the imagination.

Now let's say you don't have the resources to pick and choose doctors; like so many, you are "stuck" with a particular doctor or group. Maybe you have Medicaid and it's only accepted by certain doctors, or you have very limited doctor choices because of where you live, or you can only afford to go to the local clinic. Then, it is even more important to be aware of your needs and the treatments that are available to ensure that you receive the proper care.

It helps if you can communicate in the doctors' world, using their terms and showing them that you're educated about these things and not to be messed with. It's also a good idea to speak to your providers in a nice tone, in order to participate as a team member—not as an adversary or enemy—in your care. Now, don't laugh. Being nice can go a long way to establishing a good relationship. I have learned that if you can set aside your pride, which I can do easily, a little butt kissing, especially with doctors and nurses, can go a long way.

I have witnessed firsthand that coming across as snotty, bitchy, arrogant, or overly demanding instantly puts them on guard and on the defensive. You're not going to win anyone over or sway someone to your side by being nasty. Think about it. So, please save all of that for when it may be really needed in order to get some attention and care.

Causes Leading to a Premature Baby

When looking at over 1,000 women who delivered their babies before 28 weeks, researchers found that 40% of the babies came early due to preterm labor, 23% due to prelabor premature rupture of membranes, 18% due to preeclampsia, 11% due to placental abruption, 5% due to cervical incompetence, and 3% due to fetal indications/intrauterine growth restriction.

They concluded that the factors leading to a preterm delivery can be split into one group related to intrauterine inflammation/infection, which includes preterm labor, prelabor premature rupture of membranes, placental abruption, and IC, and another group related to abnormalities of the placenta not caused by infection, including preeclampsia, fetal indications, and intrauterine growth restriction.[37] In many women, the exact cause of their preterm birth is unknown.[3]

This book is based on the conditions listed above and seeks to answer the following questions: What are they? What are the risk factors that can cause one to "get" them? (Note: they aren't contagious.) What are my risks? How are they treated, and what treatments are available? What is my chance of having a healthy baby?

Dr. Charles Lockwood, of New York University School of Medicine, describes the paths that, either separately or together, lead to a preterm birth as including: 1) maternal or fetal stress, 2) ascending genital track or systemic infections, which cause the release of inflammatory responses and trigger labor (these include periodontal disease, pneumonia, sepsis, pancreatitis, and even asymptomatic bacterial infections[3]), 3) hemorrhage (which can lead to cervical changes and rupture of your bag of waters), and 4) expansion of the uterus (this is when your uterus stretches to an enormous size like when carrying multiple babies; the more babies, the more stretching, and the earlier you are likely to deliver).[38]

Another article concluded that within the causes of preterm birth, there are essentially two groups, one with chorioamnionitis (inflammation of the fetal membrane's amnion and choriondue to bacterial infection) and placental bacteria recovery (infection of the placenta), which are associated with preterm labor, prelabor premature rupture of membranes, placental abruption, and IC, and the second having no bacterial infection or inflammation component, but having a dysfunctional placenta, which is related to preeclampsia and fetal indication/intrauterine growth restriction.[37]

Preterm births caused by inflammation are more common in black women (likely due to genetics—sorry, ladies), while placental abruption issues are more common in older, married, educated women with other kids, and those with stress-related preterm births who tend to be pregnant for the first time, anxious, or depressed.[3]

You may hear the phrase "placenta-mediated pregnancy complications." This includes preeclampsia, placental abruption, or intrauterine growth restriction. It is estimated that a whopping one in six pregnancies is affected by these conditions, which are the number-one cause of illness or morbidity in both mothers and babies in developed countries like the U.S.[39] Before writing this book, I never realized how common these are. I thought I was the only one.

In later chapters, I break each of these down and provide the research that is currently available. No matter how you say it, experiencing any one of these conditions sucks in a major way. To experience any of these conditions is to pretty much eliminate the ability to have a normal pregnancy. Life as you know it will change, and drastically.

It could involve meds to stop contractions, avoid infection, or control your blood pressure, steroids to speed up lung development, bed rest (even hospital bed rest), numerous ultrasounds, visits to doctors,

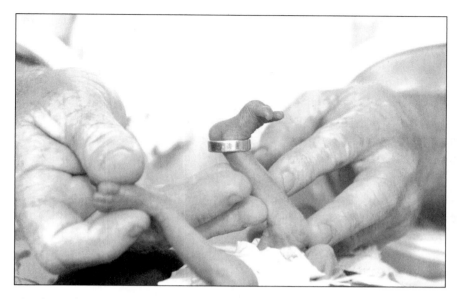

The feet of a tiny micropreemie. Even looking at this picture, it's hard to truly grasp just how small they are. (Yes, that's a wedding band.)

and monitoring (maybe even home monitoring). And this is only concerning the medical side of things. The hardest part is actually the mental anguish and range of emotions you will experience and have to deal with as a result of a difficult pregnancy.

Can Preterm Birth Be Prevented?[3]

The short answer to this question is... kind of. Sure, there's much in preterm birth that neither we as moms-to-be nor the doctors can control, but there are precursors, risk factors, and even limited tests that, yes, can be used to help prevent the early birth of our babies.

According to Dr. Jason Baxter, the author of a chapter on prevention of preterm birth in a medical textbook, one of the main problems is that a lot of the focus and money has been spent on research for treatments. By that time, the complex chain of events that controls preterm birth and leads to the baby being born early has already progressed too far. They have spent too much money on studying things beyond the point of no return, instead of looking at things earlier in the process. Dr. Baxter is stating the obvious: if you are driving at 60 miles an hour and someone slams on the brakes in front of you, and you do the same, only to find that your brakes aren't working, it's too late; you're going to have an accident. If you'd had your car checked and had your brakes fixed before you set out, you could potentially have avoided the accident.

Dr. Baxter believes prevention in all women, either before pregnancy or early in the pregnancy, is the key to successfully reducing preterm births. To him, this is a more effective approach than the one used today.

As he so eloquently puts it, "The United States healthcare system provides perverse incentives, making tertiary care more profitable than primary prevention. More money is made by the healthcare industry on tests, procedures, and drugs for PTB than is made on primary prevention of PTB enacted by policy makers, communities, schools and leaders."[3] That's telling it how it is! Sad, but true.

Some of the strategies presented by Dr. Baxter for prevention include:

- ✦ Education on preterm birth—what it is, what leads to an early birth, how common it is
  Also, better education on:
  - Plain old awareness to reduce pregnancies in teens and in older ladies (both groups have higher preterm birth rates)
  - Increasing the time between pregnancies to 18–24 months, since pregnancies close together are at a higher risk
  - The effects of alcohol, tobacco, and drug use
  - Prevention of sexually transmitted diseases
- ✦ Universal care before pregnancy to help women be in the best of health when they do become pregnant, including counseling on diet, exercise, contraception to avoid unplanned pregnancies, and ideal body mass index
- ✦ Better health policies for women to minimize extreme working conditions, including long hours spent standing or long working hours
- ✦ Reduction in the number of women who have abortions
- ✦ Reduction in multiple gestations by limiting embryo transfers in

assisted pregnancies—i.e., IVF—thereby avoiding
"Octo-mom" scenarios

Realistically, though, how many of these are going to happen? Can you imagine a system providing care for ALL women? It would be great, but the list is idealistic. In a perfect world, all of it would happen and, poof, an overall significant reduction in the preterm birth rate would be seen for the first time in many years. However, the system as it stands will never allow for these wonderful changes to occur—not in the U.S., and *definitely* not in poorer countries. Where will the money come from for education or universal care? It's too bad, because these things are simple enough to actually make a difference. So, where does that leave us? Well, the burden falls on our doctors and on us.

It's important, either prior to pregnancy or early on, to consult your doctor on any possible and potential risk factors you may have. So, what does this mean? It means we need doctors who are knowledgeable about and trained in preterm birth, right? They need to do a thorough screening on all their patients for possible risk factors, right? It would seem that way to me. It also doesn't hurt for us to be educated...hence this book.

Stillbirth

A stillbirth is when the baby dies in the womb before birth. This is an extremely devastating and heartbreaking experience. Sadly, stillbirths are more common than most people know. We typically just don't talk about it, because it's too depressing, making it an isolating experience for those who are unfortunate enough to have one.

Unbeknown to most of us, stillbirth is one of the most frequent bad outcomes of pregnancies, occurring in one in every 200 pregnancies.[40] There are estimated to be 3.2 million stillbirths worldwide each year, with 26,000 in the U.S. alone.[41] There are a lot of families out there who are suffering, most of them silently, and who are struggling to deal with the loss of their unborn baby.

After the loss of my son, people seemed to come out of nowhere to share their experiences of loss. I learned that my neighbor had suffered a late stillbirth, as had a close colleague. It helped to know that others had survived this terrible loss, and that I would as well. Take a small amount of comfort in the fact that you are not alone, and there is nothing to be ashamed of.

A study in Norway found that preterm birth, fetal growth restriction, preeclampsia, and placental abruption are associated with an increased chance of a later stillbirth. In this particular study, they found an overall stillbirth rate of only 1%. Women who delivered at 22–27 weeks were six times more likely to have a stillbirth in a later pregnancy.[42] Fetal growth restriction is a common cause of a late loss.[32]

In another study on the causes of stillbirth, the authors concluded that it's related to abnormalities in the baby, infection, medical conditions of the mom, and complications of pregnancy such as preeclampsia and placental abruption; however, a large proportion of stillbirths remains unexplained. The study confirmed what is already known, that age and smoking are related to stillbirth. Placental function is also related to late stillborn deaths, and further predictive tests are needed to help identify women at risk.[43]

Does all this sound familiar? Like the factors for preterm birth? This is scary stuff. What I need to do is remind you what all this is really saying. Again, this is just a risk...not an absolute.

It's NOT Your Fault

You may tend to blame yourself, thinking, "If only I hadn't gone on that run," or, "I shouldn't have lifted all those laundry baskets," or even, "I wish I hadn't had all that great pre-baby sex with my man." Maybe you've questioned yourself because you'd been working too hard or spending too much time on your feet. Stop right now!

It could be in your genes (preterm labor happens more often in white women, while black women suffer from more PPROM), or it could be due to risk factors or environmental factors over which you have no control or that may even be unknown. Fact is, it's *not* your fault, and although I know it's not easy to do, you need to stop blaming yourself.

A recent study looked at the pregnancy outcomes of hairdressers. We know that hairdressers are typically exposed to chemicals and spend a large part of their day on their feet. What they found was that there was no increased risk of a preterm delivery.[44]

In one study in Brazil, they concluded that "Mild physical activity during the second trimester of pregnancy, such as walking, has an independent protective effect on low birth weight, preterm birth, and intrauterine growth restriction."[45] Now let's be clear on what this is saying. You shouldn't walk or engage in physical activity if you're experiencing preterm labor, or if you are experiencing bleeding or certain other high risk conditions. Talk to your doctor first to determine what activities you should or shouldn't be doing. What it does say is that for most women, some activity is actually good for them, and may even help to reduce preterm birth.

Many of these studies only give us limited answers, and one study often conflicts with the next, but the overall consensus seems to be that working lots of hours and having to engage in very physical labor, as well as stress, probably has an effect and can lead to an early baby.[3]

One study says that "Housework and other daily activities do not seem to be associated with preterm birth." Sorry, "normal" ladies... you won't be able to get out of those chores, but those of us who know we're high risk will. This study acknowledged the need for further studies on occupational physical activity.[46] In the meantime, maybe focus on the upside—you'll probably be let off the hook with household duties. I can't say I did many chores throughout my pregnancies, so I guess that's one positive...no floors, no cooking, no vacuuming, and no toilets.

Don't beat yourself up for what's happened in the past—for example, saying things like, "I delivered early because I was pushing myself to work long hours before the baby came." Even the researchers aren't totally clear on what activities actually lead to an early delivery, so how can you be? There are certainly factors you do have control over; smoking, certain drugs, and poor nutrition can all lead to preterm delivery, so there are no excuses here. Seek help if you can't stop these behaviors.

If you are reading this book, then you probably fall into the high-risk category. For you, the rules have changed...dramatically for some of you. Many activities, like sex, housework, and a normal life, have been thrown out the window, but always remember not to beat yourself up...it's not your fault.

This Is the Hand You Were Dealt...Now Deal With It

Is it fair that you can't enjoy a normal pregnancy? No. Does it suck that you have to deal with all these aspects of a high-risk pregnancy? Definitely yes. Is it all right to bitch and whine about it and to be depressed about it at times? Of course. Really, though, you have no choice other than to deal with it and try to make the best of it. But if you're going to survive this experience without ruining who you are as a person or letting it take control of your life, you must find a way to manage that line of thinking. Keep things in check, and maybe you'll discover that you can find moments where you can actually relish your pregnancy.

You can choose to run away from the fear and decide that you're never going to have a baby in order to avoid dealing with this, and for some who make that choice, it's a reasonable decision. But many of us choose to take the risk, suck it up, and try our luck, knowing that it's going to be tough. Many of us are successful in having a child, while others are not.

Although it seems like a lifetime when you're living it, it's actually a relatively short amount of time in the grand scheme of your life. Try to keep that in perspective from day to day, as hard as that can be at times.

The Waiting Game

If you have one of the conditions leading to the chance of an early delivery, pregnancy can become nothing more than a waiting game, striving to reach all those milestones while nervously chewing at your nails. You may even find yourself crying every day because of the fear of losing your baby or of having a baby who is very sick.

I know this is scary, I know it's the pits, and I know it is very stressful, but it's important that you try to get some joy out of your pregnancy. Try to spend some time behaving like a "normal" pregnant gal, even though you may not be allowed to have sex, you may need to monitor yourself for contractions, you can't walk around, or maybe you're not even allowed to take a shower.

By this, I mean treasure your expanding belly and the movements of your baby inside you. Seek joy in picking out some baby outfits or looking at strollers. These are experiences that we get to experience but a few times during our life. I'm going to repeat this theme frequently, because I want to drill it into your head and into your subconscious mind.

If there is one thing I really regret, it's that I missed out on all of this when I was carrying my daughter. Don't lose the pregnancy experience simply because you're high risk and fear has taken over. Don't lose it even though you understand that you may not have a good ending. Always remember, it's only a maybe, not a definite.

In Summary: What Can I Do to Reduce My Risk?

You may not be able to change how your cervix, placenta, or uterus behaves, but there are a few things you can do to help reduce your chances of having an early baby.

1. Quit friggin' smoking, girls. I realize it's hard, but smoking is not only a nasty and expensive habit, quitting can unquestionably reduce your chance of a preemie baby, a very sick baby, a small baby (low birth weight, intrauterine growth restriction), early rupture of membranes, and even placenta previa and placental abruption. This one you have control over, so please quit, or at the very least, try and cut way back. Unfortunately, things like the patch or nicotine gum have not been shown to be safe in pregnancy,[3] so talk to your doctor about using them. (Quitting drug use and moderate to heavy drinking is an obvious no-brainer too. . . I hope.)

2. You lucky skinny ladies need to eat more to increase their body mass to an ideal number or to weigh more than 120 pounds before they get pregnant. And chubbies, you have to lose some weight to lower your BMI to under 35 before you get pregnant. (Not an easy task, but give it a shot.)

3. Take folic acid supplements, ideally for at least a year before you get prego. This has been shown to reduce your risk of PTB.[3]

4. If you work long hours, stand a lot, or have to lift things many times a day, unfortunately, you need to change this. For some, this will be hard, since your boss may not be too keen on changing your job duties. In these cases, it is up to you whether you want to take the risk. I have spoken to many women in high-risk situations who had to scrape to get by because they were forced to leave their job. Not an easy decision. (Look into your local state disability laws, because you may have some protection here. All you would then need is a doctor's note and some paperwork to be filled out in order to get some money to help you get by.)

5. Go to a good doctor who is knowledgeable about everything having to do with preterm birth. Make sure he/she takes a full history and asks all the right questions. If not, walk out and move on.

6. Don't get pregnant right after you've had a baby. Give it some time. (I know, sometimes shit happens, and in that case you'll just have to deal with it. Again, make sure you discuss this with your doctor, as it is a definite risk factor.)

7. If you're going through in-vitro fertilization, you should speak with your IVF doctor about limiting the number of eggs/embryos that are transferred. Otherwise, you may be faced with another not so great decision—namely, selective reduction.

8. Make sure you're screened and treated for sexually transmitted infections, as well as non-symptom-producing bacterial infections.

The majority of women who have their babies early have none of these risk factors.[3] Unfortunately, the world is full of unorganized and unknown chaos. That said, it's essential to recognize any potential risk factors and discuss them with your doc.

What Can My Doctor Do to Help Reduce My Risk?[3]

1. He/she can take the time to get a full and detailed history, as well as obtaining and looking over your old records **BEFORE** you meet. (This can be a hard one to get them to do, girls.)

2. Determine, based on discussion/review of past pregnancies and other current risk factors, the likelihood of another early baby.

3. Prescribe 17-alpha-hydroxy-progesterone caproate (P17) injections, which are injected into the muscle, usually the butt, from 16 weeks until 36 weeks if you have had a prior early birth at 20 to 36 weeks due to early rupture of membranes, preterm labor that wasn't induced, or early cervical shortening/dilation without contractions. (These are known as spontaneous preterm births, as opposed to medically indicated ones.) P17 reduces the likelihood of another early birth by about 35%. It is even more effective in those women who have had very early preterm births.

4. Place a cerclage in women who are found to have a short—i.e. less than 2.5 cm—cervix (ultrasound-indicated cerclage), or in someone who is dilated with visible membranes (emergency cerclage) if she is pre-24 weeks and has had a previous spontaneous early birth.

5. Screen for the presence of high numbers of bacteria or other sexually transmitted diseases. When high numbers of bacteria are found, they should be treated with antibiotics either before pregnancy (preferable) or throughout pregnancy.

6. If it is believed, based on various symptoms such as bleeding/spotting, a very short cervix of less than 1.5 cm, no cervix, or preterm labor, that a woman between 24 and 34 weeks who is high risk for preterm delivery will likely deliver soon, give corticosteroids to speed up the development of the baby's lungs. Give one dose and repeat in 24 hours. If she holds out for three weeks, another course can be given if an early birth still seems likely. Antenatal corticosteroids are best when used when birth is believed to be imminent within one to two

weeks, and you are not yet 34 weeks. This can be hard to determine, so giving it to all women thought to be at really high risk for delivering at 24 weeks (like those with any spotting/bleeding, cervical changes, or a positive FFN test) is an option.

References

1. Keirse MJ. The history of tocolysis. *Br J Obstet Gynaecol* 2003;110(Suppl. 20):94–97.
2. Othman M, Neilson JP, Alfirevic Z. Probiotics for preventing preterm labour. *Cochrane Database of Systematic Reviews* 2007, Issue 1. Art. No.: CD005941. (Last assessed as up to date: April 15, 2010)
3. Berghella V. *Preterm Birth: Prevention & Management*. West Sussex, UK. Wiley-Blackwell, 2010.
4. Sayres WG Jr. Preterm labor. *Am Fam Physician* 2010;81(4):477–484.
5. Joseph KS, Huang L, Lui S, et al. Reconciling the high rates of preterm birth and postterm birth in the United States. *Obstet Gynecol* 2007;109(4):813–822.
6. Martin JA, Osterman MJK, Sutton PD. Are preterm births on the decline in the United States? Recent data from the National Vital Statistics System. NCHS data brief, no 39. Hyattsville, MD: National Center for Health Statistics. 2010.
7. March of Dimes. Late preterm birth: every week matters. Medical perspectives on prematurity (3/2006). http://www.marchofdimes.com/files/MP_Late_Preterm_Birth-Every_Week_Matters_3-24-06.pdf.
8. Faye-Petersen OM. The placenta in preterm birth. *J Clin Pathol* 2008;61(12):1261–1275.
9. Goldenberg RL, Culhane JF, Iams JD, Romero R. Epidemiology and causes of preterm birth. *Lancet* 2008;371(9606):75–84.
10. Martin JA, Kirmeyer S, Osterman M, Shepherd RA. Born a bit too early: recent trends in late preterm births. *NCHS Data Brief* 2009;24:1–8.
11. Mozurkewich E, Chilimigras J, Koepke E, et al. Indications for induction of labour: a best-evidence review. *BJOG* 2009;116(5):626–636.
12. Tsourapas A, Roberts TE, Barton PM, et al. An economic evaluation of alternative test-intervention strategies to prevent spontaneous pre-term birth in singleton pregnancies. *Acta Obstet Gynecol Scand* 2009;88(12):1319–1330.
13. Ventura SJ, Martin JA, Curtain SC, Mathews TJ. Births: final data for 1997. *National Vital Statistics Report* 1999;47(18):1–96.
14. Althuisius S, Dekker G. Controversies regarding cervical incompetence, short cervix, and the need for cerclage. *Clinics in Perinatology* 2004;31:695–720.
15. Callaghan WM, MacDorman MF, Rasmussen MF, et al. The contribution of preterm birth to infant mortality rates in the United States. *Pediatrics* 2006;118(4):1566–1573.
16. Cole FS. Preventing and managing premature births: toward a national policy. *Medscape Public Health & Prevention* 2006;4(1).
17. Nabet C, Lelong N, Colombier ML, et al. Maternal periodontitis and the causes of preterm birth: the case-control Epipap study. *J Clin Periodontol* 2010;37(1):37–45.
18. Wise LA, Palmer JR, Heffner LJ, Rosenberg L. Prepregnancy body size, gestational weight gain, and risk of preterm birth in African-American women. *Epidemiology* 2010;21(2):243–252.

19. Köck K, Köck F, Klein K, et al. Diabetes mellitus and the risk of preterm birth with regard to the risk of spontaneous preterm birth. *J Matern Fetal Neonatal Med* 2010;23(9):1004–1008.

20. Rakoto-Alson S, Tenenbaum H, Davideau JL. Periodontal diseases, preterm births, and low birth weight: findings from a homogeneous cohort of women in Madagascar. *J Periodontol* 2010;81(2):205–213.

21. Aliyu MH, Lynch O, Saidu R, et al. Intrauterine exposure to tobacco and risk of medically indicated and spontaneous preterm birth. *Am J Perinatol* 2010;27(5):405–410.

22. Banerjee B, Pandey G, Dutt D, et al. Teenage pregnancy: a socially inflicted health hazard. *Indian J Community Med* 2009;34(3):227–231.

23. Goldenberg RL, Culhane JF, Iams JD, Romero R. Epidemiology and causes of preterm birth. *Lancet* 2008;371(9606):75–84.

24. Torloni MR, Betrán AP, Daher S, et al. Maternal BMI and preterm birth: a systematic review of the literature with meta-analysis. *J Matern Fetal Neonatal Med* 2009;22(11):957–970.

25. Toh S, Mitchell AA, Louik C, et al. Antidepressant use during pregnancy and the risk of preterm delivery and fetal growth restriction. *J Clin Psychopharmacol* 2009;29(6):555–560.

26. Hitti J, Garcia P, Totten P, et al. Correlates of cervical *Mycoplasma genitalium* and risk of preterm birth among Peruvian women. *Sex Transm Dis* 2010;37(2):81–85.

27. Breugelmans M, Vancutsem E, Naessens A, et al. Association of abnormal vaginal flora and Ureaplasma species as risk factors for preterm birth: a cohort study. *Acta Obstet Gynecol Scand* 2010;89(2):256–260.

28. Stephansson O, Larsson H, Pedersen L, et al. Crohn's disease is a risk factor for preterm birth. *Clin Gastroenterol Hepatol* 2010;8(6):509–515.

29. Ghosh JK, Wilhelm MH, Dunkel-Schetter C, et al. Paternal support and preterm birth, and the moderation of effects of chronic stress: a study in Los Angeles county mothers. *Arch Womens Ment Health* 2010;13(4):327–338.

30. Odibo AO, Talucci M, Berghella V. Prediction of preterm premature rupture of membranes by transvaginal ultrasound features and risk factors in a high-risk population. *Ultrasound Obstet Gynecol* 2002;20(3):245–251.

31. Altieri P, Gambineri A, Prontera O, et al. Maternal polycystic ovary syndrome may be associated with adverse pregnancy outcomes. *Eur J Obstet Gynecol Reprod Biol* 2010;149(1):31–6.

32. Fretts RC. Etiology and prevention of stillbirth. *Am J Obstet Gynecol* 2005;193(6):1923–1935.

33. Macones GA, Parry S, Nelson DB, et al. Treatment of localized periodontal disease in pregnancy does not reduce the occurrence of preterm birth: results from the periodontal infections and prematurity study (PIPS). *Am J Obstet Gynecol* 2010;202(2):147 e1–8.

34. Newnham JP, Newnham IA, Ball CL, et al. Treatment of periodontal disease during pregnancy: a randomized controlled trial. *Obstet Gynecol* 2009;114(6):1239–1248.

35. Shah PS, Balkhair T, Ohlsson A, et al. Intention to become pregnant and low birth weight and preterm birth: a systematic review. *Matern Child Health J* 2011;15(2):205–216.

36. Vogel I, Hollegaard MV, Hougaard DM, et al. Polymorphisms in the promoter region of Relaxin-2 and preterm birth: involvement of Relaxin in the etiology of preterm birth. *In Vivo* 2009;23(6):1005–1009.

37. McElrath TF, Hecht JL, Dammann O, et al. Pregnancy disorders that lead to delivery before the 28ᵗʰ week of gestation: an epidemiologic approach to classification. *Am J Epidemiol* 2008;168(9):980–989.

38. Bernstein PS. Autumn in New York—confronting preterm delivery in the 21ˢᵗ century: from molecular intervention to community action. (Conference Report) November 10–11, 2000. www.medscape.com/viewarticle/408935.

39. Rodger MA, Paidas M. Do thrombophilias cause placenta-mediated pregnancy complications? *Semin Thromb Hemost* 2007;33(6):597–603.

40. Reddy UM. Prediction and prevention of recurrent stillbirth. *Obstet Gynecol* 2007;110(5):1151–1164.

41. Reddy UM, Goldenberg R, Silver R, et al. Stillbirth classification—developing an international consensus for research: executive summary of a national institute of child health and human development workshop. *Obstet Gynecol* 2009;114(4):901–914.

42. Rasmussen S, Irgens LM, Skjaerven R, Melve KK. Prior adverse pregnancy outcome and the risk of stillbirth. *Obstet Gynecol* 2009;114(6):1259–1270.

43. Pasupathy D, Smith GC. The analysis of factors predicting antepartum stillbirth. *Minerva Ginecol* 2005;57(4):397–410.

44. Ronda E, Moen BE, Garcia AM, et al. Pregnancy outcomes in female hairdressers. *Int Arch Occup Environ Health* 2010;83(8):945–951.

45. Takito MY, Benicio MH. Physical activity during pregnancy and fetal outcomes: a case-control study. *Rev Saude Publica* 2010;44(1):90–101.

46. Domingues MR, Matijasevich A, Barros AJ. Physical activity and preterm birth: a literature review. *Sports Med* 2009;39(11):961–975.

CHAPTER 2

Preterm Birth...It Happens, and Yes, You *Can* Have a Healthy Baby

This chapter covers preterm labor, preterm premature rupture of membranes, preeclampsia, placental abruption, fetal indication, intrauterine growth restriction, and multiples.

You Have the Right to Hope

Here's an important message to keep in mind as you read through this book:

> *"Doctors are amazing, but they're human too. Statistics are for gamblers...don't get caught up in them. Statistics only matter if you are one...right now, you are NOT a statistic. Hope is a mainstay."* ~ Nicole, North Carolina (who spent 42 days at home on bed rest, then 54 days in the Trendelenburg position in the hospital, which is where she was basically upside down)

As she goes on to say about bed rest, *"96 days...but it was worth it...I have my beautiful twins."*

Preterm Labor[1]

"Preterm labor does not have to hurt. It can be anything from a backache to a slight tightening of your uterus. Mild contractions feel like someone is blowing up a small balloon in your belly, and you'll notice a 'tightening.' Usually, labor contractions are more painful, but it really depends on how far along you are."
~ Tracy, Minnesota

"Preterm labor was a tough one for me. This was in my third pregnancy, after two singleton pregnancies. I had experienced Braxton Hicks contractions and 'real' labor, preterm labor was like a combination of the two. The preterm labor contractions affected my whole uterus. There was a regularity, but most of them weren't painful at all. If I hadn't been hospitalized and monitored 24/7, I would not have realized at least half of them were occurring." ~ Angela, California (Who birthed twins in her third pregnancy at 34 weeks, after 15 weeks of bed rest, 12 of which were in the hospital. Hospital bed rest is even worse than home bed rest . . . by far.)

"This is the problem with preterm labor—I felt nothing. I had no idea I was experiencing contractions at all. If I was not using a monitor at home (my doctor gave it to me since my cervix was funneling), I would have had no idea. By the time I got to the hospital I was already 2 cm dilated." ~ Jamie Rodriguez (who spent three months on hospital bed rest to have her twins at 34 weeks)

Preterm labor is when you experience regular contractions of the uterus AND changes to your cervix before full-term gestation—i.e., 37 weeks. (Some have suggested that more than 5 contractions per hour are required for it to be considered "true" preterm labor, while others have suggested that it should be more than six.) Recently, this has been defined as having a cervical length of 2 cm or less as determined by transvaginal ultrasound or a measurement of 2 to 3 cm with a positive FFN test. Some feel that this criterion can "improve the diagnostic accuracy for preterm labor."

Doctors have found that using other ways to figure out preterm labor, like finger dilation checks or effacement estimates, lead to 40%

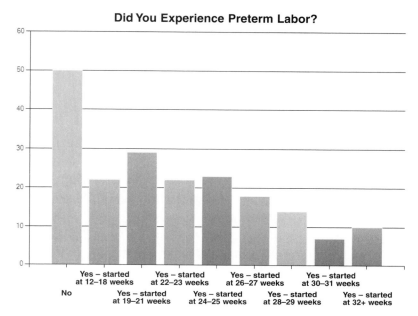

Figure 2-1. From my survey of 177 high-risk women.

more women being falsely labeled as in preterm labor. The bottom line is that transvaginal ultrasound is more accurate, reducing the chance of wrongly labeling women as being in preterm labor, thereby avoiding all that extra anxiety.

Early labor accounts for about half of all babies who are born too early. Preterm labor contractions differ from Braxton Hicks contractions, as these tend to be irregular and do NOT cause changes to your cervix. Braxton Hicks contractions are practice contractions, while preterm labor contractions are definitely not. It can be hard to tell the difference between the two, so I suggest that if you have any concerns, call your doctor. Never be embarrassed to ask, even if it's only to seek reassurance.

Preterm contractions may show themselves in many different ways. They may not always be painful, and could feel like just a tightening or even a tingling sensation in your stomach area. They can also feel like the cramps/cramping you may have experienced during periods, or even just lower back pains, which can easily be confused with normal pregnancy pains.

They can also feel like you have heaviness or pressure in your stomach, crotch, or butt area. Maybe the only sign is that there is a change in your discharge. You may even just feel a bit off, not quite able to put your finger on what's happening. These can be very hard symptoms to pinpoint, so if you are high risk, be on the lookout, and tune into your body.

How Does Labor Start?[1]

The average length of pregnancy is 38 weeks from conception … you know, sperm meets egg, and all that stuff from high-school sex ed. classes. Typically, after that amount of time has elapsed, labor is kicked off by the placenta, which releases a corticotrophin-releasing hormone (CRH). That stuff, CRH, in turn stimulates the production of another hormone in the baby that signals completion of junior's lung development. Each of these is your body's way of knowing that the time is here … normally.

What Does My Cervical Length Mean?[1]

So, you're having contractions, but what does it really mean if your cervix is 3 cm? What about if you're at 1 cm? This knowledge of your cervical length by your caregivers, particularly in women who have not yet broken their membranes, is very important information. This little number can help them to determine the best care for you and your baby, as well as how soon you are *likely* to deliver.

A really nice, comforting statistic is that more than 70% of women who suffer from preterm labor and who are at high risk of an early delivery will actually NOT deliver early, but will make it to term. I need to say that again—more than 70% of you who experience early labor will keep on baking that baby until the popper pops and the baby is ready to be born. Not so bad.

Doctors have discovered that even if you are in the throes of early labor, and your cervix is 3 cm or more, the actual chance of you having your baby within the week is only 1%. So, it's very, very unlikely. Even if your length is less than 1.5–2 cm, you're still at relatively low risk, with only a 20–50% chance of having your baby within the next seven days. Unfortunately, though, there's more than a 60% likelihood of your baby arriving before 35 weeks.

Just knowing cervical lengths has had a marked effect on the rate of premature births and has actually lessened the number of babies that are born early. So, ask for a transvaginal, not a finger, length check. Remember, 3 cm or more is an awesome length. At this length, you are most likely not having "true" preterm labor. (I'm sure it may feel like real pain, and isn't much fun, but you can rest assured.) A length of 2–3 cm is still okay, but you will have to be watched, and FFN testing will help to figure out your chances of delivering soon.

Can't They Treat and Stop Preterm Labor?

Even though medicines called tocolytics are used to stop contractions, the overall rate of preterm birth—i.e., the number of babies born before 37 weeks—has not decreased.[1] This is somewhat misleading, in that it suggests that these drugs don't work; however, that's not necessarily true. They often do work, doing the job they're supposed to do…delaying the birth just long enough.

The research may not show that they work long term—i.e., for many weeks or months—most of the time, but they do stall labor sufficiently to allow enough time for antenatal corticosteroids to be administered, a life-saving treatment for preemies. They can also allow mom to be moved to a better hospital if necessary, in order to provide the best care for her preemie. You should know that there have also been women who have taken tocolytics for longer periods of time, and then gone on to successfully carry to term.

Many doctors feel that if you have progressed to an advanced stage of preterm labor, meaning that you are dilated more than a few centimeters, you should not be treated using tocolytic drugs in an attempt to stop labor. Most likely, however, they will still be used to allow for steroid administration.

So, they may not be able to stop contractions in all women for several months, but the answer to the question above is a resounding "Yes!" Yes, there is hope to carry your baby that extra length of time to secure a chance at his/her health. Yes, there is hope that a bout of

early labor can be stopped, and not return again. Hope…Hope…
Hope. It's Possible…It's Possible…It's Possible!

How Can I Check for Contractions?

I prefer the "hardness" test, which was explained to me by a nurse
while I was in the hospital. Use your fingertip to touch the tip of your
nose. Do you feel how soft it is? This should be how your abdomen
feels. Now touch your chin and then your forehead with your fingertip. Can you feel the difference?

During a contraction, your stomach is going to feel hard, like your
forehead, and as the contraction drops off, it is going to feel more like
your chin. If this tightening is in a rhythmic pattern, about four or
more in an hour, then you may be having preterm contractions. Call
your doctor.

The most important, and the hardest thing, is figuring out if you are
really having contractions. (See Chapter 5 for a bit of help with this.)
If you notice these tightening sensations, dull aches, pains, pressure, or
just a weird feeling, take some time to lie down and monitor them.

Feel your stomach at the top of your uterus, which is up by your
boobs as you get further along, and notice if it hardens with those feelings you are having. Also, take note of what activities you were doing.
If you noticed this when you were walking around, it wouldn't hurt to
minimize or stop that activity. Bring this up with your doctor.

At around 32 weeks, I noticed that if I shopped or walked any distance, I would start contracting. It was Halloween, and so instead of
walking around door-to-door with all the kids, which is what I really
wanted to do, I had to follow them in the car, just to be safe. I didn't
want to take any chances with my cervix, even though I had a stitch.
Paranoia? Maybe. Overly cautious? Definitely. But these are the markers of a high-risk pregnancy, right?

So, if you notice any of those sensations, or you just think something seems "off," call your doctor. Drink a glass of water, too, because
dehydration has been shown to bring on contractions. Make sure you
empty your bladder frequently, because a full bladder can irritate your
uterus and possibly cause contractions as well. Lie down, preferably on

your left side to maximize blood flow to the baby, and try to relax, even though this can be damn near impossible.

Having said all that, I should note that although many doctors advise it, the science doesn't confirm the benefit of drinking water (i.e. hydrating) to reduce preterm labor. The data is limited on this, so who knows. Also, activity reduction during preterm labor has not been studied.[1] Now, who would design a study that makes some women run a marathon, while others lie down during early labor? No one. (Okay, I'm exaggerating a bit, but you get the picture. These are tough studies to actually conduct.)

Treatment typically includes a combination of bed rest or reduced activity, fluids, medicines to stop or arrest labor (tocolytics), or any mixture of these. Remember, every day makes a difference, especially between those vital weeks of around 24 to 26 weeks.

In a study of women between 24 and 34 weeks who were having contractions (symptomatic preterm labor), only 21.5% actually delivered before 37 weeks.[2] Early labor does not equal an early baby for *most* women.

Struggling with preterm labor isn't easy, that's for damn sure. The extra day-to-day stress, the drugs, their side effects, and the reality of a preemie all take a toll on you and your emotional stability. Hang in there, girls. You can do this!

The Major Issues with Preterm Labor[1]

1. It's very hard for your doctor to know with certainty that you are in "real" preterm labor (especially early preterm labor).

2. They must determine whether there are other issues causing your contractions, such as an infection.

3. Your doctor must, must, must be sure how far along you are in order to best plan treatment. In the U.S. this is not that big of a problem, since most of us have first-trimester ultrasounds. These early ultrasounds accurately determine how far along we are. Now think about elsewhere around the globe. Do you think all those women get ultrasounds early on? No way.

4. Your providers must figure out if the hospital is equipped to take care of your baby should he/she come now. Do they have access to steroids? If not, they need to figure out where you can safely go for care. (It has been shown to be better to move mom with baby still on board than to move the baby after it has been born.)

5. Now they must consider the questions, "Should I use tocolytics?" and "Which one should I use?" (Remember, they have to weigh the benefits, which is holding off birth, with the risks, because many carry nasty side effects.)

6. They need to consider, "Do I prescribe antibiotics?" Do you have signs of infection, or do they think that you may be at risk of infection because of dilation, or that you may have low-lying inflammation/infection?

Cochrane Reviews

1. There is not yet enough evidence to show that probiotics reduce preterm birth. (These are live microorganisms that provide a health benefit. Think Activia yogurt, and the claims that it helps regulate you.) The thought is that since 30 to 50% of preterm labor is believed to be due to an underlying infection in mom, probiotics would counteract the infection/inflammation. Of the two trials considered, they did find that probiotics are beneficial in treating vaginal infections during pregnancy.[3]

2. The use of preventative antibiotics in women with intact membranes and preterm labor has no "clear overall benefit." Although reduction in infections has been shown, it was not recommended for *routine* practice.[4]

"While shopping, I began to feel slightly ill and sweaty. The lady at the store said I didn't look well. I called the doctor's office and asked if I could come in, and they said they would try to squeeze me in. I waited in the lobby for approximately 30 minutes, and during that time I began to feel some cramping, like from your monthly cycle. When I was finally called, I then sat for approximately 5 to 10 minutes waiting for the doc to

come into the room. She said, 'Well, let's take a look,' and then she said, 'Oh…momma, you should have gone to the hospital!' I started to get up from the table to get dressed (the hospital was across the street), and she stopped me and said, 'I don't think you understand. If you stand up, the baby could fall out. I can see the feet.' I had to wait for the paramedics to arrive so I could be transferred by ambulance across the street." ~ Cindy, USA (had a daughter at 26 weeks after preterm labor)

"I noticed that the pain would come and go in a rhythmic fashion. It started in my back and moved around to my stomach. My tummy would get hard and then it would go away. I would relax when the pain left and brushed it off as normal pregnancy pain. No one had ever explained preterm labor to me, and I knew it was way too early for me to be in labor. Once I got home, I went to the bathroom, wiped, found a huge amount of mucus, and still thought everything would be all right. If I had only known about the signs and symptoms of preterm labor, I would have gone to the hospital earlier, and things may have turned out differently.

I again experienced all of this with my daughter, Violet, who was born at 24 weeks. My water broke at 23 weeks 3 days. The only difference this time was I recognized that I was in labor. The nurse, however, did not believe me, and I had to demand transport to Labor and Delivery because I knew. Just because my contractions were not showing up on the monitor didn't mean I wasn't having them. I most certainly was. Contractions on a 24-weeker are much different than a full-term baby, and the position of the uterus may not show them. Trust your instincts and ask questions. Don't believe everything the doctors and nurses tell you, because everyone and every pregnancy is different."
~ Melissa, Louisiana (experienced a failed transvaginal cerclage)

Preterm Premature Rupture of Membranes (PPROM)

We've all watched TV shows where the very pregnant lady happily calls out, "My water just broke. We're having a baby!" For the vast majority of women, their water breaks either just prior to labor, during labor, or, unfortunately, more often these days, with the help of a "hook" in order to speed things along. Most times this happens at or very near term. Typically, this is a joyous occasion, as this "event" signals the reality that we will be parents very soon. (In the medical world, this is called rupturing of the membranes.)

For the woman who experiences a rupture before her baby is ready to be born, however, this is an extremely critical, difficult, and stressful situation. The earlier you are in your pregnancy, the more this is true. PPROM is the rupture of your amniotic sac—i.e., membranes—before 37 weeks gestation. Even though preterm birth is on the rise, it is good to know that preterm birth as a result of early membrane rupture has decreased in women carrying one baby.[1]

PPROM can be broken down into three categories: 1) rupture before viability, which is typically considered to be around 23 weeks; 2) ruptures labeled "remote from term" (at 23–31 weeks along); and 3) rupture near term (at 32–36 weeks gestation).

The length of time you will carry your baby increases the earlier you are when your water breaks. Current studies have determined that 38% of women will deliver within one week and 69% within five weeks after PPROM near viability.[1] That means if your water breaks at, say, 23 weeks, almost 70% will deliver by 28 weeks, but 30% of women still have the chance of making it past 28 weeks. Remember, just going from 23 weeks to 28 weeks is a huge achievement for your baby's well-being.

The purpose of the amniotic sac is not only to house the amniotic fluid in which the baby lives, but even more importantly, also to provide a barrier from external microorganisms and even your body's own natural bacteria, which are found in the vagina, to keep them from infecting the membranes, fluid, placenta, and your baby. It provides a barricade to help maintain a sterile environment in which your baby can develop.

The membranes also play a role in the progression of labor. When a woman's water breaks, it causes the body to release chemicals to trigger contractions, which in turn brings on labor. This signal plays a large and mostly mysterious role in the chain of events leading up to the delivery of your baby.

The biggest problems for those who experience PPROM are: 1) infection/inflammation, and 2) the "triggering" of labor after rupturing. Managing these are both equally important in extending your pregnancy, and both can be quite challenging for doctors to treat.

Other issues that can potentially be encountered are umbilical cord prolapse, which is when the cord falls out into the vagina—essentially, it "washes" out with the rupture, which is an extremely critical situation; placental abruption (experienced by only 4–12% of women with PPROM); and, of course, issues associated with prematurity. As a reality check, early ruptures only occur in only 3% of all pregnancies.[1,5]

Genetics and gene-environment interactions have been thought as possible causes of PPROM. These may (or may not) increase vulnerability or reduce your ability to resist or fight disease.[6] Also at play, it seems, could be "programmed fetal membrane weakening prior to labor," which means that for any number of reasons, the timing is off and this weakening occurs too early.[7]

Other risk factors for an early rupture are previous preterm delivery between 25 and 30 weeks, a cerclage (cervical stitch) in your current pregnancy, bacterial vaginosis (BV), a cervical length of less than 2.5 cm, and greater than 25% funneling.[8] It should be noted, however, that according to another study, in high-risk women a length of less than 1.0 cm and funneling of greater than 75% was most predictive of PPROM.[9]

How Do They Know for Sure My Water Broke?[1]

Believe it or not, it's not always obvious that your amniotic sac has broken. Sometimes, the leak is ever so slight and can be confused with pee. (You know everyone leaks, especially during pregnancy, so you're not alone.) Always be on the lookout for any increased wetness.

A tip to help you check whether it is pee versus amniotic fluid, which you can do at home, is to use a little toilet paper to block just your pee hole (aka urethra). Stand in front of the mirror to see if any drips can still be seen emerging from the opening of your vagina. If you have ANY doubts at all, call your doctor. Believe me, a false alarm is way better than having a slow leak that is left untreated.

If your doctor checks, expect a sterile speculum exam to look for obvious leakage. If it's still unclear whether there's amniotic fluid, a quick pH check using Nitrazine™ paper will most likely then be used. Amniotic fluid pH is in the neutral range of 7.1–7.3, while typical vaginal secretions are acidic, at 4.5–6.0.

If amniotic fluid is present, the paper will turn blue. False positives are common with this test and can be caused by blood, semen, and BV. Another option is to look under the microscope for what is called "ferning." This can also be caused by things other than amniotic fluid, like cervical mucus or a lot of blood. As a last resort, they can inject a bluish die into your uterus and look for staining on a maxi pad.

Sorry Girls: PPROM = Hospital

Only 18% of women who have had an early rupture are able to go home. Techniques to seal off the leak have been explored, but as yet nothing has been found that works.[1]

One study looked at the effect of chorioamnionitis on the outcomes of babies and found that worse outcomes were experienced by babies whose moms had had an infection; in fact, there was about a 20% higher chance of a bad outcome. Infection was determined to be separate from other risk factors.[10]

This comes as no surprise, because infection is our enemy. However, these findings by no means guarantee that if you have an infection, you're going to have a very sick baby. It's true that infection can lead to poorer outcomes than no infection, but there is still hope. The statistics are far from being absolute or carved in stone. Remember that. The chance of infection is why it's important for you and your doctor to take preventative measures to fight it off. This is why hospitalization is most times mandatory, to help reduce this risk and to closely monitor you.

Infection/Inflammation

Both preterm labor and PPROM are often thought to occur due to underlying conditions, such as infection or inflammation, vascular disease, or uterine over-distension (over-expansion of your uterus, like in multiples).[11] One study has showed a strong link between interluekin-8 levels, a type of protein, and early rupture of membranes. This suggests the possibility of looking at these levels and using them as an indicator for early diagnosis of infection/inflammation, and hence the impending rupture of membranes.[12]

Many studies have looked at other proteins to see if they are linked to premature rupture of membranes, including one study that found that the BMP-2 protein in membranes is "closely related to PROM."[13] I have to admit that all this stuff is way over my head; therefore, I can't and won't, bog you down with all the details of those studies. Suffice it to say, the ultimate goal of this research is to identify "triggers" or "markers" so these can then be used for early determination and treatment.

The goal is to save more babies and to deliver healthier babies. Trust me, there are lots and lots of very smart people around the world trying to solve these mysteries. (That last study came out of China.) This is a tough challenge for scientists, as the human body is very complex, much more complex than putting a rocket ship into space… go figure.

Weighing Time Versus Risks

The gestational age of your baby will make all the difference in terms of how you are monitored and treated, as well as to your stress level. Clearly, the earlier you are, the more serious the situation is. If you are really early, you may be transferred to a hospital that is better able to care for your preemie baby, should he or she arrive.

If you are in an advanced stage of labor, have an intrauterine infection or lots of bleeding (bleeding that has stopped may be okay), or the baby's status (based on what are called "non-reassuring tests") appears to be questionable, you will be delivered. Should they find evidence that your baby's lungs are matured at 32–33 weeks, which is a possibility after treatment with steroids, the accepted treatment at this point is delivery; "…there is little to be gained from conservative management and delivery is encouraged."[1]

Types of Ruptures

It is important to also consider the type of rupture. Sometimes a small or partial rupture can self-seal, and you can go on to carry your baby for many more weeks. Although, the chance of resealing is low (this is more common after an amniocentesis), it can happen.[1]

Also, there can be slow leaks that with monitoring and, most likely, antibiotics will allow you to carry your precious cargo for longer, allowing more time to bake that baby. I'm not going to say it will be easy…it won't. Your stress level will be through the roof, and it'll feel like a long and difficult, even torturous, journey, but it CAN be done.

More Stats and Studies

One study compared babies of moms who ruptured before 24 weeks (i.e., pre-viability…I hate, hate that word) with those of moms who did not have PPROM. They found that the average duration after the rupture was 45 days (or more than 6 weeks) for membranes that had broken, on average, at 21 weeks. I can't even imagine what it would be like to suffer ruptured membranes at 21 weeks, but the authors concluded that, "The survival rate for infants born at less than 32 weeks following PPROM at pre-viable age has improved significantly; however, these infants had a higher rate of adverse composite neonatal outcome."[14]

In another study, they found that the survival rate was 43% when ROM occurred before 22 weeks and 52% when it occurred at 26 weeks. After 26 weeks, this number went way up to an almost 85% rate of survival and reached 97.5% when ruptures occurred after 30 weeks. The authors acknowledged that the most important factor for survival of babies to moms with PPROM is really how far along mom is when she delivers, NOT when she ruptures.[15]

Another study looked at antibiotics, amniotic volume, and pregnancy outcomes of women with PPROM at 24 to 32 weeks. Fluid of less than 5 cm, measured by the amniotic fluid index, was found in 67% of these women, and 63% of the deliveries occurred within 1 week, while 82% were within 2 weeks. This is plenty long enough to administer steroids. The difference in survival and health of your preemie after an additional week or two baking time, along with steroids, is huge.

It was found that low fluid levels were NOT linked to a higher incidence of infection. They also discovered that the women who received antibiotics had a LONGER period until delivery, and the babies had fewer issues with sepsis (widespread inflammation/infection).[16] Antibiotics have been shown to increase the length of time the baby stays inside the womb, while also reducing the common complications that premature babies face.[1]

The use of injections of 17 hydroxyprogesterone caproate (17P) into the muscle, or daily progesterone in the form of suppositories inserted into the vagina, is thought to reduce repeated early birth due to preterm labor or PROM in high risk women.[1]

So, what's the point of all this? Even though many women who have had a PPROM will go into labor in the near future, some will remain pregnant for a long time, several weeks or even months. There are also steroids available that can do wonders for our little guys and girls. As the authors of *Preterm Birth: Prevention & Management* point out, the earlier you are when your waters break, the greater the chance you have of carrying your baby longer.[1] A double-edged sword, yes…but it's good to know and worth repeating.

If you are going through this, remember my words, despite all these scary figures being thrown around. Beyond the medicines, machines, tears, and fears there is hope…and you have to hold onto it. You absolutely have got to have hope. I've seen my friend, who ruptured at 25 weeks, delivered at 26 weeks to the day (they sectioned her), and then was able to bring home her precious healthy baby with no tubes, oxygen, or monitors three months later. It happens. Yes, I also know many will leave the hospital with empty arms, barren bellies, and broken hearts. You *can* believe in miracles (or a good outcome)…it's okay, go ahead, give it a try.

Who's at Risk?[1]

Women who:

+ Have had a previous preterm birth.
+ Are at an economic disadvantage (the poor).
+ Are very skinny—i.e., have a low body mass index.
+ Have had a cerclage or have had biopsy procedures to their cervix. (PPROM affects 25% of those with a cerclage and 50% of those who receive a physical-exam-indicated cerclage.)
+ Are experiencing early labor or contractions in their current pregnancy.

✦ Have a urinary tract infection or a sexually transmitted disease.

✦ Suffer from an overextended uterus due to multiples or excess amniotic fluid (polyhydramnios).

✦ Have had an amniocentesis.

✦ Are experiencing vaginal bleeding.

✦ Are smokers!

Just Say No

Infection is the most common hurdle after an early rupture. If you're being cared for using a "conservative" approach, which is minimal intervention and no antibiotics, your risk of infection is further amplified by 13–60%.[1]

My advice in order to limit potential exposure and to minimize your chances of getting an infection is to just say "No!" to internal examinations...period. We know that after your membranes rupture, infection is now your biggest and sneakiest enemy, and putting anything into your cooter can introduce bacteria and lead to an infection. A good doctor will not continuously examine a woman with prematurely ruptured membranes. Hell, even with a full-term rupture, examinations should be kept to a minimum.

Why do they really need to know the status of our cervix? What's the benefit of knowing if you are 2 cm dilated? Is this worth the risk of infection? NO! Any time you can buy to extend your pregnancy helps. If they really need to see what's going on, ask for an EXTERNAL ultrasound; alternatively, even an internal ultrasound using a sterile cover is better than manual checks, and it's more accurate. Limit any checks, even these.

Even in this high-risk situation, it seems everybody and their mom wants to put their fingers in your crotch to see what's going on in there. There are the nurses, doctors, med students, and residents...WHY? This doesn't make sense. When I was being transferred from my little local hospital to the big hospital that was better able to care for me, being 6 cm dilated at 22 weeks, a wise nurse whispered in my ear, "It is your right to say 'No' to being examined internally. You can say 'No' to anybody. You should know there will be a lot of people wanting to check you out. Say 'No.'" If only I'd taken that bit of advice, maybe things would be different today.

This may go against everything you were raised to believe in—speaking out against your providers—but you must. You don't need to be rude or nasty. You can simply say something like, "I prefer you don't examine me internally, as I wish to reduce the risk of introducing an infection," or you can say, "Please keep your fingers and probes out of my vajayjay." Say it however you prefer, but make it clear.

This same bit of advice holds true for those women with intact membranes who are dilated, and especially for those with exposed membranes, like in IC or advanced preterm labor. The internals are OFF LIMITS. Oh, and you should be getting large doses of intravenous antibiotics as well, to help ward off infection.

What If My Water Breaks and I Have a Cerclage?

The question here becomes, "Do I leave my cerclage in, or should it be taken out?"

One study looked at the timing for removal of cerclages after PPROM: immediately—i.e., less than 24 hours after the rupture—or delayed—i.e., more than 24 hours after the rupture. They found that leaving the cerclage in caused a significant increase in the length of pregnancy, but found little difference in the overall outcomes of both mom and baby. With delayed removal, 56% of women were still pregnant seven days later, versus only 24% of those who had their cerclages removed immediately.[17]

You should note that this study was in women who did not have an infection and who were not experiencing active labor (i.e. regular contractions). If I was in this situation, I would say just leave it in. That's not just based on the previously cited study, either…it just makes sense.

To avoid the chance of stirring up or irritating anything down there or of introducing an infection, it makes sense to just let it be until there is no other option but to take it out. These could include signs of infection—whereupon, depending on how far along you were, they would weigh whether to deliver the baby immediately—or if your body switched into labor mode. You don't want to go into active labor with a cerclage still in place, because of the very real possibility of damaging your cervix.

What Can I Expect If My Water Breaks Early?[1]

1. Confirmation of the rupture. Is your sac really broken?

2. To spend time in the hospital. You will not be going home until your baby comes.

3. Hospital bed rest. Bummer. Along with that, expect those leg compression things to avoid issues associated with bed rest.

4. Daily monitoring of the baby's well-being (heart-rate monitoring, non-stress tests, biophysical profile). They will be looking for signs of distress, like heart-rate dips or jumps.

5. Routine checks for infection, fever, uterine tenderness, chills, even changes in vaginal discharge, possibly even an amniocentesis to look at white blood cell counts.

6. Antibiotics. (They have been shown to increase the time women carry their babies; some studies even showed an extension of three weeks, reduced infection rates, and decreased problems for the baby.)

7. Monitoring for contractions and tocolysis to stop them if present (even though this hasn't been shown to improve the baby's outcome for certain).

8. Discussions of delivery versus risks. (Not delivering immediately will not be an option for certain issues like heavy bleeding, infection, etc.)

9. Antenatal corticosteroids if it's believed you will deliver within seven days.

10. A check for lung maturity.

11. When you make it to 34 weeks, get ready for baby. You should be delivered at this time, as there is no benefit in keeping baby in any longer with ruptured membranes.

"I didn't get any contractions, just a gush of water. Each time the little ones held on for a while, but then I would feel the cord coming out, so labor would be speeded up." ~ Olivia, London, UK

"Trust your instincts. We were told to terminate when my water broke at 18 weeks. I laid in a hospital bed for 10 weeks. Our little man held on till 28 weeks. He spent three months in the NICU. Against all odds, he is a happy and healthy 10-month-old." ~ Nicole, Wisconsin

Cochrane Reviews

1. There is not enough evidence to show that amnioinfusion, where a solution is used to refill the uterine cavity, is beneficial to babies after PROM (for example, to reduce umbilical-cord compression). Based on this, it should not be routinely performed in women suffering early ruptures.[18]

2. Certain antibiotics can help women with early ruptures to extend their baking time, and reduce infection and potential developmental issues, though it has not been observed to save more babies. One antibiotic, co-amoxiclav, should NOT be used, as it increases the likelihood of a rare bowel condition. The recommended antibiotic is erythromycin.[19]

3. "There is insufficient evidence to guide clinical practice on the benefits and harms of immediate delivery compared with expectant management for women with PPROM." This is because the trials so far have been inadequate and/or have a poor design. (Expectant management is when they wait for labor/contractions to happen naturally after the water has broken before full term.)[20]

Parting Words of Advice

"This is such a scary time, and the best thing you can do is to try to remain calm and take good care of yourself. It is so hard to do that when you're worried all the time, but you can't always trust the statistics anyway—one of my twins ruptured at 22 weeks, but I was able to carry him and his sister to 29 weeks… nothing short of a miracle. Do your best to stay positive, and do all the fun pregnancy things you can do—even if you have to shower in the hospital, or bed rest, like me!" ~ Tracy, Minnesota

What to Expect After PPROM

o Dr. will go over risk factors and possible cause of the rupture.

o Rupture will be confirmed (pooling, ferning, or with nitrazine strips).

o Group B strep culture performed, treatment with antibiotics if needed.

o Gestational age of the baby will be confirmed (via ultrasound).

o Expect counseling on baby outcomes. (This all depends on how far along you are, presence of infection, etc.)

Do you have?

o Intrauterine Infection (IUI)

o Non-reassuring fetal testing (NRFT)

o Advanced labor (AL)

o Significant bleeding (SB)

NO   **YES**

Less than 23 weeks along:
Dr. (and you) will consider delivery vs. waiting it out to see what happens.

DELIVER

Between 23 and 31 weeks along:
Expect conservative management, which includes:

o Hospitalization. (Ideally in a hospital equipped to care for your preemie if baby comes now.)

o Corticosteroids for lung development.

o Broad spectrum antibiotics, like erythromycin or ampicillin.

o Delivery of the baby if any of the above is seen (IUI, NRFT, AL, SB) or when the baby's lungs are developed or you reach 34 weeks.

Between 32 and 33 weeks:

o Baby's lung maturity can be checked, if mature, baby should be delivered.

o Delivery of baby after the steroids do their job or at 34 weeks or more.

o If you're being managed conservatively, see above.

34 or more weeks = deliver. (No point in risking infection or other problems if you're at this gestation!)

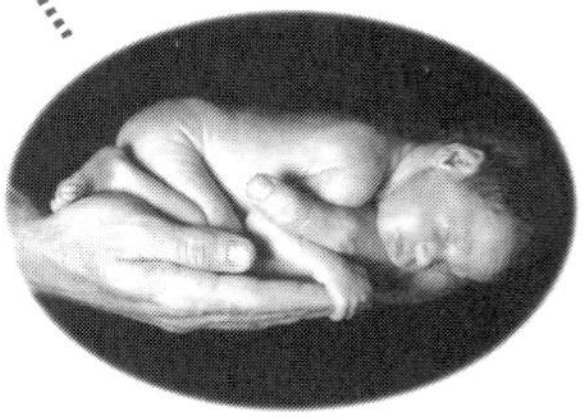

Figure 2-2. Chart Adapted from *Preterm Birth: Prevention & Management.*[1]

Preeclampsia[21]

Most of this information is from the Preeclampsia Foundation, an organization dedicated to providing education about and supporting research into this condition. To donate money to help support research on this and related conditions, please visit their website, www.preeclampsia.org. (This website also has a ton of stories from others who've been through this.)

This condition only affects women and their unborn babies during pregnancy, typically after 20 weeks, or during the six-week period after birth, even then it's still a major problem for mom. Preeclampsia is present in about 5–8% of ALL pregnancies and is more common in first-time pregnancies and older moms (another source states that up to 10% of pregnancies are affected[22]). Typically, it is resolved within 48 hours after birth.

This condition may develop quickly and leads to high blood pressure and protein in the urine. Symptoms include swelling (especially in the face and feet), sudden weight gain, headaches, and changes in vision. Some women don't display any of these symptoms but still end up with preeclampsia.

Regular prenatal visits are mandatory to enable doctors to track and manage the possible onset of preeclampsia; this is one reason why you get your blood pressure, weight checked, and your urine tested for the presence of protein at each visit. Worldwide, more than 76,000 deaths of the mom and more than 500,000 deaths of the baby are caused by this and other hypertensive disorders each year, and it is also a major contributor to preterm birth.

How Will I Know If I Develop This?

According to the Preeclampsia Foundation, "High blood pressure is a silent killer. Oftentimes, women diagnosed with preeclampsia do not feel sick. Many signs and symptoms of preeclampsia mirror other 'normal' effects of pregnancy on your body. Women diagnosed with preeclampsia may feel frustrated when prescribed bed rest because they feel fine. If you feel fine, it may be hard for you or your partner to appreciate that preeclampsia is a serious condition."

But it is a serious condition…like preterm labor or PPROM, which can lead to an early delivery. In preeclampsia, early delivery is most often determined by your doctor in order to stop the condition from getting worse, in order to protect you.

Here are the warning signs:

+ Hypertension (high blood pressure) is a blood pressure of 140/90 or greater, observed twice within a six-hour period. Some women who typically have lower blood pressures can still develop preeclampsia, even if their numbers don't get that high. A rise in the diastolic (lower number) of 15 degrees or more or a rise in the systolic (upper number) of 30 degrees or more is cause for concern, especially if you have other symptoms. So, the Preeclampsia Foundation highly recommends being aware of your normal blood pressure, especially those of you who tend to run on the low side.

+ Edema (swelling), especially in your hands and face. Hello, puffy eyes. This could be a sign of a problem. Look for indentations when you push on the swollen regions, or discoloration in your legs. Note: some swelling is very common in pregnancy, but talk to your doctor about any noticeable changes, especially in these regions. Most pregnant women soon find they can't squeeze into any of their rings, even though they don't have preeclampsia, but talk to your doctor if anything feels "off."

+ Protein in your urine (proteinuria). The pee sample you provide to your doctor at each visit is used for testing for abnormally high protein levels using a dip strip. This happens when the small blood vessels in your kidneys become damaged, leading to leaking of protein into the urine.

  • The result on the strip is either "trace" (which is common and not a problem), or 1+, 2+, etc. A 1+ or higher could mean the start of preeclampsia, even if your blood pressure is below the threshold. A 2+ is a major red flag. Sometimes, a 24-hour urine collection test will be required to thoroughly evaluate what's going on. That's not much fun, especially if you have to go every hour on the hour.

✦ Sudden weight gain of more than two pounds in a week or six pounds in a month. Let's face it though; how many pregnant women experience "growth spurts" and gain more than two pounds in a week? That's right, lots. Just be sure you keep your eye on this.

✦ Migraine-like headaches that just don't seem to go away, even when treated in the normal manner. This is another tough one, being a common pregnancy symptom, especially in women who are prone to migraines. I had terrible headaches in my second trimester, especially in my first pregnancy, and my midwives had me come in during one of those headaches to check my blood pressure, which was fine. Needless to say, I was lucky, but you can never be certain. Headaches can be the result of high blood pressure, hormones, allergies, etc. The point is, let your doctor know if you're having any headaches so they can rule out preeclampsia.

✦ Nausea and/or vomiting in the second or third trimester. (Not to be confused with a stomach bug or food poisoning…so have your doctor check your blood pressure and urine for protein.)

✦ Changes in vision, such as temporary loss of vision, a sensation of flashing lights, heightened sensitivity to light, blurred vision, or spots before the eyes. This is a very serious symptom and should be checked out immediately, even if it means a late-night hospital trip.

✦ Signs of high blood pressure could also include a racing pulse, mental confusion (although this is also common with sugar problems, like diabetes), a feeling of high anxiety, or difficulty catching your breath (another vague symptom that is common if baby is pressing on your diaphragm).

✦ Stomach pain, beneath your ribs on the right side of your body, and/or right shoulder pain. This can be mistaken for heartburn, indigestion, or kicks from the baby.

✦ Sudden and specific lower back pain, different from the normal aching in the lower back that one invariably experiences when pregnant. This could be a sign of HELLP or some other liver problem, especially if you're displaying other symptoms of preeclampsia.

+ Overly strong reflex reactions in situations such as when you're accidentally bumped. (This is called hyperreflexia.)

Who's at Risk?

+ The main risk factor is having had the condition before, especially if it developed before the third trimester. The earlier you developed it previously, the higher the risk you'll have it again; and the worse you had it before, again, the higher the risk in your next pregnancy. (The risk of having it again varies widely, from 5 to 80%, so they really don't know. More research is needed.)

+ Women with a BMI of 30 or higher.

+ Women with a history of chronic high blood pressure, diabetes, or a kidney disorder.

+ Those with a family history of the disorder (i.e., a mother, sister, grandmother, or aunt who had it).

+ Women who are carrying multiple babies.

+ Those over 40 or under 18 years of age.

+ Women with polycystic ovarian syndrome (PCOS).[23]

+ Those with lupus or other autoimmune disorders, such as rheumatoid arthritis, sarcoidosis, or MS.

What Are the Treatment Options?

+ The #1 treatment is to have your baby (along with a course of corticosteroids to speed up lung maturity, if needed). They will try to keep the baby baking as long as possible, until the point at which the risk to mom and baby is believed to be too high. Then, mom is either induced or a C-section is performed. (Michelle Duggar, from the show *19 Kids and Counting* on TLC, developed this condition and had to deliver her baby, Josie, at 25 weeks. Josie is doing great now, even though she only weighed 1 pound 6 ounces at birth.)

- According to one article I found, the best approach to treatment is "preconception evaluation and counseling, early antenatal care, frequent monitoring of maternal and fetal well-being, and timely delivery."[24] You want to be in the best possible health before you become pregnant to further reduce your risk of developing preeclampsia.

✦ Acetylsalicylic acid (aspirin)

- One review found that aspirin therapy started before 16 weeks, after women identified as having an abnormal placenta via uterine artery studies, showed a large reduction in the incidence of severe preeclampsia, gestational high blood pressure, and IUGR.[25]

- Another review found that aspirin reduced the number of baby deaths and preeclampsia in women with risk factors. They concluded that, "Given the importance of these outcomes and the safety and low cost of aspirin, aspirin therapy should be considered in women with historical risk factors."[26]

✦ The other main treatment is bed rest—especially hospital bed rest, so they can keep a closer eye on you. Yeah, how exciting. Lying on the left side in an attempt to optimize blood flow may be recommended, even though there is no proof for or against its effectiveness, but it can't hurt. The theory is that when you lie flat on your back, the weight of your uterus presses on the vein that supplies blood to your heart.

✦ When swelling is a problem, it is recommended that you should drink plenty of water, believe it or not, and keep your feet up. You should also avoid sitting still for long periods.

✦ Medication can be used to keep high blood pressure under control.

- Giving magnesium sulfate to all women with preeclampsia in the world's 143 least developed countries could prevent as many as 35,000 cases of eclampsia each year. The World Health Organization (WHO) includes magnesium sulfate on its essential drugs list, but only about half the world's countries have it listed. It should be noted that this drug can cause quite a range of side effects and must be used with caution. (Historically, it has been used to prevent eclamptic fits.)

◆ And for a final word, "Supplementation with fish oil, calcium, or vitamin C and E and the use of antihypertensives have been shown to be ineffective in the prevention of recurrent preeclampsia and are not recommended."[24]

Toxemia, PET, HELLP, and PIH? What's All That About?

These are all related hypertensive (high blood pressure) disorders of pregnancy. Toxemia and preeclamptic toxemia (PET) are outdated terms based on the belief that this condition was due to toxins in the blood. Pregnancy-induced hypertension, or PIH, is another term used to describe this condition. Technically, they're each a little different, at least to those in the medical world, but they all fall under the general category of preeclampsia.

The danger with preeclampsia is that it can lead to a more serious condition called eclampsia. This can cause a woman to have seizures and possibly even end up in a coma. Yikes! You should know, however, that this condition is quite rare and is treatable. Research has shown that "more women die from preeclampsia than eclampsia, and one is not necessarily more serious than the other."[21]

HELLP syndrome and eclampsia are also related conditions. This is where red blood cells break down (hemolysis, H), causing high or elevated liver enzymes (E) and low platelet levels (LLP). Interestingly, black women tend to develop seizures more often, while white women are more likely to get HELLP Syndrome.

HELLP occurs in a small number of women who have preeclampsia (4–12%) and is a major problem, usually affecting the liver. It can actually appear at any time, not necessarily only after the appearance of preeclampsia symptoms, and is often mistaken for the flu or for gallbladder problems.

A proven treatment is the use of magnesium sulfate. Yes, this is the same magnesium sulfate used to stop contractions. You will see in the chapter on tocolytics that there are serious side effects with many of these drugs, and magnesium sulfate is no exception, but when weighing your options—magnesium sulfate or serious complications as a result of this condition—the answer is clear.

The Causes of Preeclampsia

Again, this information is from the Preeclampsia Foundation (www.preeclampsia.org).

There are a number of theories, ranging from too much blood flow to too little. Some current theories include:

Medical Description	Layperson's Description
Uterine ischemia/ underperfusion	Damage to the lining of the blood vessels.
Prostacyclin/thromboxane imbalance (ASA)	Disruption to the balance of hormones that maintain the width of blood vessels.
Endothelial activation and dysfunction	Damage to the lining of the blood vessels that regulate the width, which in turn keeps fluid and protein inside and stops blood from clotting.
Calcium deficiency	Calcium helps maintain width of vessels, so a deficiency would impair the function of this (see above).
Hemodynamic vascular injury	Injury to blood vessels caused by too much blood flow.
Preexisting maternal conditions	Undiagnosed high blood pressure or other pre-existing problems, such as diabetes, lupus, sickle cell disorder, hyperthyroidism, kidney disorder, etc.
Immunological activation	The immune system thinks that damage has occurred to the blood vessel, and in trying to fix the "injury" actually makes the problem worse (like scar tissue).
Nutritional problems/ poor diet	Insufficient protein, excessive protein, not enough fresh fruit and vegetables (antioxidants).
High body fat	High body fat may be a symptom of a tendency toward developing this disorder, which is linked to the genetic predisposition for high blood pressure, diabetes, and insulin resistance.

What Are the Problems for Baby?

+ Prematurity and related problems from being born too early.
+ Intrauterine growth restriction (IUGR) from decreased blood flow.

✦ Acidosis, whereby blood flow is restricted from the limbs, kidney, and stomach to preserve the vital supply to the brain and heart. In extreme circumstances, a poisonous waste product, lactic acid, is produced. If too much acid is produced, the baby loses consciousness, and delivery must occur immediately.

✦ Possible increased risk of high blood pressure and diabetes later on.

✦ Death. (There are about 1,200 such deaths each year in the U.S. alone, and the rate is higher in those countries not able to care for preemies.)

Preeclampsia and Heart Problems[21,27]

It is important to know that if you develop preeclampsia (and/or other placental dysfunction issues), you run the chance of developing "long-term cardiovascular complications." These include coronary heart disease, stroke, and general heart disease. The risk of suffering heart problems has been found to be highest in women who develop placenta-related conditions and whose babies also have issues related to the placenta.

This would include a woman who has high blood pressure and protein in her urine *and* whose baby is found to have IUGR, especially if her baby is born early. This is relatively rare, and most women return to normal either soon after delivery or within a few weeks of giving birth.

What Can I Do to Prevent Possible Later Heart Issues?

First, you can take care of yourself before, during, and after pregnancy. Being obese and dealing with the complications of being overweight only increases the chance of suffering these problems later. Watch what you eat, maintain a healthy diet, and of course, exercise. (I'm sure you've never heard this before.)

Now, I'm not talking about taking on a raw-food diet or some other crazy strict diet like many of the stars seem to do…just use your common sense. A bacon, egg, and cheese bagel for breakfast, a hamburger and French fries for lunch, and pizza followed by a sundae for dinner is not a healthy diet. Talk to your doctor or a dietician if you need help with dietary changes.

I'm also not talking about training for an iron-man competition, either. Twenty-one minutes of brisk walking every day and two brief muscle-strengthening sessions per week is all that is recommended by the Center for Disease Control and Prevention.[28]

Oh, and one more thing…quit smoking. Duh!

It's essential that you work with a doctor who is knowledgeable about this condition and the possibility of later heart problems, so you can be monitored properly.

Fear of Another Pregnancy

After suffering a traumatic pregnancy, this is to be expected, as can be said for many of the "conditions" talked about in this chapter. Preeclampsia can be a bit different, as it can come on very, very suddenly, leading to an immediate delivery of the baby and a very sick mom. I've heard of women waking up in the Intensive Care Unit days after they've had their baby and having no idea what was happening or had happened.

You may also have been told not to get pregnant again. We now know that your risk is highest if you've had preeclampsia before, so the easy solution is to say, "Hey, no more kids." Well, not so fast. Maybe you want more children, and just maybe it won't be the same the next time around. Before you give up hope for another baby, see a perinatologist for a second opinion. Talk about your options, consider preventative aspirin, and seek support from other women, like from Sidelines volunteers, if you decide to go for it.

> *"My husband and I are planning on trying for a second baby while our daughter is still very young. I've been a little worried about trying so soon because I developed preeclampsia with her, but I realized that no matter when I get pregnant again, the worry will still be there. The best thing I can do is hope and pray for another healthy outcome to any subsequent pregnancies."* ~ Sarah, Texas

Cochrane Reviews

1. Low doses of aspirin, an antiplatelet agent, help to prevent preeclampsia and some of the complications associated with it.[29]

2. There is not enough evidence to prove the benefits of plasma volume expansion for women with preeclampsia. (The thought is that this treatment will have a beneficial/counteracting effect as plasma volume is reduced in women with this condition.)[30]

3. There is not enough evidence to show that progesterone prevents preeclampsia or its complications, and it "should not be used for this purpose in clinical practice at present." (In the past it was used for this.)[31]

4. "Daily rest, with or without nutrient supplementation, may reduce the risk of preeclampsia for women with normal blood pressure.... Current evidence is insufficient to support recommending rest or reduced activity to women for preventing preeclampsia and its complications. Whether women rest during pregnancy should therefore be a matter of personal choice."[32] (Okay, so this is saying what? Should we or shouldn't we?)

5. Taking vitamins before getting pregnant or early on in pregnancy may have the benefit of reducing the development of preeclampsia and may even make you more likely to have a multiple pregnancy. It does not reduce miscarriage or stillbirths.[33]

6. Nitric oxide has not been shown to prevent preeclampsia.[34]

7. "Magnesium sulphate helps prevent eclamptic fits in pregnant women at increased risk."[35]

Placental Abruption[1,36,37,38,39]

Placental abruption is when the placenta separates from the uterus due to internal bleeding sometime between the twentieth week and when the baby is born. A hematoma, or collection of blood, further separates the placenta from the uterine wall, causing compression and compromise of the blood supply to the baby. If you have vaginal bleeding in MORE than one trimester, you have about a 50% chance of your water breaking early.

The Basics

Some amount of placental separation prior to delivery occurs in about 1 out of 150 deliveries. The severe form, which results in fetal death, only occurs in about 1 out of 500 to 750 deliveries. Overall, this only occurs in around 1% of all pregnancies throughout the world. Tests to determine this include abdominal ultrasound, complete blood count, pelvic exam, fibrinogen level, partial thromboplastin time, and pro-thrombin time. (The last three tests have to do with coagulation of blood.)

Placental abruption is suspected when a pregnant mother has sudden localized abdominal pain with or without bleeding. The top of the uterus, the fundus, may have to be monitored, as a rising fundus can indicate bleeding.

Treatment depends on the amount of blood loss and the age of the baby. If the baby is less than 36 weeks, and neither you nor the baby is in any distress, then you may just be monitored in the hospital until either a change is observed or the baby is old enough to be born safely, whichever comes first.

Immediate delivery of the baby may be required if the baby is ready, or if either of you is in trouble. Blood replacement and maintenance of your blood pressure may be needed. Vaginal birth is usually preferred over C-section, unless the baby is showing signs of problems.

The mother rarely dies from this condition; however, these factors have been shown to increase the risk of death in both mother and baby: the absence of labor, a closed cervix, delayed diagnosis and treatment, excessive blood loss resulting in shock, and hidden vaginal bleeding in pregnancy. Excessive loss of blood is not good and can lead to shock and possible death in either the mom, the baby, or both.

Problems with the baby appear early in only about half of all women with this condition. The mortality rate for babies is about 15%, and those who do survive have a 40–50% chance of further complications, which range from mild to severe.

Early recognition and proper management are key. Controlling diabetes and high blood pressure also decreases the risk of placental abruption.

Symptoms of Placental Abruption

- ✦ 80% have vaginal bleeding. (Although sometimes this is not obvious, as blood pools behind the placenta.)
- ✦ 70% have abdominal or back pain and uterine tenderness.
- ✦ 60% of the babies show fetal distress.
- ✦ 35% have abnormal uterine contractions.
- ✦ 25% experience premature labor.

Types of Abruptions

Classification is based on the extent of separation of the placenta (partial vs. complete) and the location of the separation [marginal (side) vs. central].

- ✦ Grade 0: No symptoms present and is only diagnosed through postpartum examination of the placenta.
- ✦ Grade 1: The mother may have vaginal bleeding with mild uterine tenderness, but there is no distress to the mother or her baby. (Approximately 48% of all cases.)
- ✦ Grade 2: The mother has symptoms, but she is not in shock. There is some evidence that the baby is in distress with fetal heart-rate monitoring. (About 27% of all cases.)
- ✦ Grade 3: Mom has severe bleeding, which leads to shock and the death of the baby.

What Can I Expect?

Typical treatments are IV fluids and blood transfusions. You'll be carefully monitored for symptoms of shock, and your baby will be watched for signs of distress, including an abnormal heart rate.

An emergency C-section may become necessary. In cases of complete separation of the placenta, this is mandatory if the baby is to be saved. If it's very early in your pregnancy and there is only a small separation, you'll be kept in the hospital for observation and released after a few days if your condition remains stable. If the baby is at a good gestational age, vaginal delivery is still an option if both you and baby are doing well, so don't completely rule out your dream of a vaginal birth.

What Could Happen to Me?

✦ A significant loss of blood may require blood transfusions and intensive care after delivery.

✦ The uterus may not contract properly after delivery, so the mother may need medication to help her uterus contract.

✦ Mothers may have problems with blood clotting for a few days after giving birth.

✦ If the mother's blood does not clot (particularly during a C-section), and too many transfusions are required, the doctor may consider a hysterectomy.

✦ A severe case of shock can affect other organs, such as the liver, kidney, and pituitary gland. Diffuse cortical necrosis in the kidney is a serious and often fatal complication.

✦ In some cases where the abruption is high up in the uterus or is slight, there is no bleeding, although these women experience extreme pain.

What About My Baby?

✦ If a large amount of the placenta separates from the uterus, the baby will probably be in danger until delivery and may die *in utero*, leading to a stillbirth.

✦ Your baby may be premature and need specialized care.

✦ If the baby is in distress in the uterus, he or she may have a low level of oxygen in the blood after birth.

✦ Your baby may have low blood pressure or a low blood count.

✦ If the separation is severe enough, the baby could suffer brain damage or even die.

Causes

The exact causes of a placental abruption are often unknown. "Direct" causes, though infrequent, include:

✦ Maternal hypertension (high blood pressure)—the most common cause of abruption, occurring in about 44% of all cases.

+ Injury to the abdominal area from a fall or automobile accident (1.5–9.4% of all cases).

+ Smoking. (Let's be clear, this is not a few cigs here or there if you're having trouble quitting, but heavy-duty chain smoking.)

+ Alcohol consumption, drinking more than 14 alcoholic drinks per week while pregnant. (Obviously not good.)

+ Cocaine use.

+ An abnormally short umbilical cord.

+ Sudden decompression of the uterus (e.g., premature rupture of membranes, delivery of the first twin).

+ Prolonged rupture of membranes (>24 hours).

+ Uterine fibroids located behind the placenta.

+ Bleeding in the placenta from a needle puncture, like after an amniocentesis.

+ Maternal age-women who are younger than 20 or older than 35 are at a greater risk.

+ Abnormalities of uterine blood vessels and the uterine lining (decidua).

+ Diabetes.

+ Previous abruption-women who have had an abruption in previous pregnancies are at greater risk.

+ Increased uterine expansion, which may occur with multiple pregnancies or an abnormally large volume of amniotic fluid, or following a large number of prior deliveries.

+ Some infections are also diagnosed as a cause.

+ Genetics has also been suggested.[40]

If you would like to better understand placenta abruption via pictures (I'm a picture person), you can visit the following websites:

+ www.childrenscentralcal.org/HealthE/P02461/P02482/Pages/P02437.aspx

+ www.i-am-pregnant.com/encyclopedia/Pregnancy/Placenta/Placental-Abruption

+ www.allina.com/mdex/nd0289g.htm

"I was put on bed rest every time I had bleeding, which was several times during my first pregnancy, and was told to stay lying down for at least 48 hours after it subsided. When things were going along normally I tried to have rest periods during the day, as it seemed like the bleeding episodes were connected to overdoing things." ~ Carol, Ohio

"Even though bleeding can be a common occurrence in some pregnancies, you should always contact your doctor as soon as possible. Even if it's nothing, it's better safe than sorry. Even if you have bled a dozen times and it's the same as before, let your doctor know. Also, take bed rest seriously. If the doctor tells you to stay in bed, stay in bed. Even if you think you're OK."
~ Corrine, location unknown (Her 26-weeker is now nearly 8 months old, weighs 14 pounds, and is doing great. She started bleeding at 11 weeks and had to have blood transfusions.)

Cochrane Review

1. "There is no evidence from trials to show the best way to help pregnant women and babies when there is a placental abruption. The clinical management of placental abruption has to rely on knowledge other than that obtained through randomised clinical trials."[41] (Big help this is.)

Fetal Indication and Intrauterine Growth Restriction

Better Off Outside the Womb: Fetal Indications

Problems with the baby are another cause of early deliveries, except in these cases, it's because the doctor believes that it is better for the baby to be born now. They have to weigh the circumstances before coming to the conclusion that it's now better for the baby to be outside than inside.

There are many factors and situations that can lead the doctor to believe that your baby would do better if she/he were to be delivered early. Examples include issues with the placenta, which may not be providing enough nutrients or functioning properly, or a suspected infection.

IUGR

Intrauterine growth restriction (formerly known as Intrauterine Growth Retardation), or IUGR, is exactly what it sounds like. This is when the baby fails to grow at a "normal" rate. Newborns are considered to have had restricted growth when their birth weight and/or length is below the 10th percentile for their gestational age, and they have an abdominal circumference below the 2.5th percentile.[42]

So, what does this mean? If your baby is in the 9th percentile for his/her gestational age, it means that 91% of babies born at the same age are bigger. It's important to remember that the weight "guidelines" vary depending on how far along you are, so the weight necessary to be ranked below the 10th percentile, and therefore the determination of IUGR, is different at, say, 30 weeks than 34 weeks (see Figure 2-3). Often, you won't know your baby has suffered IUGR until he or she is actually born.

The growth of a developing baby is either:

1. Appropriate for gestational age
2. Large for gestational age
3. Small for gestational age
4. Intrauterine growth restricted

Doctors use these terms in order to better communicate and to prepare for the care of the baby after birth. Will the baby need special nutrition? Monitoring? According to one article, "Size matters when it comes to the health and welfare of neonates."[43]

Risk Factors

IUGR has been described as "a complicated perinatal condition, with multiple causes."[44] IUGR is caused by maternal, fetal, placental, and external factors. Often, it is the result of a placental problem, but not always, as issues with the baby are sometimes to blame. These include genetic diseases, congenital malformations, infection (such as rubella, cytomegalovirus, toxoplasmosis, or syphilis), multiple babies, and cord defects.[45]

Issues in the mom can also lead to restricted growth: decreased blood flow, low blood volume, depleted levels of oxygen transport, poor nutrition status, teratogens (something that effects the development of an embryo or baby), a short timeframe between pregnancies, race, age, or low socioeconomic status.[46] Other possible causes are heart disease, high altitudes, and preeclampsia/eclampsia. Unfortunately, the cause is often unknown.

There are, however, several well-known risk factors that can lead to IUGR that can easily be addressed by mom, either before pregnancy or early on, so suck it up and, for the sake of your wee one, avoid:

+ Alcohol abuse
+ Drug addiction
+ Poor nutrition
+ Smoking

Growth of the baby is dependent on the nutrients supplied by mom through the placenta and on into the umbilical cord. In IUGR, the baby lacks the proper nutrients, specifically amino acids, needed to grow, because of either metabolism issues in the placenta or inadequate transport from mama to baby.[47] This condition also affects the growth and development of the kidneys, liver, and heart, as these are the developing organs with the highest cell-turnover rates.[48]

The exact mechanisms at work are way beyond the scope of this book, and you really don't need to know that level of detail. Save that for the researchers. Believe me, you really don't want to read it. I have, and it's far from fascinating. According to the Fetal Diagnostic Center, "One of the most common risks for IUGR is inadequate blood flow to the uterus, which results from either abnormal vessels within the uterus and placenta, maternal fatigue, or maternal stress."[49]

How Will I Know My Baby Has IUGR?

It is often found during ultrasounds, when the baby doesn't appear to be achieving the desired size or weight. However, a lower than normal weight gain is *not* a good determinant for diagnosing. Sometimes, it's discovered during routine measuring of the fundal height of the uterus, where the height appears to be off from the gestational age.

As a rough guide, if you're 28 weeks, you should measure 28 cm from the top of your uterus to your pubic bone, while if you're 32 weeks, this measurement should be 32 cm. This measurement doesn't work until after 20 weeks and isn't always accurate, particularly for very heavy women. (An ultrasound is always better.) There is also variability depending on how the baby is lying, as well as on the skills of the person doing the measuring—specifically his or her ability to correctly identify the top of the fundus.

Ultrasounds for diagnosis and delivery of the baby at the right time, not too early and not too late, are the key to effective treatment in pregnancies affected by IUGR.[44]

Usually, they test to ensure that the baby is free from structural and/or chromosomal abnormalities, as well as looking at the circulation of the mother and baby to pick up any placental problems and to rule out genetic problems and intrauterine infections.[50]

It is recommended that Doppler velocity waveform ultrasound analysis is used to look at the fetal vessels and estimate the baby's weight, as well as the abdominal circumference, to best identify and evaluate IUGR. If it is identified, monitoring should then include vessel analysis and biophysical testing every week or two, depending on your situation.[51]

There are a lot of different practices among providers on the frequency/types of tests they run to watch the baby for signs of distress. These include fetal movement monitoring, fetal heart rate, growth scans, Doppler ultrasounds to look at blood flow, and changes in the baby's heart rate with movement checks.

It has been determined that in early pregnancy, higher diastolic blood pressure, the bottom number, and higher hematocrit blood levels, were found to be linked to smaller babies, as were moms who smoked and didn't take folic acid supplements.

First-trimester growth restriction leads to a higher chance of preterm birth, low birth weight, and small size for gestational age at birth.[52] Low-risk women who had a larger "notch" depth (something very specific researchers looked for and way beyond our understanding) in their uterine arteries (these carry blood and exchange oxygen) at 20–23 weeks had a 41.8% rate of adverse outcomes, which included small babies (at or below the 5th percentile), preeclampsia, delivery before 33 weeks, placental abruption, or death of the baby, compared to a rate of only 4.6% for those without this notch. (To put things in perspective, the overall rate of these problems was only 5.3%, so keep in mind the fact that all of this is rare.)[53]

The researchers' hope is that knowledge of the notch depth can help doctors consider the best approach to minimizing problems and determining appropriate treatments.

Where Does Your Baby Fall? (SGA ≠ IUGR)

Low Birth Weight (LBW) babies weigh between 2500 g and 1500 g (3 lb 5 oz), Very Low Birth Weight (VLBW) babies weigh less than 1,500 g, and Extremely Low Birth Weight (ELBW) babies weigh less than 1,000 g (2 lb 3 oz). Normal weight at term delivery is around 2,500–4,200 g (5 lb 8 oz to 9 lb 4 oz).

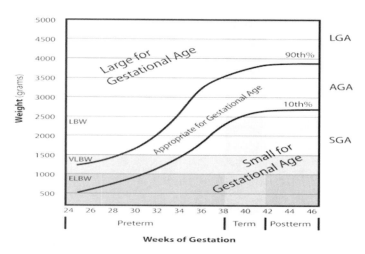

Figure 2-3. LGA = Large for Gestational Age (above the 90th percentile, more than 2,500 g or 5 lb 8 oz), AGA = Appropriate for Gestational Age (above the 10th and below the 90th percentile), SGA = Small for Gestational Age (below the 10th percentile). *Reference: Wikipedia.*

Types of Growth Restriction[49,54]

Symmetrical Growth Restriction (less commonly known as global growth restriction) is where the baby has developed slowly throughout the entire pregnancy, having been affected very early. The head circumference of a newborn who has experienced this type of growth restriction is in proportion to the rest of the body. This affects 25% of IUGR babies and presents a 25% risk of chromosomal abnormalities (e.g., Down syndrome, trisomy 13, trisomy 18).

Common causes include:

+ Early intrauterine infections, such as cytomegalovirus, rubella, or toxoplasmosis
+ Chromosomal abnormalities
+ Anemia
+ Maternal substance abuse

Asymmetrical Growth Restriction occurs when the baby has grown normally for the first two trimesters but encounters difficulties in the final trimester of development, usually secondary to preeclampsia. These babies have a smaller head circumference relative to their birth weight. They have a small, thin body, out of proportion with their head, and appear "long and skinny." Other symptoms include dry, peeling skin and an overly thin umbilical cord.

Common causes include:

+ Chronic high blood pressure
+ Severe malnutrition.

The treatment is either delivery or improved blood flow to the uterus (via bed rest).

What Problems Can I Expect for My Baby?

IUGR babies can suffer both short- and long-term problems, and some even die. Complications from birth and trouble adjusting after birth include such things as perinatal acidosis (high acid in the baby's body fluids), hypoglycemia (low blood sugar), hypothermia (low body temperature), coagulation problems, certain immunologic deficiencies, and issues related to prematurity. Kids could suffer shortness, cognitive delays, and a slightly higher chance of neurologic disorders as they grow older.[55]

Other Problems Your Baby MAY Encounter[49]

Intrapartum Asphyxia—this occurs when the baby is unable to handle the stress of labor as well as a healthy baby, specifically during contractions, when oxygen is reduced. This in turn can lead to acidosis.

Neonatal Hypoglycemia and Hypocalcemia—low blood sugar and calcium.

Meconium Aspiration—when a baby is stressed in utero, it sometimes has its first poop, called meconium, which is a sticky, tar-like substance. When the baby poops while it's still in the womb, it can then breathe it in, leading to all sorts of problems.

Neurodevelopmental Delay—studies have shown that babies with bad IUGR are more likely to experience developmental delays, cardiovascular disease, and other problems later in life.

In summary: IUGR = bed rest. Sorry, ladies.

Types of Surveillance Tests[49]

Non-Stress Test—Doctors watch the changes in the baby's heart rate as the baby moves. If the heart rate increases more than 15 beats for more than 15 seconds, this is considered to be a reactive response, which is normal. If the heart rate does not increase, remains flat, or decreases, this is an abnormal response.

Amniotic Fluid Index—The amniotic fluid (of the four pockets) is measured to obtain a number. Doctors are looking for a reduction in the number over time, as this could indicate IUGR.

Doppler of the Umbilical Artery—This is an ultrasound that looks at the baby's blood flow through the placenta and at whether there is any resistance. If resistance is seen, then this is a clue as to why the baby is having growth problems.

Biophysical Profile—This test combines a non-stress test and the amniotic fluid index with fetal movement, breathing, and muscle tone. "While the biophysical profile is a useful test, when it becomes abnormal, the fetus may have already suffered some damage."[49]

Cochrane Reviews

1. It is not clear whether or not the use of abdominal decompression, which involves a hard dome placed over your belly that uses pressure, works in cases of impaired fetal growth and preeclampsia.[56]

2. There is no evidence (i.e., no studies have been done) showing that the use of transcutaneous electrical nerve stimulation (TENS) therapy helps blood flow through the placenta in women with placental insufficiency.[57]

3. There is too little evidence to prove whether the use of betamimetic drugs improves the growth of the developing baby who is smaller than average. More research is needed.[58]

4. There is not enough evidence to evaluate the benefits and risks of maternal oxygen therapy for suspected impaired fetal growth. [59] They found only three studies, each with a small sample size, so you guessed right...more research is needed!

5. There is not enough evidence to show whether nutrient therapy helps women who are carrying smaller than expected babies.[60]

6. There is not enough evidence to prove the benefits of extra plasma for slow-growing babies.[61] (There were NO studies included!)

Summary: Cochrane Reviews in this area don't say, or seem to know, jack. They're of little help.

Multiples

I've included multiples in this chapter because this is a big risk factor for delivering early. Only 23% of all pregnancies are multiples, but they lead to 15–20% of all early births. Almost 60% of twins arrive too soon. Forty percent of them will come early due to spontaneous labor caused by PPROM.[1] About 8% of twins are born before 32 weeks, or what is considered very preterm, while 48% are born between 32 to 36 weeks, and 44% at term or later.[62]

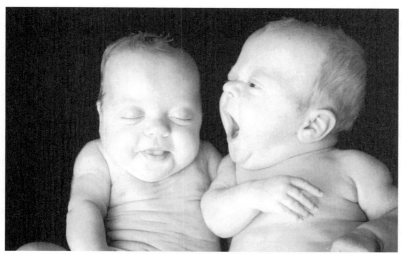

Three month premature twins at 4 months old (1 month adjusted).

Preterm twins have been on the rise over the last couple decades; therefore, the need for respiratory support for these babies has also increased. The good news is that death rates in twins have decreased over that same period. Even though they're coming earlier, they have a higher chance of surviving today than they did 20 years ago.[62]

Regrettably for you ladies carrying multiple babies, common treatments such as 17P injections have not been proven effective in reducing preterm birth. There seem to be other factors at work that are causing you to have your babies early. As the authors of a medical text state, "Currently, the only proven effective approach to prevention of PTB (preterm birth) in multiple gestations is avoidance of multiple gestations."[1] That's not much help.

That could be seen as kind of a depressing statement, but you don't have to see it that way. Many, many women carrying multiples have either made it to term or had early babies who are now healthy, active kids.

Now for the good news: For those of you carrying twins who are in preterm labor, only 20% of you will actually have your babies within seven days. To determine whether you are in "true" versus "false" labor, a cervical length of less than 2.5 cm is the cut-off point for concluding that you are having "real" (productive) contractions. A length of 3.0 cm or more, along with a negative FFN swab, at 24 weeks means only about a 5% chance of having your babies before 32 weeks.[1]

The phenomenon I spoke of previously in regards to the actual stretching of the uterus causing early birth is shown in the fact that the more babies you're carrying, the bigger your stomach will be, and the less time you will most likely carry these babies. The average carrying time of twins is 35.3 weeks, and this drops to 29.9 weeks with quads.[63]

All I can say to you ladies is, "YOU GO, GIRL!" How amazing are you, growing not only one baby, but two, three, or four? So, you really have to hang in there. Back pain, weight gain compounded by multiple babies, all on top of a high-risk pregnancy: you really deserve a gold medal. (And some diamonds, a vacation, and maybe even a car from your significant other.)

These are not suggested for multiple pregnancies, as they have not been shown to help reduce early births:[1]

+ Preventative contraction-stopping medications (i.e. tocolytics) (they are linked to more side effects in women with multiples)
+ Progesterone
+ Bed rest
+ Cerclage
+ Home uterine monitoring for contractions
+ Cervical length checks in women with NO symptoms

What should always be considered, however, are:[1]

+ Antenatal corticosteroids for any woman thought to be in preterm labor or who has experienced preterm premature rupture of membranes (PPROM) at 24 to 34 weeks, no matter how many babies she is carrying.
  • Steroids have been proven to reduce the incidence of death of the baby, respiratory distress syndrome, cerebroventricular hemorrhage (a common type of brain bleed in preemies), necrotizing enterocolitis (where the intestine dies), and infection within the first 48 hours after birth.

If you're carrying a higher number of multiples, you may be forced to make a tough decision and "reduce" the number of babies you're carrying. Then, not only will you have to choose to reduce, if that is your choice, but on top of a high-risk pregnancy, you will also have to grieve the loss of your other baby (or babies). This will surely be a difficult decision, one that only you and your spouse/significant other can make. Make sure you are clear on the exact risks for the number of babies you're carrying and the consequences of your decision.

> *"I had a multi-fetal reduction from quadruplets to twins because I was advised that the quadruplet pregnancy would not have been viable without the reduction."* ~ Margaret, Hong Kong

Cochrane Review

---

1. "There is currently not enough evidence to support a policy of routine hospitalization for bed rest in multiple pregnancy. No reduction in the risk of preterm birth or perinatal death is evident, although there is a suggestion that fetal growth is improved. For women with an uncomplicated twin pregnancy, the results of this review suggest that it may be harmful in that the risk of very preterm birth is increased. Until further evidence is available to the contrary, the policy cannot be recommended for routine clinical practice."[64]

Twin-to-Twin Transfusion Syndrome (TTTS)[65]

So you may wonder why I included this in a book about conditions that lead to preterm birth. First, I got several requests to include this information, so as a promise to them, here it is. Also, women carrying multiples are at a higher risk for preterm birth, and some of them have to deal with this too, so it does apply.

This condition affects monochorionic twin pregnancies, or identical twins, which occurs in about 1 in 320 pregnancies. Weekly monitoring is suggested in identical twin pregnancies. Twins sometime share the same placenta and blood flow, which usually doesn't cause a problem, as it's equally shared. This syndrome happens when the blood flow is uneven and goes through one twin, the donor, then to the other twin, the recipient.

The donor twin typically has very little amniotic fluid and often doesn't grow well. The recipient twin has lots of fluid, causing a swollen bladder among other issues. A bladder that is bigger in one baby on ultrasound is an early sign. The risk of death for both babies is very high, at about 80% WITHOUT treatment. Fifteen weeks' gestation is considered an important time to get checked in order to predict, with accuracy, whether your babies will suffer from this. The most severe cases typically develop between 16 and 18 weeks. If the babies survive there's the chance of physical or neurological damage.

Treatments include:

+ Amnioreduction, or the removal of excess amniotic fluid continually throughout pregnancy.

+ Laser treatment of the abnormal vessels in the placenta (endoscopic laser surgery).

+ Puncture of the membrane between the babies (septostomy).

+ Allowing one twin to die (selective feticide).

One study found that a laparoscopy-assisted technique for laser photocoagulation (which causes the tissue around a point of blood leak to coagulate and seal it off) was linked to better survival of the babies with TTTS who had a complete anterior placenta (a placenta located in the front of the uterus).[66] This was shown to be a very promising treatment for babies.

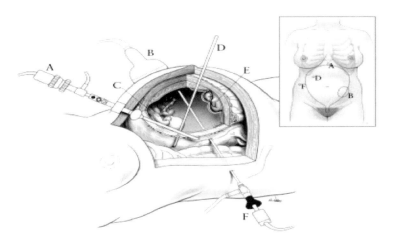

Figure 2-4. Diagram of laparoscopy-guided fetoscopy with an anterior placenta. A, laparoscope; B, ultrasound probe; C, recipient baby in its sac; D, blunt probe; E, donor baby or "stuck twin"; F, fetoscope. (I know it looks intimidating, but this saves TTTS babies.)

Summary: Multiples and TTTS

♦ All woman carrying identical twins need to be screened for this at around 15 weeks.

♦ If you are showing signs of this condition, doctors who perform this surgery can be hard to come by. Do your research, contact multiples support groups for references, and know you may have to travel. Many healthy babies have been born after TTTS, especially with a skilled doctor experienced in doing this surgery.

My Struggle with TTTS

By Jenni

"February 23, 2007 was one of the worst days of my life. I was 23 weeks pregnant with identical twin boys. That morning, I sat in a hospital room with my husband as the doctor told us that there was a very good chance that we were going to lose both our babies. That was the moment that I began praying for a miracle.

We had only been trying for a short time, which was surprising given that I had been diagnosed with Polycystic Ovarian Syndrome (PCOS) and was told that it might take us "a while" to conceive. "Do you see two heartbeats?" he asked at our nine-week sonogram. All we could do was laugh. We were overjoyed, unbelievably excited, and also completely terrified. The thought of one baby was overwhelming enough. What were we going to do with two? "Two college tuitions," my husband, Tom, kept saying over and over as we left the doctor's office.

At our first visit with the perinatologist, she briefly mentioned a condition that occurs in 15% of twin pregnancies, called Twin-to-Twin Transfusion Syndrome. She told us that if it was to occur, "not much can be done," and that current treatments were "very experimental." Tom and I left the office slightly concerned, but we dismissed most of our fears due to an 85% chance that our babies would be just fine. I did a little bit of research on TTTS and then put it out of my mind.

We started planning for the arrival of our boys. I was told that I would probably be on some amount of bed rest due to being pregnant with twins, so I began researching baby items. I registered at Babies 'R Us. We bought a house with a backyard big enough for two boys to run around and play. We purchased two cribs and painted stencils on the babies' bedroom wall to match the quilt that my mother-in-law, who had passed away a year earlier, made for her future grandchildren. I left my job when we moved, so that I could be a full-time mom to my two baby boys. I switched medical practices and met the doctors who would eventually help us fight to save the lives of our precious boys.

My new doctors monitored me very closely, and, at 19 weeks, when there was a slight discrepancy in the babies' amniotic fluid (a possible early sign of TTTS), I began having weekly sonograms. My doctor told me that TTTS occurs when identical twins share a placenta, and one twin starts to get more nutrients and amniotic fluid than the other. The recipient twin gets more placental blood flow, which causes increased blood in the baby's body and increased urine output, which causes increased amniotic fluid. The increased blood volume (too much blood in the baby's body) can lead to heart failure. The donor twin has decreased placental blood flow and decreased blood volume, which causes poor growth and development, as well as decreased amniotic fluid, which causes further growth retardation. He said that there are treatments for TTTS, including an amniotic fluid reduction, which decreases fluid in one amniotic sac with the hope that the levels will even out. The other treatment is laser surgery, in which they separate the blood vessels in the placenta, thereby essentially giving each baby his own placenta from which to nourish himself.

When my fluid levels were slightly off, my doctor was concerned but also confident. He said that there wasn't much to worry about right now, and if things worsened, they would send me to Philadelphia for surgery, which he said was no longer considered "experimental," as my previous doctor had suggested. His confidence helped to ease my nerves; however, *when I did my own research, I learned the scary truth about TTTS. There is an extremely high chance of "fetal demise," but in the mind of a pregnant mother, you call this the death of both of your tiny, helpless babies. The laser surgery is somewhat new, and there are strict criteria you must meet in order to qualify for it.*

Finally, on my third week in a row of the babies' fluid levels being "slightly" off, they evened out to a stable level. The doctor told me that I could "take next week off" and skip the sonogram. Tom and I were so relieved, and we spent the weekend with my family. Toward the end of the weekend, I began to experience heaviness in my abdomen but assumed it was just what being pregnant felt like. That Wednesday, I went to a Broadway show with my mother. She called it my "last hurrah," meaning that I would soon be a mother and have much less free time. Neither of us had any idea that her statement was more true that we ever imagined.

I was continuing to experience the abdominal heaviness, and on the advice of my mother, I called the doctor just to "check it out." They told me to come in for a sonogram. I asked if I could come the next day, since I was meeting a friend in the area. The doctor said he would prefer if I came that afternoon. I told my husband I'd be back in an hour or two and went to the doctor appointment that would change my life forever. It was then that I was diagnosed with TTTS. The babies' fluid levels were dramatically different, and baby B was heading toward heart failure. I had an immediate amniotic fluid reduction. My parents came that night to be there with me, as they have always been throughout my life. I was admitted to the hospital for observation after the fluid reduction.

It was the next morning that we were told by our doctor that our babies would probably not survive. The amniotic reduction had not helped as much as he had hoped, and baby B was even closer to experiencing heart failure. My husband and I sat and listened to him, but all I could think about was doing whatever was necessary to give my boys a chance to live. The doctor put in a cerclage to try to avoid an early birth, but was concerned that the procedure could cause contractions because of the unstable uterine environment. The contractions came, but then they lessened, and we managed to make it through another day.

I spent the weekend waiting at the hospital. The plan was to send me to Children's Hospital of Philadelphia for laser surgery to separate the blood vessels in the placenta. But first I had to make it through the weekend without going into labor. It was then that I began the first of many days to be spent in bed. I was very fortunate to have such supportive friends and family to help distract me and get me through that first weekend and the weeks to come. The weekend passed with fewer contractions, thanks in part to a terbutaline pump (intravenous medication to stop the contractions), which made me feel awful but was well worth it.

I sat in my father's car for an hour to get to the hospital in Philadelphia, praying at each bump in the road, that this wouldn't be the one that would send me into labor. We checked into a hotel and waited to meet with the doctors. The first day at the hospital consisted of many tests to prepare for the upcoming laser surgery. Toward the end of the day, we were met with more bad news. Our doctor explained that there was an unusual measurement in baby B's brain that might indicate brain damage due to the TTTS. They recommended an MRI to confirm this and told us that we had something to think about that evening. They explained that if baby B did in fact have brain damage, we had the option to "clamp the cord" in order to give baby A a higher chance of survival. Tom and I discussed it somewhat, but it was just too much for me. I said that I needed to wait and see what the MRI would show before considering this possibility.

The next day, the MRI took 45 minutes. Possibly the longest 45 minutes of my life. The results came back that afternoon, and we were told that baby B did not have any brain damage, and we could go ahead with the surgery as planned. The relief we felt was immense, but we still had an enormous hurdle in front of us.

The following day we met with the doctors as well as a hospital social worker. The doctors explained that even with the surgery, there was only a 60% chance that both babies would survive. They also said that if we were lucky, they would make it to 28 weeks, which would increase their chance of survival but still carries the risk of problems related to prematurity. We were informed that there was a possibility that the surgery would send me into preterm labor and the babies would have to be delivered. The social worker asked me if this was to happen, would I like to hold them and say goodbye? I broke down at this point and immediately said, "No." The social worker recommended doing this for the purpose of closure, but I could not imagine being able to live through such a heart-wrenching experience. I can't even begin to imagine the feelings of a mother who has to go through something like this, and my heart goes out to anyone who had to endure such pain.

Finally, the day of the surgery came. It was quick for me, of course, but my husband, his father and my parents waited anxiously in the waiting room for several hours. When they brought me out of surgery, I began having very intense contractions. I remember the look of concern on my husband's face, but he did not tell me at the time how upset he truly was. I found out later that he left the room and began to cry in the hallway, with his father comforting him. He truly was my strength, and I never could have gotten through those weeks without him.

The contractions eventually subsided, and a day later, the doctors declared the surgery a success. They reminded me, however, that there was still an extremely high risk of preterm labor and put me on bed rest at home. Then, all we could do was wait.

I stayed in bed all day long, only allowed to get up to use the bathroom or to go to my weekly doctor appointments. My parents visited every weekend, and we played way too many games of bedside poker. Each week, Tom would mark my accomplishment by writing the week number in blueberries on my morning waffle. Days turned to weeks, weeks turned to months, and I stayed in bed. Twenty-eight weeks came and went, with only a few episodes of contractions that required medication. The babies continued to grow, and baby B's heart continued to improve. I was in bed for a total of 13 weeks.

Finally, on May 28th, 2007, at 5:30 in the evening, I went into labor. We had made it to 36 weeks and were completely overjoyed. Thomas Jacob was born at 10:06 pm, Aidan Scott at 10:07 pm. Two completely healthy baby boys who required no NICU stay at all. Four days later, Tom and I took our miracle babies home and began our life as the parents of newborn twins.

Today my boys are happy, healthy, active three-year-olds. My experience with TTTS seems like a lifetime ago, but it will always be with me. Tommy and Aidan have added incredible meaning and happiness to my life. They are my whole world. Tom and I went through such a painful and difficult pregnancy, but we wouldn't change a thing. Our boys are everything to us, and to change our experience would be to change who they are. We couldn't imagine our life any other way.

We supported each other, we hoped, we bargained, we put our faith in our doctors and followed every single instruction they gave us. But there are parents who did exactly what we did who have lost their babies. Sometimes things turn out the way you hope for, and sometimes they don't. I believe that we were extremely lucky. And I try to always remember just how lucky we are.

For me, this experience has strengthened a belief that I think every mother has: children are a precious gift, and each day with them should be treasured. Whether you've had a difficult pregnancy or an easy one; twins, triplets, or a single baby; boys, girls or both, becoming a mother is a life-altering experience. Of course, there will be times when we are frustrated, exhausted, or overwhelmed. But I plan to always do my best to cherish as many moments with my boys as I possibly can. Each moment that a mother spends with her child, making him smile, watching him play, helping him find his way in the world, is truly miraculous."

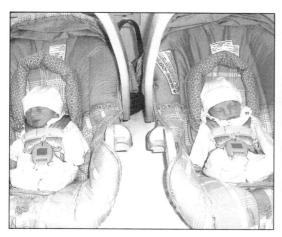 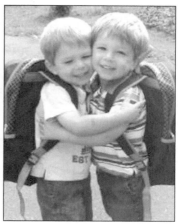

Cochrane Review

1. "Limited evidence suggests the best way to save babies with twin-to-twin transfusion syndrome is to perform laser treatment to the placenta," when compared to removing excess fluid. Since this is such a specialized area, the authors point out that if there is no expertise with laser surgery, "amnioreduction is then the treatment of choice."[67]

Things That Work…and Things That Don't

Folic Acid

Folic acid is commonly taken pre-pregnancy and during early pregnancy to prevent neural-tube defects. Researchers wondered whether women who continued taking folic acid vitamin supplements beyond the first trimester would promote fetal growth and reduce preterm birth. They found that preterm birth was reduced significantly in the folic acid group, 7.6% vs. 11.8%.[68] I guess this is just another reason to take your vitamins.

Omega-3 a Cure-All?

One study looked at whether Omega-3 fatty acid supplements could prevent preterm birth in women who had already had a spontaneous prior preterm birth and who were also receiving 17 alpha-hydroxy-progesterone caproate (aka P-17, or progesterone). They found that it had no impact and did not reduce the rates of preterm delivery.[69]

Metronidazole

Metronidazole is an antibiotic that's used mostly for anaerobic bacteria and protozoa [think bacterial vaginosis (BV) infections]. Some scientists wondered if this drug would help reduce early preterm labor in asymptomatic high-risk women with positive fetal fibronectin in the second trimester. Unfortunately, the opposite happened, and it actually increased preterm birth before 30 weeks. The study was canned before it was concluded, because it was clear that the intended benefit was not being achieved, but up to that point the preterm birth rate almost doubled in women taking the drug.[70] Not good…so, *do not* take this drug.

Initially, the scientists had very good reasons to believe that this antibiotic would help women at risk, because we know that an underlying infection can often be blamed for an early delivery, but now that this information has been published, we should all hope that no doctor will prescribe this drug for a woman at risk of an early delivery. The scary thing for me, as I wrote this, is that I realized that I took this drug, Flagyl, as it is commonly known, early in my pregnancy with my second son due to a suspected BV infection. Scary.

Cochrane Review

"Taking zinc while pregnant can help to reduce preterm birth, but not other problems, such as low birthweight babies. It is not completely clear whether this effect was due to nutritional issues in the women involved in the studies."[71]

References

1. Berghella V. *Preterm Birth: Prevention & Management.* West Sussex, UK. Wiley-Blackwell, 2010.
2. Mateus J, Pereira L, Baxter J, et al. Effectiveness of fetal fibronectin testing compared with digital cervical assessment of women with preterm contractions. *Am J Perinatol* 2007;24(6):381–385.

3. Othman M, Neilson JP, Alfirevic Z. Probiotics for preventing preterm labour. *Cochrane Database of Systematic Reviews* 2007, Issue 1. Art. No.: CD005941. (Last assessed as up-to-date: April 15, 2010)

4. King JF, Flenady V, Murray L. Prophylactic antibiotics for inhibiting preterm labour with intact membranes. *Cochrane Database of Systematic Reviews* 2002, Issue 4. Art. No.: CD000246. (Last assessed as up-to-date: April 15, 2010)

5. Medina TM, Hill DA. Preterm premature rupture of membranes: diagnosis and management. *Am Fam Physician* 2006;73(4):659–664.

6. Mingione MJ, Pressman EK, Woods JR. Prevention of PPROM: current and future strategies. *J Matern Fetal Neonatal Med* 2006;19(12):783–789.

7. Moore RM, Mansour JM, Redline RW, et al. The physiology of fetal membrane rupture: insight gained from the determination of physical properties. *Placenta* 2006;27(11–12):1037–1051.

8. Odibo AO, Talucci M, Berghella V. Prediction of preterm premature rupture of membranes by transvaginal ultrasound features and risk factors in a high-risk population. *Ultrasound Obstet Gynecol* 2002;20(3):245–251.

9. Odibo AO, Berghella V, Reddy U, et al. Does transvaginal ultrasound of the cervix predict preterm premature rupture of membranes in a high-risk population? *Ultrasound Obstet Gynecol* 2001;18(3):223–227.

10. Oboro VO, Adekanie BA, Apantaku BD, Onadipe OA. Pre-term pre-labour rupture of membranes: effect of chorioamnionitis on overall neonatal outcome. 2006;26(8):740–743.

11. Goldenberg RL, Culhane JF, Iams JD, Romero R. Epidemiology and causes of preterm birth. *Lancet* 2008;371(9606):75–84.

12. Najati N, Rafeey M, Melekian T. Comparison of umbilical cord interlukin-8 in low birth weight infants with premature rupture of membranes and intact membranes. *Pak J Biol Sci* 2009;12(15):1094–1097.

13. Li QS, Qi HB. Expression of bone morphogenetic protein-2 in fetal membranes from pregnant women with premature rupture of membranes and its clinic significance. *Zhonghua Fu Chan Ke Za Zhi* 2009;44(6):405–408.

14. Soylu H, Jefferies A, Diambomba Y, et al. Rupture of membranes before the age of viability and birth after the age of viability: comparison of outcomes in a matched cohort study. *J Perinatol* 2010;30(10);645–649.

15. Paumier A, Gras-Leguen C, Branger B, et al. Premature rupture of membranes before 32 weeks of gestation: prenatal prognosis factors. *Gynecol Obstet Fertil* 2008;36(7–8):748–756.

16. Mercer BM, Rabello YA, Thurnau GR, et al. The NICHD-MFMU antibiotic treatment of preterm PROM study: impact of initial amniotic fluid volume of pregnancy outcome. *Am J Obstet Gynecol* 2006;194(2):438–445.

17. Jenkins TM, Berghella V, Shlossman PA, et al. Timing of cerclage removal after preterm premature rupture of membranes: maternal and neonatal outcomes. *Am J Obstet Gynecol* 2000;183(4):847–852.

18. Hofmeyr GJ. Amnioinfusion for preterm rupture of membranes. *Cochrane Database of Systematic Reviews* 1998, Issue 1. Art. No.: CD000942. (Last assessed as up-to-date: April 15, 2010.)

19. Kenyon S, Boulvain M, Neilson JP. Antibiotics for preterm rupture of membranes. *Cochrane Database of Systematic Reviews* 2003, Issue 2. Art. No.: CD001058. (Last assessed as up-to-date: April 15, 2010.)

20. Buchanan SL, Crowther CA, Levett KM, et al. Planned early birth versus expectant management for women with preterm prelabour rupture of membranes prior to 37 weeks' gestation for improving pregnancy outcome. *Cochrane Database of Systematic Reviews* 2010, Issue 3. Art. No.: CD004735. (Last assessed as up-to-date: April 15, 2010.)

21. Preeclampsia Foundation, www.preeclampsia.org.

22. Grujić I, Milasinović L. Hypertension, pre-eclampsia and eclampsia-monitoring and outcome of pregnancy. *Med Pregl* 2006;59(11–12):556–559.

23. Boomsma CM, Fauser BC, Mackion NS. Pregnancy complications in women with polycystic ovary syndrome. *Semin Reprod Med* 2008;26(1):72–84.

24. Barton JR, Sibai BM. Prediction and prevention of recurrent preeclampsia. *Obstet Gynecol* 2008;112(2 pt 1):359–372.

25. Bujold E, Morency AM, Roberge S, et al. Acetylsalicylic acid for the prevention of preeclampsia and intra-uterine growth restriction in women with abnormal uterine artery Doppler: a systematic review and meta-analysis. *J Obstet Gynaecol Can* 2009;31(9):818–826.

26. Coomarasamy A, Honest H, Papaioannou S, et al. Aspirin for prevention of preeclampsia in women with historical risk factors: a systematic review. *Obstet Gynecol* 2003;101(6):1319–1332.

27. Newstead J, von Dadelszen P, Magee LA. Preeclampsia and future cardiovascular risk. *Expert Rev Cardiovasc Ther* 2007;5(2):283–294.

28. Center for Disease Control and Prevention, http://www.cdc.gov/physicalactivity/everyone/guidelines/adults.html.

29. Duley L, Henderson-Smart DJ, Meher S, King JF. Antiplatelet agents for preventing pre-eclampsia and its complications. *Cochrane Database of Systematic Reviews* 2007, Issue 2. Art. No.: CD004659. (Last assessed as up-to-date: April 15, 2010.)

30. Duley L, Williams J, Henderson-Smart DJ. Plasma volume expansion for treatment of pre-eclampsia. *Cochrane Database of Systematic Reviews* 1999, Issue 4. Art. No.: CD001805. (Last assessed as up-to-date: April 15, 2010.)

31. Meher S, Duley L. Progesterone for preventing pre-eclampsia and its complications. *Cochrane Database of Systematic Reviews* 2006, Issue 4. Art. No.: CD006175. (Last assessed as up-to-date: April 15, 2010.)

32. Meher S, Duley L. Rest during pregnancy for preventing pre-eclampsia and its complications in women with normal blood pressure. *Cochrane Database of Systematic Reviews* 2006, Issue 2. Art. No.: CD005939. (Last assessed as up-to-date: April 15, 2010.)

33. Rumbold A, Middleton P, Crowther CA. Vitamin supplementation for preventing miscarriage. *Cochrane Database of Systematic Reviews* 2005, Issue 2. Art. No.: CD004073. (Last assessed as up-to-date: April 15, 2010.)

34. Meher S, Duley L. Nitric oxide for preventing pre-eclampsia and its complications. *Cochrane Database of Systematic Reviews* 2007, Issue 2. Art. No.: CD006490. (Last assessed as up-to-date: April 15, 2010.)

35. Duley L, Gülmezoglu AM, Henderson-Smart DJ. Magnesium sulphate and other anticonvulsants for women with pre-eclampsia. *Cochrane Database of Systematic Reviews* 2003, Issue 2. Art. No.: CD000025. (Last assessed as up-to-date: April 15, 2010.)

36. Google Health, Placenta Abruptio, https://health.google.com/health/ref/Placenta+abruptio

37. Gaufberg SV. Abruptio placentae in emergency medicine. Emedicine (from WebMD), Dec 12, 2008, http://emedicine.medscape.com/article/795514-overview.

38. Wikipedia, Placental abruption, http://en.wikipedia.org/wiki/Placental_abruption.

39. Medline Plus, U.S. National Library of Medicine, National Institutes of Health, Placenta abruptio, http://www.nlm.nih.gov/medlineplus/ency/article/000901.htm.

40. Zdoukopoulos N, Zintzaras E. Genetic risk factors for placental abruption: a HuGE review and meta-analysis. *Epidemiology* 2008;19(2):309–323.

41. Neilson JP. Interventions for treating placental abruption. *Cochrane Database of Systematic Reviews* 2003, Issue 1. Art. No.: CD003247. (Last assessed as up-to-date: April 29, 2009.)

42. Valsamakis G, Kanaka-Gantenbein C, Malamitsi-Puchner A, Mastorakos G. Causes of intrauterine growth restriction and the postnatal development of the metabolic syndrome. *Ann N Y Acad Sci* 2006;1092:138–147.

43. Lawrence EJ. Part 1: A matter of size: evaluating the growth-restricted neonate. *Adv Neonatal Care* 2006;6(6):313–322.

44. Kinzler WL, Vintzileos AM. Fetal growth restriction: a modern approach. *Curr Opin Obstet Gynecol* 2008;20(2):125–131.

45. Medline Plus, National Institutes of Health, Intrauterine Growth Restriction, http://www.nlm.nih.gov/medlineplus/ency/article/001500.htm.

46. Hendrix N, Berghella V. Non-placental causes of intrauterine growth restriction. *Semin Perinatol* 2008;32(3):161–165.

47. Cetin I, Alvino G. Intrauterine growth restriction: implications for placental metabolism and transport. A review. *Placenta* 2009;30(Suppl. A):S77–82.

48. Platz E, Newman R. Diagnosis of IUGR: traditional biometry. *Semin Perinatol* 2008;32(3):140–147. http://www.fetal.com/IUGR/treatment.html.

49. Fetal Diagnostic Centers, Dr. Greggory R. DeVore M.D. (located in Pasadena and Tarzana, California).

50. Rizzo G, Arduini D. Intrauterine growth restriction: diagnosis and management—a review. *Minerva Ginecol* 2009;61(5):411–420.

51. Ott WJ. Sonographic diagnosis of fetal growth restriction. *Clin Obstet Gynecol* 2006;49(2):295–307.

52. Mook-Kanamori DO, Steegers EA, Eilers PH, et al. Risk factors and outcomes associated with first-trimester fetal growth restriction. *JAMA* 2010;303(6):527–534.

53. Becker R, Vonk R. Doppler sonography of uterine arteries at 20–23 weeks: depth of notch gives information on probability of adverse pregnancy outcome and degree of fetal growth restriction in a low-risk population. *Fetal Diagn Ther* 2010;27(2):78–86.

54. Wikipedia, Small for gestational age, http://en.wikipedia.org/wiki/Small_for_gestational_age.

55. Pallotto EK, Kilbride HW. Perinatal outcome and later implications of intrauterine growth restriction. *Clin Obstet Gynecol* 2006;49(2):257–269.

56. Hofmeyr GJ. Abdominal decompression for suspected fetal compromise/pre-eclampsia. *Cochrane Database of Systematic Reviews* 1996, Issue 1. Art. No.: CD000004. (Last assessed as up-to-date: April 15, 2010.)

57. Say L, Gülmezoglu AM, Hofmeyr GJ. Transcutaneous electrostimulation for suspected placental insufficiency (Diagnosed by Doppler Studies). *Cochrane Database of Systematic Reviews* 1995, Issue 1. Art. No.: CD000079. (Last assessed as up-to-date: April 15, 2010.)

58. Say L, Gülmezoglu AM, Hofmeyr GJ. Betamimetics for suspected impaired fetal growth. *Cochrane Database of Systematic Reviews* 2001, Issue 4. Art. No.: CD000036. (Last assessed as up-to-date: June 23, 2009.)

59. Say L, Gülmezoglu AM, Hofmeyr GJ. Maternal oxygen administration for suspected impaired fetal growth. *Cochrane Database of Systematic Reviews* 2003, Issue 1. Art. No.: CD000137. (Last assessed as up-to-date: April 15, 2010.)

60. Say L, Gülmezoglu AM, Hofmeyr GJ. Maternal nutrient supplementation for suspected impaired fetal growth. *Cochrane Database of Systematic Reviews* 2003, Issue 1. Art. No.: CD000148. (Last assessed as up-to-date: April 15, 2010.)

61. Say L, Gülmezoglu AM, Hofmeyr GJ. Plasma volume expansion for suspected impaired fetal growth. *Cochrane Database of Systematic Reviews* 1996, Issue 3. Art. No.: CD000167. (Last assessed as up-to-date: April 15, 2010.)

62. Hartley RS, Hitti J. Increasing rates of preterm births coincide with improving twin pair survival. *J Perinat Med* 2010;38(3):297–303.

63. Goldenberg RL, Culhane JF, Iams JD, Romero R. Epidemiology and causes of preterm birth. *Lancet* 2008;371(9606):75–84.

64. Crowther CA. Hospitalisation and bed rest for multiple pregnancy. *Cochrane Database of Systematic Reviews* 2001, Issue 1. Art. No.: CD000110. (Published 2009.)

65. The University of Maryland Medical Center, www.umm.edu/ttts, High-Risk and Twin Pregnancies, with Dr. Ahmet Baschat.

66. Papanna R, Johnson A, Ivey RT, et al. Laparoscopy-assisted fetoscopy for laser surgery in twin-twin transfusion syndrome with anterior placentation. *Ultrasound Obstet Gynecol* 2010;35(1):65-70.

67. Roberts D, Neilson JP, Kilby M, Gates S. Interventions for the treatment of twin-twin transfusion syndrome. *Cochrane Database of Systematic Reviews* 2008, Issue 1. Art. No.: CD002073. (Last assessed as up-to-date: January 30, 2008.)

68. Czeizel AE, Puhó EH, Langmar Z, et al. Possible association of folic acid supplementation during pregnancy with reduction of preterm birth: a population-based study. *Eur J Obstet Gynecol Reprod Biol* 2010;148(2):135–140.

69. Harper M, Thom E, Klebanoff MA, et al. Omega-3 fatty acid supplementation to prevent recurrent preterm birth: a randomized controlled trial. *Obstet Gynecol* 2010;115(2 pt 1):234–242.

70. Shennan A, Crawshaw S, Briley A, et al. A randomized controlled trial of metronidazole for the prevention of preterm birth in women positive for cervicovaginal fetal fibronectin: the PREMET study. *BJOG* 2006;113(1):65–74.

71. Mahomed K, Bhutta ZA, Middleton P. Zinc supplementation for improving pregnancy and infant outcome. *Cochrane Database of Systematic Reviews* 2007, Issue 2. Art. No.: CD000230. (Last assessed as up-to-date: April 15, 2010.)

CHAPTER 3

Incompe . . . What? More Than You Ever Wanted to Know About Your Cervix

Incompetent cervix, weak cervix, cervical incompetence, cervical insufficiency . . . these are all terms you will hear to describe this "condition" (for lack of a better word). I call it IC, for incompetent cervix, simply because this is the term that I heard first, and it stuck, but I have no preference for any particular terminology. It is what it is.

Many people now frown on the use of this term because it's "negative" and tends to suggest a fault within the woman. Instead, they support the use of "cervical insufficiency." Is this really a softer term? Incompetent . . . insufficient . . . what's the difference? The point is, it all sucks having to deal with it, so I couldn't care less what you call it. Using softer words to describe it doesn't lessen what it really is . . . a real pain in the ass . . . or should I say, a real pain in the cervix. (Really, there's no physical pain at all involved.)

If you're like me, prior to your pregnancy or loss, you'd probably never even heard about IC or thought anything like this could happen to you. The term "incompetent" can imply something faulty with us, which is so far from the truth. How about if, instead, we call our cervices defective, nonexistent (for some of us), or just plain annoying? Because really, how many pregnant women, before labor sets in or they want to be in labor, give two hoots about their cervix or how long it is? I'll tell you…NONE!

How many women spend week after week wondering how long their cervix is, or if it shrunk? NONE. How many women freak if their cervices lose even 1 millimeter of length? Again, NONE. In reality, you will come to find out that, in the grand scheme of all pregnancies, only a small number of women suffer from IC.

Coming to terms with this was far from easy for me. I cursed my body after I lost my baby boy. I hated myself. I was way beyond angry and sad. I felt that I'd let my husband down, that I was somehow defective, and that he should get another wife who could carry his baby.

I cursed women who carried babies without a care in the world. I was so jealous of their easy pregnancies…blah back ache…blah I'm getting fat…blah I'm nauseous. My hidden thoughts were that I hated them, although I would never say anything mean to someone, because that's not me. It wasn't their fault I had IC.

I thought about giving up ever knowing and treasuring what pregnancy and birthing a live baby would be like, and considered adoption. (I should point out here that I am absolutely NOT against adoption. We had many discussions about our various options, and we just decided that it wasn't right for us at that time.) I spent hours crying in the shower so no one would hear me or know that I was crying…again. It was a very lonely time.

Slowly, however, I came around and found life to be fun again. I started laughing again. I started making it one day, then a couple days, then weeks without crying. Maybe you can say I came to terms with my loss because I later had a healthy child. Yes, I admit that definitely helped…lots. Had I lost my daughter—and there were many days where we weren't sure—that might have pushed me over the edge. I might have given up, and not be here today writing this book.

The dream of writing this book to help women who are in the same place as I was has saved me and helped me to come to terms with all that has happened. Volunteering for Sidelines and supporting other women has been a great outlet for me and has enabled me to channel my energy in a positive way. I am just lucky that I was able to turn to these outlets, and not to alcohol or drugs (not that I was a saint there either).

During pregnancy, we are unique in that we live and breathe our cervix, its length (or loss of length), the presence of funneling, or the status of our cervical stitch, aka cerclage, as it is known throughout the medical community, and whether it's holding strong. (Cerclages will be discussed in detail in a later chapter.) For us, our cervix is the cause of a huge amount of stress, concern, heartbreak, and fear. Please stay closed and long. Please hold my baby in.

A cervix is essential to the normal process of birth. As we all know, you need to dilate to 10 cm in order to deliver your baby. With this in mind, the cervix also plays a large role in the causes of an early baby, and also has the potential to be a big player in the prevention of early birth.

An incompetent cervix is one of the causes of preterm delivery. Over the years, and hundreds of studies later, it has been shown that cervical shortening, dilation of the *internal* cervical opening, and funneling, observed before term, are signs of an early delivery...possibly. Remember the whole odds thing? There's plenty of room for hope.

The simplest description of this "condition" is when the cervix is too weak to stay closed during pregnancy, often resulting in the extremely premature birth of your baby. Traditionally, it is defined as recurrent (i.e., three or more) second-trimester losses in the absence of true labor.

Current definitions have clarified this previous definition, stating that it is when you have had a prior preterm birth and/or loss(es) in the second trimester, AND shortening or dilation of your cervix before 24 weeks in your CURRENT pregnancy.[1]

Recent opinion is that the "AND" stated above is very important in considering how this condition is treated. Changes in thinking, which were driven by the research, have meant that, to possibly avoid unnecessary surgery—i.e., cerclage—many providers prefer to observe cervical changes before a cerclage is even offered. You will see less and less early cerclages, called preventative or history-indicated cerclages, today compared to the past. This is the "wait-and-see approach," which is discussed in the chapter on cerclages.

In this condition, the cervix thins and dilates in the absence of pain, contractions, ruptured membranes, or blood loss. (This is an important differentiation from premature labor). Preterm delivery is most likely to occur if there is no interference (i.e., treatment), for example with a cerclage.

This process of cervical thinning, leading ultimately to dilation and then delivery of the baby, is often slow and gradual and has been observed to take months in many women. With the use of proper techniques, namely transvaginal ultrasonography, early changes can be detected and treatment initiated (cerclage, progesterone, bed rest).[1]

Unlike the glucose test for diabetes or a blood test for HIV, there are no tests available for IC, so diagnosing it can be quite challenging. It is often only discovered after a loss or, if you're one of the lucky ones, after observation of shortening during your pregnancy in time to "catch" it.

The cervix is mostly made up of fibrous connective tissue (70% being type 1 collagen). With IC, the collagen can decrease to only about 67%, which makes the cervix structurally weaker.[1] Based on this, some have questioned whether it would be possible to measure amounts of cervical collagen using a noninvasive tool called a Collascope to provide a better way of diagnosing IC or determining outcomes.

They have shown that the reading obtained is much lower in women with IC. In simple terms, the lower the reading, the weaker your cervix is and the earlier your baby will come, theoretically.[2]

Hey wouldn't that be something? Before we even became pregnant, they could simply scan our cervix and produce a reading letting you know whether or not you had a good, strong cervix. Then, we wouldn't have to lose a baby to know that we need to be monitored and treated for this condition, which, sadly, is often the case now. So much anguish after a difficult pregnancy or loss could be avoided.

Often, the only symptoms a women experiences are an increase or change in her discharge and/or vaginal pressure (with very little bleeding). Some blood-tinged mucus from the loss of the mucous plug is also a warning sign of cervical dilation.

Dilation causes the amniotic sac (i.e., bag of water) to drop down into the vagina, causing the feeling of pressure. Often, this drop eventually causes the membranes to rupture—i.e., your water to break.

(*Cervix* is Latin for "neck." It is located in the lower, narrow portion of your uterus where it joins with the top of the vagina. It is cylindrical or conical in shape and protrudes through the upper frontal portion of the vaginal wall.)

Increased discharge was the only symptom I had, and I thought little of it when I placed that fateful call to my midwife, who wanted to see me to play it safe. (Increased discharge or a small amount of blood is usually your mucous plug coming out, which, just to drive the point home, is a sign that your cervix is dilating. Obviously, if you are near term, there is no need to worry about it, but I was only 21 weeks and a few days.)

I had been having increased discharge for about two days, which I thought was normal during pregnancy, since I'd had discharge all along. I was attending a two-day meeting, and I remember going to the bathroom and looking down after I'd peed to see a long, boogery string of discharge. I was a bit taken aback but thought, "Uhh, gross… this is what happens to you when you're pregnant?"

The next day, I felt a bit off and the weather was bad, so I called in sick and slept all day. I didn't notice much discharge, as being off my feet had probably taken pressure off my cervix. It wasn't until the following day, after I'd had sex and noticed even more discharge, that I started looking into it.

Since then, I have learned to always pay attention to any changes and to question them. It wasn't until I read a passage in *What to Expect When You're Expecting*,[3] which mentions that discharge could be a sign of premature labor, that I thought to call my midwife. For me, it was the signal that my whole world was about to be thrown upside down.

Thinking back, the only other symptoms I experienced were low kicks, almost in my coochie area. Just prior to this time, I finally felt my baby's first kicks, which were really low. It wasn't until later pregnancies, when I felt the baby kick up around and below my belly button, that I realized that what I'd experienced before wasn't normal, but was a sign that my son had "fallen" into my vagina. It was my first pregnancy, so how was I to know that kicks weren't supposed to be that low?

After I was admitted to the hospital, the first thing they saw when they put the speculum in to examine me were "fetal parts." "We have fetal parts here" is all I remember them saying. They could see his feet dangling low into my vagina.

It's often hard to differentiate IC from premature labor. In many cases, it's the chicken and the egg argument… did IC cause the cervix to open, in turn causing the waters to break/membranes to become exposed/infection, or did infection/contractions cause the cervix to open? It is these situations that can make IC difficult to diagnose. Not to mention that it only occurs in less than 1 to 2% of pregnancies.[4]

There were about 4.1 million recorded births in the U.S. in 2004,[5] so presumably; approximately 82,000 of these women had IC. This means that many doctors have never seen, or maybe even heard of, a case of IC, so finding the right doctor with experience can be quite a challenge.

According to one review article, "Cervical incompetence is still one of the most controversial obstetric entities." The same author concludes that, "Cervical incompetence and preterm labor are not distinct entities, but rather part of a spectrum leading to preterm delivery."[6]

Another article discusses the fact that there is no clear diagnosis. This, together with the lack of indisputable evidence for the effectiveness of cerclages, leads to confusion about how patients with IC should be cared for, and an increase in medical/legal disagreements surrounding appropriate treatments. The authors even point out that instead of clearing up these questions, cervical ultrasonography has actually done the opposite. It has increased confusion as to when/how to diagnose IC and further muddied the waters as to under what circumstances treatment becomes necessary.[7] For conditions such as diabetes or high cholesterol, there is a set standard of care and treatment. The same cannot be said for IC.

When looking at 1,006 women who delivered before 28 weeks, researchers found the following percentages: preterm labor 40%, prelabor premature rupture of membranes 23%, preeclampsia 18%, placental abruption 11%, cervical incompetence 5%, and fetal indication/intrauterine growth restriction 3%,[8] making this condition the second least common of those leading to preterm delivery.

Lucky you... you won the lottery of a rare pregnancy "condition." And that's not all. It's one that is tremendously challenging to diagnose and treat. In addition to that, many will even have to lose a baby or two in order for it to be figured out that they are in this shitty situation. Yeah, lucky us, right? (Yes, I have been told I'm sarcastic.)

Unfortunately, the reality is that a lot of us without a prior history or with some of the risk factors described below will suffer horribly from the loss of a baby or from a highly stressful pregnancy and the very real possibility of a preterm baby. Like it or not, this is the card we have been dealt.

In reality, the exact cause of IC, and preterm birth for that matter, is largely unknown. This uncertainty about the cause of IC is due to several reasons, including the fact that the exact biological and physical causes are not well understood. IC does not always show itself with each pregnancy, and the presence of a shortened cervix does not mean for certain that the result will be an early birth. Atypical cervical functioning has been shown to be a considerable part of the overall dilemma of preterm birth.[9]

Uterus and Uterine tubes

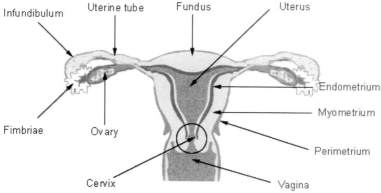

Figure 3-1. Internal view of female reproductive system. *Diagram courtesy of Wikipedia.*

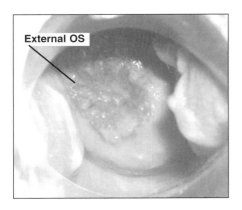

This is an approximately 1cm (i.e., one fingertip) dilated cervix. The area you can see around the outside opening (os), is a shallow, vascular, mucus-producing endocervical epithelium (which is usually on the inside) that has grown out onto the exterior portion of the cervix. This is called an ectropian cervix. This is normal in some women and often expands during pregnancy.
(Courtesy of the "Beautiful Cervix Project" www.beautifulcervix.com)

IC Is Different than Premature Labor

Many in the medical community recognize both IC and preterm labor as parts of a set of events that leads to early delivery of your baby. "True" IC, in fact, is not preterm labor, in that, as I've said before, no contractions are necessary. The events that can lead to the early delivery of your baby are painless and can be described as "silent."

Some women have both IC and a weak/short cervix, and also experience early labor. This is a delicate situation that requires careful monitoring and treatment in order to help you carry your baby into a safer zone. When you already have a fragile cervix, and you add in early contractions, well…you know what can happen.

So, even though IC is different from preterm labor, it is not entirely known whether the mechanisms for both have certain similar biological triggers or similarities.

One study found significant contractions in 64% of women who had cerclages.[10] So, what does this all say? It says that a lot of us with IC are having contractions, too. Is this number correct? Probably not exactly, as maybe some of those cerclages were placed in women who didn't have "true IC."

As you may recall, preterm birth is the number-one cause of infant illness and death. It has been estimated that 20–25% of all second-trimester losses are the result of IC and 16–20% of premature deliveries are caused by this. [11]

Risk Factors for IC

There are some women who have known risk factors. These include those women who have had:

✦ DES (Diethylstilbestrol) exposure while they were in their mom's womb (becoming increasingly rare, as DES has not been in use for a long time).

✦ Previous cervical surgery, including laser cone biopsy, cold-knife conization, or Loop Electrosurgical Excision Procedure (LEEP).
  • However, one small study concluded that LEEP was not considered a risk for delivery before 32 weeks. (Technically, anything earlier than 37 weeks, not 32 weeks, is considered preterm.)[12]

✦ Damage from a previous traumatic birth.

✦ A malformed cervix or uterus—i.e., an anatomical abnormality (congenital Mullerian anomalies).[13]

✦ Previous trauma on the cervix from D&C (dilation and curettage), multiple abortions (specifically over-dilation of the cervix during an abortion).[13]

✦ Deficiencies in cervical collagen and elastin.[13]

✦ Genetic susceptibility/environmental factors.[9]
  • Infection
  • Inflammation
  • Uterine activity
  • Abnormal implantation
  • Gene-environment interactions

And last but not least:

✦ NO RISK FACTORS AT ALL…it just happens.

If you have any of the above risk factors, it does not automatically mean you will have IC; however, it is advisable that prior to pregnancy, or early on in pregnancy, you seek the advice of a perinatologist (an OB who specializes in high-risk pregnancies) or an OB/GYN who is experienced with it to discuss your situation and devise a plan on how to monitor your pregnancy.

> *"We terminated a pregnancy due to neural tube defect last*
> *September; this is what I think weakened my cervix."*
> ~ Alison, California

More about Specific Risk Factors

DES (Diethylstilbestol) Exposure[14]

DES is a synthetic estrogen that was developed to supplement a woman's natural estrogen production. It was first prescribed in 1938 for women who experienced miscarriages or premature deliveries. It was originally considered effective and safe for both the pregnant woman and her baby, and from 1938 to 1971 about 5 to 10 million moms and babies were exposed to DES. In 1971, the Food and Drug Administration (FDA) advised physicians to stop prescribing this to pregnant women because it had been linked to a rare vaginal cancer in the female babies.

More than 30 years of research have confirmed that there are health risks associated with exposure. However, not all exposed persons will experience these health problems.

It has been shown that:

✦ Women prescribed DES while pregnant are at a modestly increased risk for breast cancer.

✦ Men exposed to DES before birth (in the womb), known as DES Sons, are at an increased risk for noncancerous epididymal cysts.

DES Daughters (women exposed in the womb) are at an increased risk for:

✦ Clear cell adenocarcinoma (CCA), a rare kind of vaginal and cervical cancer.

✦ Reproductive-tract structural differences (for example, a T-shaped uterus).

+ Pregnancy complications, including ectopic (tubal) pregnancy and preterm delivery.
+ Infertility.

Research has found that preterm births were more common in DES-exposed daughters compared to nonexposed women. They have found that it is hard to differentiate preterm labor versus IC in exposed women.[15]

Previous Cervical Surgery

My advice to any woman who has had any sort of surgery on their cervix, or a portion of her cervix removed, is to seek the advice and care of an experienced doctor during (or before) pregnancy. Also, demand observation of your cervix with at least weekly or biweekly length measurements. The extent of damage or the amount of retained length of cervix should be evaluated, and whether a cerclage and/or bed rest/reduced activity is recommended. (Or consider a transabdominal cerclage to further improve your chances should you have a very short, or no, cervix.)

Ladies, take the reins on this. If there's one thing I hope you will take away from this book, it's this . . . become your own pregnancy advocate. Don't EVER be afraid to speak up and ask questions. I've had women tell me their doctors dismissed the fact that they had cervical surgery, and they later suffered because of this oversight.

You should always seek to understand what is happening or could happen, and question, question, question everything. Always seek answers, and while you need to remember that there won't always be concrete answers, there's nothing wrong with asking questions.

In a study of 109 women who had a previous cone biopsy and whose cervical lengths were monitored between 16 and 24 weeks, they found that 28% had a short cervix of less than 2.5 cm, and only 30% of those with a short cervix (nine women) actually had their baby before 35 weeks. Of the women who didn't have a short cervix, 6% (five women) had their babies before 35 weeks.[16]

I find these odds to be quite reassuring for you ladies who have had cone biopsies. Still, it can't be a bad thing to be on the safe side and see a doctor with experience in this area to be extra sure.

One study recommended the use of photodynamic therapy (PDT) as opposed to cold-knife conization, as PDT causes no significant cervical tissue damage, unlike cold-knife conization, which leads to the risk of IC. The PDT method was shown to be as effective as cold-knife conization in the treatment of preinvasive cervical lesions due to HPV infection.[17]

Procedures such as laser vaporization, cryotheraphy (where suspected cancerous or precancerous cells are frozen off), and the majority of removals by cutting are not linked to an early birth. Obviously, however, removing the cervix, or trachelectomy, carries a very large risk of leading to a preterm baby.[1]

Another study found that increasing the cone depth during LEEP is linked to an increased risk of preterm delivery. They estimated that for each additional millimeter of tissue removed, the risk went up 6%. This risk also increases with the number of LEEP procedures performed.[18] So, the more they take off your cervix, the greater the chance you will deliver early. This makes sense. To me, it says: LEEP equals tell your doctor, so you can take action to prevent a preterm birth.

Another study published in 2010 confirmed the previous study. They found that the chance of having an early delivery increased after one cervical surgery (a 4.9-fold increase in extreme prematurity) and increased even more following two cervical surgeries, up to a ten-fold increase.[19]

To further confuse you, a study was done to explore whether LEEP surgery is related to preterm birth. They looked at women who had LEEP and then went on to become pregnant, and also at women who had babies and then went on to have LEEPs. When they compared the preterm birth rates with those of the general population, they found no increased risk of preterm birth for either group of ladies.[20]

Unfortunately, it's not as easy as 1 + 1 = 2. My advice is simple. You've had a LEEP (or other cervical surgery), so you know you may be more likely to have an issue (i.e., a preemie) because of it. Make sure that when you meet with your doctor, you bring this up and say, "So, what is your policy on women with a history of cervical procedures?"

Then you wait to see if you're happy with the answer. I would expect a response like, "We would place a preventative cerclage, as you already have a short cervix, just to be sure." Or, "Well, we know women with LEEPs are most likely at a higher risk of delivering early, so I make sure to monitor your cervix with weekly/biweekly checks from 16 weeks to 24 weeks and place a cerclage if indicated." A blank stare or no answer means a quick dash out the door and a call to another doctor.

Damage from a Previous Birth

Often, the diagnosis of IC due to a second-trimester loss or detection of a short or dilated cervix in the second trimester can come as quite a surprise. Many women have already carried one or more babies to term with no problems before they developed IC.

One study looked at which risk factors place women who had a previous term delivery at risk for cervical insufficiency in a subsequent pregnancy. They found that a previous history of curettage, precipitous delivery, or a prolonged second stage (pushing stage) were independent predictors. (A precipitous delivery is a rapid, spontaneous delivery less than three hours after the onset of labor.)[13]

Previous Trauma on the Cervix from D&C (Dilation and Curettage) or Multiple Abortions

One study has shown that there is a trend towards preterm delivery in women who have had previous abortions; the higher the number of abortions, the higher the rate of early delivery. Also, IC seems to be more common in women who've had abortions.[21]

Another study that included 65 women who'd had more than one previous abortion found that 23% of them had a cervix of less than 2.5 cm between 14 and 24 weeks. They also found that these women had more early babies, in that 47% of those with a short cervix delivered early.[22] Even one abortion was shown to slightly increase your risk.[1] Again, this is only risk, and a small risk at that, so the numbers are still on your side.

This section wasn't included to make anyone feel bad or think that they deserve to have problems in their pregnancies because they've had abortions. You mustn't beat yourself up over the past. Chances are, everything will be fine when you decide the time is right for you to have a baby. My goal is only to make you aware of the possibility of IC, so that you can address this. Never, under any circumstances, blame yourself for a part of your body you can't control. IC is never anyone's fault.

Genetic Susceptibility/Environmental Factors[9]

Recent research has found that there is most likely a genetic component that plays a role in cervical incompetence. They have figured out that the genes that control connective tissue functioning, inflammation, uterine contractility, and placental function have been associated with preterm birth. The first two, connective tissue functioning and inflammation, are linked specifically to IC. They cite research that discovered that women with IC have less of a certain proteinogenic amino acid called hydroxyproline (which is a component of collagen, the main protein of connective tissue), as well as having fewer elastin fibers than women without IC.

The cervices of pregnant and non-pregnant women have also been studied (they'll study absolutely anything), and it was discovered that there are differences between the actual structure of the connective tissue in "normal" women and in those of us with IC.

I guess this makes sense, since your genetic makeup controls and dictates the "structure" of your body. If there is a defect of some sort in the gene that regulates the form and function of your cervical tissue, as well as the sub-makeup—i.e., amino acids/proteins and such—then it would make sense that this could lead to weakness in the tissue that's meant to hold your baby in until you reach term. Are you confused yet?

Other studies have found that more than one-quarter of women with IC had a close relative who also had it. This also suggests the possibility of a genetic component.

You think you're doomed if you have bad genes or an aunt with IC? Not so fast. Researchers are quick to point out that the interaction of genetic factors AND the environment is essential when determining the risk for preterm birth.

Inflammation/Infection[9]

Based on numerous studies, it has been well documented that inflammation and infection play a substantial part in causing preterm birth. Proof that IC is linked to increased inflammation has been gaining momentum over the past several years, so much so that there is a whole chapter dedicated to this area later.

IC…Despite What You May Think, It's Not All or Nothing[4,6]

IC is not necessarily a condition that, just because you have it during one pregnancy, repeats itself during each subsequent pregnancy in the same manner. The idea that it is not an "all or nothing" phenomenon is discussed in several review articles. (Review articles look at, analyze, and compile much of the research performed on a topic into one summary paper.)

Also important to consider is that not all women have the same degree of cervical weakness. For example, one woman's cervix may not "hold" beyond 18 weeks, but another might find it possible to "hold" until much later, like 35 weeks.

Furthermore, each pregnancy can be different in the same woman. A woman with IC could deliver at different gestational ages with each of her children. Having a short cervix does not always mean that you have IC, or that it will lead to a preterm baby.

One retrospective study published way back in 1962 (yes, they were even looking at this stuff back then) looked at subsequent pregnancies of women who'd had two or more second-trimester losses and who'd been diagnosed as having IC. Of their next pregnancies that were managed conservatively, 60% also ended as second-trimester losses.[23] (Conservatively managed means no treatment, such as a cerclage or bed rest, was given during the pregnancy.)

Aside from the ethical concerns I have with not treating these women who have known risk factors for IC, it says that 40% of the women went on to carry their babies after previous losses. This reiterates the fact that our cervix doesn't act in a consistent manner for each of our pregnancies. We are not necessarily doomed to lose the next baby even if we suffered a loss in our previous pregnancy. Yes, we are at a higher risk, but now that you know this, you can seek the best of care.

Another study showed a preterm delivery rate of 81% in women with a previous history of painless dilation followed by rupture of the membranes and delivery between 20 and 32 weeks. In the following pregnancies, which were initially handled conservatively, the preterm delivery rate was reduced to 38%.[24] Wow!

Research has suggested that women who get ultrasound-indicated cerclages may be more likely to carry to term, or near term, if they've already had a full-term baby, even if they've also had a premature baby. They saw that women who had not given birth to a full-term baby were more likely to have another preemie.[25]

You should consider all this information if you need a lift; you can recall it when you hit that milestone where a loss or losses occurred before, just to help get you over the hump. Tell yourself, "I am not doomed to the same fate," over and over until you believe it.

To me, this means that just because you had a loss before, there is hope that this time, you can carry your baby to a healthier gestation, especially with the right care. There is absolutely, positively, hope. So, if like me, you lost your baby or your cervix gave way at, say, 23 weeks before, it DOES NOT mean that you are doomed to repeat it this time around. Hopefully, your cervix will be stronger this time.

In this day and age, all of us with IC can stand assured that we will never be part of research where doctors would manage our pregnancies "conservatively" with a history of second-trimester losses—for example, a study in which you would not get a cerclage or get transvaginal length measurements with no treatment upon shortening.

The whole reason for writing this book is to help you understand that if you have a questionable history, and your doctor says, "You'll be fine this time around," and doesn't at least suggest cervical length measurements, you should fire him/her and look for another provider to care for you.

The IC Banned List

When you have IC, there are things you just know you can't do, and normal daily activities you can't partake in. Even though this is a major bummer, I have learned to take advantage of some of the "not allowed" activities, like vacuuming.

Here is a partial list of IC *"Can't Dos"* (talk to your doctor about the specifics of your situation, as every case is different):

+ NO lifting, as this can cause pressure on the cervix. This includes everything from a full gallon of milk or a laundry basket to your two-year-old (as hard as that can be). (I actually ended up waiting until my daughter was three to have another child because of this—until she was able to get up and down by herself and better understand things. I'm not going to lie; sometimes I was forced to lift her, but I tried really, really hard not to.)

+ Anything inserted into the vagina. This includes items for sexual pleasure, such as a penis, finger, dildo, etc., as well as tampons, douching, etc. The fear is that sexual intercourse and orgasm can trigger contractions and further shortening of the cervix, and that objects can introduce infection into the womb, which is especially problematic if you are dilated even a tiny bit.

+ For some, depending on the condition of your cervix, sitting up, using the toilet, and showering are on the "not allowed list" or the "very limited list"; time spent in a vertical position can be a big no. Let me tell you, I know how much it sucks to eat lying down. It's just not the same. I found eating a great big meal way less enjoyable, not to mention messy. Spaghetti was just not pretty, and I ruined many outfits. Oh, and the heartburn! Thank god for Tums.

+ Excessive standing and walking. This means leisurely shopping trips to the mall or walks on the beach. Remember, the high-risk period for IC is somewhere around 16 or so weeks to around 30 weeks. This is the time when the baby is getting heavier, and therefore putting weight directly onto your cervix, right up to when the baby is big enough to rest on your pubic bones. It is especially important to be cautious about undertaking too much activity during this period, as the extra weight could burden your cervix. Note: the restrictions vary from woman to woman, and according to various doctors' preferences. With my daughter, I did nothing. With my son, after a preventative—i.e., history-indicated cerclage—I was allowed to work for most of my pregnancy. I just had to rest when I got home, as well as try to stay off my feet as much as possible while at work. I did the least amount of activity outside of work as I could.

✦ Housework…many activities like vacuuming, carrying laundry, scrubbing floors, etc. are a no-go for us. Depending on how you look at this, it can be a good thing. Ideally, it would be nice to hire someone to help during our pregnancies if we had the money. I didn't, and I survived. Occasionally, that nesting thing would take control of my brain, and I would try to do some housework. Time to lower your standards.

Signs and Symptoms of IC

The signs of IC are often quite subtle. Sometimes, but not all the time, the only symptoms you may notice are an increase in discharge (from dilation and loss of your mucus plug), an increase in pressure or heaviness, low kicks in the vagina area (meaning you are dilated and the baby has dropped), or maybe you just feel a bit off or have a nagging feeling that something just ain't right. Early/slight changes to your cervix most often go unnoticed by you, and that is why transvaginal ultrasounds are key to detecting these early warning signs. Most times the symptoms I described previously don't occur until the later stages, where dilation is already occurring. Often, women will have preterm labor, signs of infection, or an early rupture, which is a sign that something is wrong.

They found that more than 40% of the women with cervical dilation didn't realize that something was off and didn't go to the doctor until their amniotic sac had dropped into the lower cervical opening.

Fifteen percent didn't go in to see their doctors until their membranes, or their baby, usually the feet, had dropped into the vagina.[1] That latter situation included me, unfortunately.

So, what are you supposed to do? First, don't ignore anything, even gut feelings. Even if you're wrong, oh well. Pay attention, and tune into your body. If you notice a change in your discharge, or you notice a change in the feelings down below, call your doc. Most of the time it will be nothing, so the only thing you lose is a little time and money. (Hopefully, you can afford to waste a little of both of those.)

The other main thing you can do is, if you have a history of problems or some of the risk factors described previously, get serial cervical length checks. If you're not, then you may want to consider switching practices. A cervical length check can catch changes early, much earlier than a hand check can. A length of less than 2.5 cm should send up red flags.

> *"For about one week prior to my 20-week ultrasound (where my cervix was funneled to less than 1 cm), I felt an 'open' or heavy feeling high up in my vagina…like I needed to do Kegels to keep everything 'up there' and in place…really, a very odd sensation…"* ~Anonymous (She had an emergency cerclage at 20 weeks and delivered her baby AT TERM following 17 weeks of bed rest. Ladies it does happen; you can make it.)

Don't Let IC or Any Other High-Risk Condition Take Away the Joy of YOUR Pregnancy

One thing all of us who have IC, or fear of an early birth, have in common is that the joy and happiness of pregnancy can quickly be replaced by anxiety, fear, loneliness, frustration, isolation, depression, sadness… the list of emotions is endless.

My greatest hope is to present information to help reduce some of these feelings and help you to educate yourself so you can take back your pregnancy. Ask questions and demand clear answers from your doctors. Enjoy the ride (as much as is possible), and step back and admire your body and the miracle you are creating.

This is one thing I regret from my pregnancy with my daughter. I did not share my pregnancy with more than a few people. I was afraid to tell people or to "get too attached" to the baby growing inside. I tried to rush through pregnancy just to make it to those critical milestones…24, 28, 30, and 32 weeks.

Even though I was so focused on being and staying pregnant, I wasn't even close to focused on the other important aspects of pregnancy, if that makes sense. It wasn't until the very end, the "safe zone," that I actually sat back and enjoyed being pregnant. I feel like I lost so much time in an experience that really only happens a couple times in your life.

So even though we have IC or any of these problems that can lead to an early birth, and even though pregnancy for us is extremely stressful (this is an understatement), I urge you to step back and treasure and relish your pregnancies. Don't rush to the end; enjoy the adventure leading up to motherhood.

References

1. Berghella V. *Preterm Birth: Prevention & Management.* West Sussex, UK, Wiley-Blackwell, 2010.
2. Schlembach D, Mackay L, Shi L, et al. Cervical ripening and insufficiency: from biochemical and molecular studies to in vivo clinical examination. *Eur J Obstet Gynecol Reprod Biol* 2009;144(Suppl. 1):S70–76.
3. Murkoff H, Mazel S. *What to Expect When You're Expecting.* 3rd Edition. New York, New York. Workman Publishing Company Inc., 2002.
4. Althuisius S, Dekker G. Controversies regarding cervical incompetence, short cervix, and the need for cerclage. *Clinics in Perinatology* 2004;31:695–720.
5. Martin JA, Hamilton BE, Sutton PD, et al. Births: final data for 2004. *Natl Vital Stat Rep* 2006;55(1):1–101.
6. Althuisius SM, Dekker GA, VanGeijn HP. Cervical incompetence: a reappraisal of an obstetric controversy. *Obstetrical and Gynecological Survey* 2002;57(6):377–387.
7. Romero R, Espinoza J, Erez O, Hassan S. The role of cervical cerclage in obstetric practice: Can the patient who could benefit from this procedure be identified? *Am J Obstet Gynecol* 2006;194:1–9.
8. McElrath TF, Hecht JL, Dammann O, et al. Pregnancy disorders that lead to delivery before the 28th week of gestation: an epidemiologic approach to classification. *Am J Epidemiol* 2008;168(9):980–989.
9. Warren J, Silver R. Genetics of the cervix in relation to preterm birth. *Seminars in Perinatology* 2009;33:308–311.
10. Ayers JW, DeGrood RM, Compton AA, et al. Sonographic evaluation of cervical length in pregnancy: diagnosis and management of preterm cervical effacement in patients at high risk for premature delivery. *Obstet Gynecol* 1988;71:939–944.

11. Grzonka DT, Kamierczak W, Cholewa D, Radzioch J. Herbich cervical pessary—method of therapy for cervical incompetence and prophylaxis of prematurity. *Wiadomości lekarskie* 2004;57(1):105–107.

12. Althuisius SM, Schornagel IJ, Dekker GA, et al. Loop electrosurgical excision procedure of the cervix and time of delivery in subsequent pregnancy. *International Journal of Gynaecological Obstetrics* 2001;72(1):31–34.

13. Vyas NA, Vink JS, Ghidini A, et al. Risk factors for cervical insufficiency after term delivery. *American Journal of Obstetrics and Gynecology* 2006;195(3):787–791.

14. Centers for Disease Control and Prevention (CDC), DES Update: Consumers, http://www.cdc.gov/DES/consumers/about/index.html.

15. Hammes B, Laitman CJ. Diethylstilbestrol (DES) update: recommendations for identification and management of DES-exposed individuals. *Journal of Midwifery Womens Health* 2003;48(1):19–29.

16. Berghella V, Pereira L, Gariepy A, Simonazzi G. Prior cone biopsy: prediction of preterm birth by cervical ultrasound. *Am J Obstet Gynecol* 2004;191(4):1393–1397.

17. Bodner K, Bodner-Adler B, Wierrani F, et al. Cold-knife conization versus photodynamic therapy with topical 5-aminolevulinic acid (5-ALA) in cervical intraepithelial neoplasia (CIN) II with associated human papillomavirus infection: a comparison of preliminary results. *Anticancer Res* 2003;23(2C):1785–1788.

18. Noehr B, Jensen A, Frederiksen K, et al. Depth of cervical cone removed by loop electrosurgical excision procedure and subsequent risk of spontaneous preterm delivery. *Obstet Gynecol* 2009;114(6):1232–1238.

19. Ortoft G, Henriksen T, Hansen E, Petersen L. After conisation of the cervix, the perinatal mortality as a result of preterm delivery increases in subsequent pregnancy. *BJOG* 2010;117(3):258–267.

20. Werner CL, Lo JY, Heffernan T, et al. Loop electrosurgical excision procedure and risk of preterm birth. *Obstet Gynecol* 2010;115(3):605–608.

21. Voigt M, Henrich W, Zygmunt M, et al. Is induced abortion a risk factor in subsequent pregnancy? *J Perinat Med* 2009;37(2):144–149.

22. Visintine J, Berghella V, Henning D, Baxter J. Cervical length for prediction of preterm birth in women with multiple prior induced abortions. *Ultrasound Obstet Gynecol* 2008;31(2):198–200.

23. Dunn LJ, Dans P. Subsequent obstetrical performance of patients meeting the historical criteria for cervical incompetence. *Bull Sloane Hosp Women* 1962;7:43–45.

24. Socol ML, Dooley SL, Tamura RK, et al. Perinatal outcome following prior delivery in the late second or early third trimester. *Am J Obstet Gynecol* 1984;150:228–231.

25. Poggi SH, Vyas N, Pezzullo JC, et al. Therapeutic cerclage may be more efficacious in women who develop cervical insufficiency after a term delivery. *Am J Obstet Gynecol* 2009;200(1):68 e1–e3.

CHAPTER 4

The Link Between Infection/Inflammation and Early Birth

I've already told you about the well-known link between infection and inflammatory responses and preterm delivery. Typically, the area where the baby grows within you, your uterus, the amniotic sac, and such, is a sterile environment (i.e., no bacteria are present). Under certain conditions, however, bacteria invade and cause havoc. This is a potentially lethal situation for your baby, depending on how far along you are and other factors, such as the extent of the infection.

Infection is present in 25% of all early births, and these women typically show no obvious signs of having an infection. The natural rate of infection in the pregnant population has been shown to be 0.4% in women who get amnios, a procedure where amniotic fluid is removed. Unfortunately, infection in itself is an indication for a potentially bad outcome. The good news is, women have been successfully treated with antibiotics, which have worked to clear up the infection, enabling them to deliver their baby at term.[1]

If you have ruptured membranes, the chance of getting an infection increases greatly. Seventy-five percent of women who experience premature rupture of their membranes have positive amniotic fluid cultures, meaning they find bacteria in their amniotic fluid. In women who have an incompetent cervix, with dilation or funneling, more than half have bacteria. This number drops to only 9% in women who have a cervical length of about 2.5 cm upon ultrasound examination. So, dilation/funneling means an increased risk of infection. Makes sense, really. The barrier that blocks bacteria from getting in there is now gone. Not so good.

One study determined that placental inflammation was linked to poor neonatal growth.[2] Inflammation, which could be due to an underlying infection, actually causes the growth of your baby to slow down.

Having an infection in the amniotic cavity, as determined by a positive amniotic fluid culture, is not a good sign. Your chance of a sick baby, or worse, increases greatly, from about 12% for negative cultures to 50% for a positive culture. Researchers have found that this is not something that happens overnight, but rather has been brewing for weeks. Babies born to moms with infections are often found to have bacteria in their blood, as well as higher rates of death and illness.[1]

Women who are prone to vaginal infections should be monitored and observed for signs of possible infections. Infection is the devil. Unfortunately, there is little you can do to prevent it. What we can do, however, is stay tuned into our bodies and, most importantly, our discharge. Changes can be a signal of infection.

Interleukin…A Marker for Infection?

Over the past several years, interleukins have been getting more attention as a possible "signal" of infection and inflammation. Interleukins are a group of cytokines, which are secreted proteins/signaling molecules that are released by a range of cells, including the well-known white blood cells.

One study determined that elevated levels of interleukin-6 and C-reactive protein in the mom are risk factors for preterm birth before 32 weeks, and for the baby to have intraventricular hemorrhage.[3]

Studies have looked at the presence of these proteins in amniotic fluid as a means to determining the likelihood of infection and inflammation and subsequent preterm birth. In one study, they looked at interleukin-18 (IL-18) to determine the presence of bacteria in the amnion region during genetic amniocentesis testing. They found that those women who delivered early (at less than 37 weeks) had much higher levels of IL-18 in their amniotic fluid compared to women who delivered at term. This level was also higher in fluid samples that came back positive for microorganisms (by standard culturing) than in those that were negative. They concluded that increased levels of interleukin-18 can help identify women who are at risk of infection and spontaneous preterm birth.[4]

Nonexistent Cervix (Acute IC) and Infection

Those of us who suffer from a nonexistent cervix, meaning dilation and possibly even bulging of the membranes into the vagina, fear infection the most. Researchers looked at women with acute IC whose cervices were dilated to at least 1.5 cm or more and who weren't having regular contractions for infection as well as for markers of inflammation (metalloproteinase-8). What they found was high levels of intraamniotic inflammation in 81% of these women, whereas a positive culture for bacteria was found in only 8%. Preterm delivery within seven days happened in 50% of all the women with positive inflammation markers (negative cultures), and 84% delivered before 34 weeks. The authors concluded that intraamniotic inflammation is, on its own, a serious risk factor for preterm delivery and bad outcomes.[5]

One study looked at detecting microorganisms, specifically a common but often difficult-to-detect organism called ureaplasmas, in amniotic fluid by culturing (standard microbiological techniques) and polymerase chain reaction (PCR) (a molecular technique based on DNA analysis) in women who had cervical incompetence. The women were dilated 1.5 cm or more, had intact membranes, and didn't have regular contractions at 16 to 29 weeks. They found that standard culturing techniques for these microorganisms didn't detect their presence in most of the women, meaning the amniotic fluid came back negative 91% of the time, while PCR was able to detect the microorganism. Those who had a negative amniotic fluid culture but were found to be positive on PCR analysis were at risk for inflammation and spontaneous preterm birth.[6]

Often, using standard microbiology techniques isn't enough to pick up the presence of these little buggers. This is yet another issue for the medical establishment to cope with when it comes to infection. Not only are they unsure how to stop it or why some women have it, they also can't detect it all the time. When making decisions, they often have to depend on other signals, such as increased white blood cell counts or fever, to help them to understand what's going on.

Like I said, unfortunately, I have firsthand experience with this. In order to determine whether I was a candidate for an emergency cerclage (I was 5–6 cm dilated with no contractions), they removed some amniotic fluid for culturing. Initial testing showed that I was negative for microorganisms, but later my white blood cell count was found to be very high. (An increased white blood cell count indicates infection in the body.) Based on that information, I was no longer able to get an emergency cerclage.

Later, after I had delivered my son and pathology had been performed, they found that I did have invasion/infection of bacteria. Unfortunately, infection/inflammation responses that lead to a preterm delivery is our body's way of trying to save us…the mothers.

Now, I know all this may be hard to hear. Sure, we would like outcomes to all be good, even with infection, but unfortunately, they're not. I know that these studies represent many moms who've lost their precious babies and gone through hell. I understand; I was one of them.

You need to remember that I want to provide you with all the information that's available so that you're 100% informed. Some of the material I present will be positive and promising, while some of it will not. You need to come out of this knowing that there are lots and lots of women who've been there, and who've gone on to have healthy babies. Think glass half-full; that 50% chance of a bad outcome after a positive culture means that half of the women and their precious cargo are fine.

I think it's safe to say that acute IC is one of the most ominous situations in all of obstetrics. At the time I found myself in this situation, I believed that my chance of a good outcome was less than 1%—i.e., pretty much none. Now, after writing this, I know that this is not the case. In these studies, there were babies who not only made it to 28 weeks, but who also went on to term or almost to term. You need to understand the reality of the situation, but at the same time, try to think positive, knowing that there's hope.

In reality, very few women will ever experience this situation. My goal is to educate both doctors and women in understanding the issues around early birth, the risk factors, and the treatment options to help avoid it. Unfortunately, for some, this won't be possible, and you will lose your baby because things weren't detected until it was too late. Should you try to have another baby, however, you will be prepared with a wealth of knowledge to help you on your journey.

Genital Infections and Bacterial Vaginosis (BV)[1]

The most common cause of very early preterm birth—i.e., between 20 and 24 weeks—is inflammation of the genital tract; this has been identified in over half of these women. They also know that having bacterial vaginosis (BV) is linked to spontaneous preterm birth, and even more so when it's found at less than 16 weeks.

Even though the majority of the bacteria found in women who deliver early due to inflammation-associated reasons have a low ability to cause physical sickness/symptoms (low pathogenicity), it's not the actual presence of the microorganisms that causes the preterm birth, but inflammation and the inflammatory response that really triggers it. In other words, it's not the bacteria themselves that cause the labor to start, because they're relatively harmless at that point; it's the body's defense mechanisms that cause our babies to come early.

Intrauterine/Intramniotic Infections (Those That Occur in the Uterus)[1]

These are trouble, and cause anywhere from 25% to 40% of all early births. This is probably even an underestimate of the actual number, as standard microbiology techniques often can't detect them, as I've said before. The earlier you show up with preterm labor, the more likely it is that you have this problem. It's a common cause for very early births, and is only discovered in 10% of late preterm, non-medically assisted births (at 35 to 36 weeks).

Doctors look for two or more of the following to identify whether you may have an infection: tenderness in your uterine area, a fever of 100.4°F (38°C) or more, or high heart rates in either you or the baby. Many women show no signs of infection; however, roughly 15–20% of women who experience preterm labor have an infection. If you do have an infection, the doctor must consider whether to induce immediate delivery, to avoid further risk to you or the baby as a result of the infection, or to extend your pregnancy, knowing the risks.

How Do They Know If I Have an Infection?[1]

There are several common signs that let us know when something is off in our body, including fever, fatigue, and maybe even some pain. When we're talking problems in the female area, this could be an increased amount of discharge, varying color, as well as a foul odor. The problem is that pregnant women with intrauterine infection and inflammation often have no symptoms. When blood is drawn, there may be an increase in white blood cells, which is a signal that the body is on the defensive against invaders. The issue with relying on white blood cell counts alone, however, is that pregnant women often have inherently higher levels, so a slight increase really doesn't tell us too much.

The best methods for detecting infection are standard microbiological culturing techniques, and even these have limitations. A Gram stain, where various stains are used to detect the presence and type of bacteria in the amniotic fluid, is often used, as well as an amniotic fluid white blood cell count and sugar level concentrations. Molecular techniques are now becoming more popular. These methods are faster to run and to get results from, and they are better able to detect bacteria. These work by detecting even the slightest number of DNA molecules. (This is called PCR or polymerase chain reaction, if you really want to know.) False negatives using classical microbiological techniques are common. Interleukin detection as a marker for inflammation is a potential new avenue for testing.

Every hospital should have the ability to check your white blood cell count, which is a very simple test. As white blood cells are not typically found in amniotic fluid, a level of 50 cells/mm^3 or above is cause for concern and indicative of inflammation or infection. In women with early ruptured membranes, that level is lowered to 30 or more cells/mm^3.

I believe that my level was nearing 500, so even though I didn't realize then that I had a problem, because I felt fine and my culture was negative, I now know that a storm was brewing inside my body. I was angry and thought they were wrong, but now I sadly know better.

Even if your lab culture comes back negative, that doesn't mean you're out of the woods. Unfortunately, as I have said, some of the most common microorganisms, known as mycoplasmas, are not culturable. The good news is that it has been shown that some infections can be successfully cleared up, and the woman can go on to carry to term and birth a healthy baby.

Another easy test you may hear about is a check of your glucose, or the sugar level of your amniotic fluid. A low level (less than 14 milligrams/deciliter) signals the presence of bacteria in women with unbroken membranes and preterm labor. The red flag in women whose membranes have broken is less than 10 mg/dl. Bacteria use sugar as a food source, and so a low level means the presence of bacteria, because they're using it up.

A newer test being used to detect the presence of inflammation involves using markers of inflammation, namely interleukin-6 (IL-6). A level of 2.6 nanograms/milliliter or more is a sign of inflammation, with the threat of a positive culture for bacteria and an early delivery. Those with amniotic infection have been shown to have higher levels of this stuff. This test is more complex and technological (it uses an ELISA assay, if you care), and may not be available in all hospitals. The results are available very quickly, usually in about three hours, whereas results from standard culturing techniques can take three days to a week.

Another similar and cutting-edge test not readily available in many hospitals is the test for MMP-8 (matrix metalloproteinase 8). Like IL-6, it appears to be a superior test in its sensitivity. Many have proposed that the best way to determine and then figure out treatment options in women with preterm labor or early ruptured membranes is to test for inflammation, rather than trying to find actual microorganisms. This MMP-8 test is a quick 15-minute test and simple to administer, being similar to the standard pregnancy kit you can get at the pharmacy, with high reliability.

Women with positive tests were found to have a shorter period to delivery than those with negative tests, and were in danger of delivery within either 48 hours, 7 days, or 14 days. This is good information for your doctor to have, so her or she can respond appropriately. Should you get steroids and/or antibiotics, or should you be moved to a hospital better able to care for your tiny baby? So, why can't all hospitals use this test? It's simple…money.

How Can I Avoid This?[1]

We know that infection is not a good sign. Unfortunately, some of you are genetically predisposed to being more likely to suffer from it. Your body automatically responds with a hyped-up inflammation response, which is bad when you're carrying a baby. Now for the good news; the risk of repeating this in your next pregnancy is only 15%.

The shorter your cervix, the more chance you have of getting an infection. This is because it's easier for the bacteria that are normally present in the vagina to travel up into the uterine area. This risk is still low, though—only 19% of women with a length of less than 2.5 cm. To make sure you do all you can to retain length and thus to keep your risk low, work with your doctor if you have a history or risk factors. Talk about possible options such as progesterone, ultrasound length monitoring, and even pelvic rest and lifting restrictions.

Many doctors recommend not using tocolysis to stop labor in women with confirmed inflammation or infection, as it most likely won't work. Giving steroids to speed up lung maturity is advised to help the baby, should he or she be born too early. Also, they have been shown to help minimize the baby's own inflammation response.

In women whose amniotic sac has already broken, treatment will depend on how far along you are. Having ruptured membranes puts you at greater risk of an even more severe infection. Being under good care, in a good of hospital, with a great NICU is important. Let's face it, an excellent hospital is better equipped and staffed to handle the very tiniest of babies.

You can't really avoid infection, but you can help yourself and your baby. Research the hospital you wish to use. Knowing you are higher risk, you should be more concerned than the average woman as to the type of NICU available and how good they are overall. Yes, this may mean more of an inconvenience, since you may have to travel further, but you can always switch back to somewhere local when you make it to a better gestation.

If you're at a higher gestation of, say, 32, 33, or 34 weeks when you rupture or when you have a confirmed or even a suspected infection/inflammation, then your baby will probably be delivered immediately. If you're less than 32 weeks when your water breaks, they're more likely to try to extend your gestation, while keeping a very close eye on you. Again, research has shown that it IS possible to get rid of amniotic infection in women whose waters have broken early, and in women with a short cervix, with the use of antibiotics. Their use has also been shown to delay delivery.

Another area where you can help yourself is by knowing your body. Discharge in pregnancy is normal, and changes to your discharge throughout pregnancy is also normal. However, sometimes changes can be a sign of dilation, loss of your mucous plug, preterm labor, or infection. I can't stress it enough: MONITOR YOUR DISCHARGE and call your doctor if you notice anything! Maybe it'll be a waste of time, and everything is all right...but so what. Remember, there's nothing wrong with being a little overly cautious. You're paying them, so don't be embarrassed about asking to be checked out if you feel something isn't right.

If you notice any bleeding, pressure, cramping, back pain, water leaking (it can be as little as slow drips), or you just feel off, go get checked right away. The sooner they catch something and get you on antibiotics, the better. I waited almost three days before I called my doctor, and by that time I was 6 cm dilated, infection had already set in. Don't be like me, please. I carried so much guilt because of this mistake.

If you're dilated, or if you have a short cervix, limit internal checks or procedures to help reduce the likelihood of getting an accidental infection. The most common way of getting an infection is what is known as the "ascending route," up from the vagina and into the uterine cavity. The best way to limit your risk is to be under the care of a good doctor who will monitor your cervical length, catch any changes early, and act if necessary, like with the placement of a cerclage.

Oh, and one more thing...don't douche. Douching can disrupt the natural pH of your vagina, allowing the wrong bacteria to thrive and take over the "good" bacteria. It can also potentially push up the bacteria found in your vagina, which could then colonize and cause intraamniotic infection. Douching has been linked to preterm birth as well.

Can't I Just Take Antibiotics, Then?

It would seem to make sense that treating high-risk women with preventative antibiotics would prevent infection, right? Well, no, actually. In several studies, treatment with routine antibiotics has been shown to have no effect on the preterm birth rates.[7,8]

So, it would seem that there is more at play here than the typical bacterial infections we get, like in a sinus infection. It's not as simple as taking an antibiotic every day to prevent preterm birth. Bummer. It would be awesome if it was.

Summary

Infection…bad. Not much you can do to prevent it…bad. Watch your discharge, and have a good doctor/hospital knowledgeable in your risk factors and treatment . . . good. Pay attention to your body for other signs, like contractions (may be very slight), fever, uterine tenderness, etc. Many women with infection have gone on to have healthy babies… awesome! And so can you.

References

1. Berghella V. *Preterm Birth: Prevention & Management*. West Sussex, UK. Wiley-Blackwell, 2010.
2. Mestan K, Yu Y, Matoba N, et al. Placental inflammatory response is associated with poor neonatal growth: preterm birth cohort study. *Pediatrics* 2010;125(4):e891–898.
3. Sorokin Y, Romero R, Mele L, et al. Maternal serum interleukin-6, C-reactive protein, and matrix metalloproteinase-9 concentrations as risk factors for preterm birth <32 weeks and adverse neonatal outcomes. *Am J Perinatol* 2010;27(8):631–640.
4. Daskalakis G, Thomakos N, Papapanagiotou A, et al. Amniotic fluid interleukin-18 at mid-trimester genetic amniocentesis: relationship to intraamniotic microbial invasion and preterm delivery. *BJOG* 2009;116(13):1743–1748.
5. Lee SE, Romero R, Park CW, et al. The frequency and significance of intraamniotic inflammation in patients with cervical insufficiency. *Am J Obstet Gynecol* 2008;198(6):e1–8.
6. Oh KJ, Lee SE, Jung H, et al. Detection of Ureaplasmas by the polymerase chain reaction in the amniotic fluid of patients with cervical insufficiency. *J Perinat Med* 2010;38(3):261–268.
7. van den Broek NR, White SA, Goodall M, et al. The APPLe study: A randomized, community-based, placebo-controlled trial of Azithromycin for the prevention of preterm birth, with meta-analysis. *PLoS Med* 2009;6(12):e1000191.
8. Andrews WW, Sibai BM, Thom EA, et al. Randomized clinical trial of Metronidazol plus Erythromycin to prevent spontaneous preterm delivery in fetal fibronectin-positive women. *Obstet Gynecol* 2003;101(5 pt 1):847–855.

CHAPTER 5

Is It or Isn't It? What the Heck Does a Contraction Really Feel Like?

Often, we just don't know, and can't tell, if what we are experiencing/feeling are the normal twinges and pains of just being pregnant or something else, like preterm labor. Even if you've already had a baby, every pregnancy and each labor experience can behave and feel very differently. And then there is that little phenomenon called the "amnesia factor," whereby most every mom, sooner or later, forgets the pain of labor and what those contractions actually felt like.

If this is your first pregnancy, it can be especially tricky trying to figure out whether you're really having contractions. Your doctor may be quick to say it's this or that, stretching, normal back pains from the extra weight, blah, blah. Hey, they don't always know either. Every woman and every body is different. It helps if you've had friends who've had babies recently, but not everyone has someone like that to go to. In this chapter, I've included input from dozens of women on what it really felt like to them.

Preterm labor can be a bit trickier to figure out than normal full-term labor. In preterm labor, it can be less obvious that you're having contractions. In part, this is due to the fact that the earlier you are, the smaller your uterus/baby is, so the less "force" this muscle is able to apply, so the less you may feel. The key with preterm contractions is being able to identify them EARLY, so they can be stopped.

> *"Once I realized what it was, I realized I'd been having them for a month before my water broke at 32 weeks with my first baby. My contractions were a tightening of the entire stomach muscles when I was in labor, but my preterm contractions were a much milder tightening that started to come regularly, almost like my baby was pushing against one side of my belly. (At least, this is what I thought they were!)"* ~ Ashley, Tennessee

> *"It took my breath away, and I needed to sit down on the floor or hang on to the back of a chair. It was not painful."* ~ Tessa, Arizona

> *"My experience with preterm labor was horrible. It felt like someone was kicking me in the back and trying to pull the organs in my midsection out with a sharp object."* ~ Unknown

Research has shown that 85% of women who had no obvious symptoms of preterm labor (they were asymptomatic), but who had short cervices between 14 and 24 weeks, were having an average of four contractions an hour when they were monitored.[1] So, the majority of women with short cervices don't know and can't feel that they're having contractions. Just great.

When comparing the frequency of contractions in asymptomatic women at 22–24 weeks with or without a short cervix, only 13% of them had a short cervix and averaged 1.6 contractions per hour, whereas those with longer cervices averaged 1.2 contractions per hour. Not much difference, is it?

Based on these observations, they concluded that the occurrence of contractions was NOT related to cervical length. Yet in the women with short cervices, there was a two-fold increased risk of preterm birth when they observed four or more contractions per hour.[2] What this says to me is that you aren't doomed to deliver immediately, even if you're having four or more contractions per hour. You just need to be watched closely.

A diagnosis of preterm labor is routinely based on a couple things going on at the same time, one being the presence of *regular* uterine contractions before 37 weeks, and the other being progressive cervical changes, either observed shortening of the cervix over time with contractions, dilation of 2 cm or more, or cervical thinning of 80% or more.[3]

How better to tell you what a contraction feels like than to use the words of those who have experienced them. *Hint:* they aren't always as painful as we're led to believe.

> *"Pain, pressure, feeling like a wave. I thought it was the baby kicking and turning around. Uncomfortable expansion of my rib cage. Not really acutely painful."* ~ Anonymous

> *"I was pregnant with twins and this was my second pregnancy. I didn't really feel the contractions at all, but I did feel a pain around my belly button. It felt very shallow, like my skin hurt. I was told to go to the hospital to have it checked out, and sure enough, I was having contractions."* ~ Erin, Florida

Do I Need to Poo?

> *"I thought I was constipated until I felt my water bulging outside me."* ~ Anonymous

> *"In my first pregnancy, my contractions just felt like I was severely constipated. There was pressure in my extreme lower back, right above my butt. I went into the clinic the next day and found out that I was dilated to 2 cm and one of our twin's amniotic sacs was bulging into the birth canal. In my second pregnancy, until the day of delivery, my contractions felt like how Braxton Hicks are described on the Internet, hardening of the entire abdomen, and were worse when standing upright. I thought this was a normal part of pregnancy, until I was at a non-stress test at 32 weeks, 5 days, when I was told I was having contractions about one minute apart. These contractions were not painful at all and, obviously, not extremely noticeable. The contractions I had on the day of delivery just felt like EXTREME rectal pressure accompanied by the urge to push."* ~ Brianna, Wisconsin

"Initially I thought I had really bad diarrhea. Then it felt like the worst cramps." ~ Michelle, Massachusetts

"I had what I think were random contractions from 16 weeks till the day I learned I was dilated, at around 19 weeks. They felt like severe gas pains. Because I'm chubby, I couldn't tell if my tummy was tightening or not." ~ Courtney, Ohio

"My contractions felt like I needed to have a bowel movement." ~ Danielle, Pennsylvania

"Just a squeeze and then it relaxed, almost like flatulence. It didn't hurt either." ~ Deb, location unknown

"I felt like my labor was gas pains. Labor started, I thought it was gas, but when I got to the hospital, I was 8 cm dilated. I delivered that night." ~ Diane, Georgia (Has a micropreemie)

Gosh, I'm Pregnant—How Can I Be Getting My Period?

"My preterm contractions started off as mild menstrual cramps that felt deep inside, then they seemed to gradually increase over time and would slowly move around to my back." ~ Laura, Canada

"I had back labor. All of my contractions were in my lower back. They felt like very intense period cramps." ~ Anonymous

"It was not what I expected. Everyone told me that I would feel a hardening in my abdomen. It was more cramping in my abdomen similar to a bad period and pressure in my vagina." ~ Kristen, Minnesota

"I did not know I was in labor. I had what felt like bad cramps and a backache. My periods have always been painful, and it never occurred to me that my 'cramps' and the tightness I was feeling was actual labor." ~ Lana, New Mexico

"I was having a lot of cramping, like heavy period cramps, but my doctor said this was normal." ~ Jessica, California (Had a premature baby after "normal" cramps)

Trust Your Gut

"With my stillbirth, I had slight cramps in the morning, but nothing I thought was 'major.' As the day progressed, my pain got worse to the point where I felt like I had to have a bowel movement. I went to the bathroom and sat on the toilet; I felt a huge amount of pressure and then my water broke. I immediately started having contractions after that. Contractions started out feeling like severe menstrual cramps that got more horrible until I delivered. With my preemie, I had pressure in my hips the day before and told my doc. He brushed it off, saying it was just the weight of my growing baby. (ALWAYS trust your gut!) I thought he knew better than me, so I went home. The next day, I didn't feel my baby move too much, so I called my husband and asked him to come home from work to take me to the hospital. By the time he came home and I got in the car, the contractions had started. When I got to the hospital, I could barely walk through the pain." ~ Nicole, Germany

"Both of my preterm labors were different from each other... but I distinctly remember thinking, 'This isn't right.'"
~ Anonymous (She had a 27-weeker after 10 weeks of bed rest and then went on to have a full-term baby at 40 weeks after 23 weeks of bed rest.)

"One day I was sitting watching TV after a long work day, and I got a bizarre cramp in my abdomen. It was tiny, barely uncomfortable, but it really startled me. I was told it was probably uterine expansion, so I didn't worry. It happened four more times in the next couple days, then started being more consistent. It felt like someone was trying to squeeze my lower tummy so I could zip up my jeans. It turned into more of a 'doubled over in the shower' pain, and the doc still told me I was just experiencing normal cramps from the uterus. They told me if I started bleeding to call back. By the time I went to the emergency room, I'd been contracting for two weeks. They were less than an hour apart, and my cervix was 'disintegrated,' as the doctor so brutally stated." ~ Chanel, California

"There is nothing more terrifying than finding out that something is wrong when you are expecting a child. Listen to your body. If you feel that something is wrong, tell your doctor. NEVER worry about seeming paranoid or overly sensitive. I saved my baby's life by going to the doctor because my stomach felt 'funny'. I was 6 months pregnant and didn't realize that these 'funny' feelings were actually contractions. My baby was born healthy (and full term) thanks to an early intervention and is now 15 years old. Had I not listened to my body my baby probably wouldn't have made it. You know your body better than anyone…listen to what it is telling you!" ~ Deborah, Colorado

"One midwife told me one thing, another doctor said it was another. A high-risk doctor said something different, and then to top it off, now my current doctor has a different opinion. I guess since you are writing this for women who have not experienced contractions in the past, my advice would be to get checked out and maybe even insist on their cervix being measured via ultrasound." ~ Jen, Alaska

"My older daughter was born at 34 weeks, 2 days after a doctor appointment showed I was 2 cm dilated and the amniotic sac was bulging out. I didn't have contractions until my water broke (about two hours before she was actually born), but I felt 'leaky' for weeks before that. I guess I was walking around dilated for weeks. Moral of the story if something feels weird, call your practitioner." ~ Alison, Massachusetts

What Is This Pressure…Damn Pregnancy Backache or Not?

"I woke up feeling the intense need to go to the bathroom. It was different from any feeling I'd felt before. It wasn't painful, but it was very intense pressure. My stomach didn't tighten, and it wasn't what I thought contractions would feel like. I called my doctor, and they told me to go to the hospital. I delivered my twins an hour and a half later." ~ Maggie, Ohio (had her

twins at 29 weeks and 2 days after an emergency cerclage, which was placed between 20 and 21 weeks)

"I never really felt anything when my cervix started to change early on, just maybe pressure, but it was constant. Once I was further along, I felt sharp pains that lasted about five seconds and would come and go when I got up to walk to the bathroom." ~ Tara, Virginia

"With my first baby, I was walking and felt twinges in my back, almost like pinches. I just assumed it was normally body growing changes. Later that day, I kept going to the bathroom every five minutes. I called my doctor because I thought maybe I had a bladder infection, but as I came to find out, I was not passing urine but fluid." ~ Lynn, Pennsylvania

Tightening. . . Is This Feeling Just My Baby Moving Around?

"Tightening in my lower abdomen, feels like the baby moving, but tight for over 30 seconds." ~ Amy, location unknown

"I felt occasional tightening of the abdomen, but for the most part I did not know I was having preterm labor until I had a contraction during a routine checkup with my OB/GYN." ~ Jessica, location unknown

"With my first pregnancy...in hindsight...I had been telling my husband for almost a week to 'feel...the baby is pushing out... right here'...as my tummy got hard. No pain, no cramping, no sore lower back, no pressure, no bleeding, no leaking of fluid, just my tummy getting tight. It was not until it was every four minutes on the nose that I had that 'aha!' moment and realized they were contractions." ~ Melinda, California

"I would feel my stomach 'ball up' or 'tighten up.' I would not experience this as painful or even uncomfortable; in fact, if I wasn't touching my stomach sometimes, I was clueless that I was having them." ~ Klea, California

I Think I'm Having Contractions! Now What?

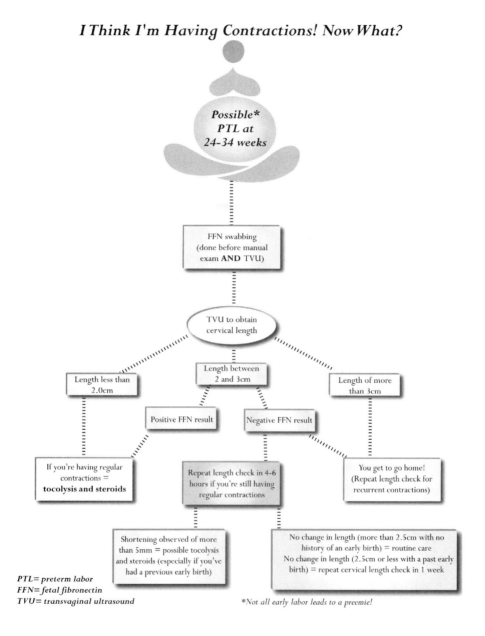

Possible*
PTL at
24-34 weeks

FFN swabbing
(done before manual
exam AND TVU)

TVU to obtain
cervical length

Length less than
2.0cm

Length between
2 and 3cm

Length of more
than 3cm

Positive FFN result

Negative FFN result

If you're having regular
contractions =
tocolysis and steroids

Repeat length check in 4-6
hours if you're still having
regular contractions

You get to go home!
(Repeat length check for
recurrent contractions)

Shortening observed of more
than 5mm = possible tocolysis
and steroids (especially if you've
had a previous early birth)

No change in length (more than 2.5cm with no
history of an early birth) = routine care
No change in length (2.5cm or less with a past early
birth) = repeat cervical length check in 1 week

PTL= preterm labor
FFN= fetal fibronectin
TVU= transvaginal ultrasound

*Not all early labor leads to a preemie!

Figure 5-1. Chart adapted from *Preterm Birth: Prevention & Management.*[4]

"Before I was told I was in preterm labor, I had been having contractions for about four weeks...I just didn't know it. I thought that my twins were stretching and fighting for space, since I hadn't gained much weight. My entire abdomen felt tight, but there wasn't much discomfort. It just felt odd to have my stomach feel that hard and stretched. Once I was actually in preterm labor, I still wasn't sure what was happening. It took my husband and me five hours before we thought to time my stomach cramps, just in case I was in labor. By the time we got to the hospital, my contractions were two minutes apart. I still really didn't think I was in labor; I had no idea." ~ Shannon, Illinois

"My contractions felt like Braxton Hicks contractions; they squeezed my belly where my baby's bum was always poking out." ~ Ashley, Pennsylvania (made it through laser surgery for twin-to-twin-transfusion syndrome, PPROM, and preterm labor to have her twin boys)

"I did not feel any pain in my preterm labour, which started at 23 weeks. My tummy would go hard for 30 seconds and then soft again; this would repeat itself after four minutes, gradually getting closer together. I was in labour when these continued for 4–5 hours, and then it started to get painful." ~ Jennie, United Kingdom

Is There a Difference Between Preterm Labor and Full-Term Labor?

"Preterm contractions: my whole belly got as hard as a rock. It felt like a giant squeeze, but no pain. It was often uncomfortable, but I could always talk through them. Actual labor: my toes curled, it was so painful. They felt like someone had reached into my uterus through my skin and was trying to rip it out of me. Big difference!" ~ Janine, Pennsylvania

"The contractions I felt before I was put on bed rest were painful. I felt cramps during most of my pregnancy, but this particular night I was trying to get to sleep and I was in intense

pain. Scared, I woke up my husband, and we shot right over to the hospital. But preterm labor had nothing on actual labor. When I delivered my daughter at 31 weeks and 6 days, the pain was like nothing I had felt. Six months later, I had kidney stones, and you could compare the pain of kidney stones to labor. Both are extremely intense!" ~ Maureen, Pennsylvania

"My contractions felt different at different stages of my pregnancy. The earliest contractions I felt were at 15 or 16 weeks, and they felt like my uterus was 'balling up' or tightening. My belly would feel firm to the touch, but often only below my belly button. I often had to instruct the nurses in triage where to place the monitor to pick up my contractions. They always wanted to place it by my belly button, but my contractions always picked up lower than that, especially early in the pregnancy. Contractions don't go away when you change position or re-position the baby…they persist." ~ Becky, California (Endured 11.5 weeks of bed rest after preterm labor started at 23 weeks, on her side and on magnesium sulfate, to have her baby. At the time of writing she was pregnant again, with preterm labor that had started at 17 weeks, and was 12.5 weeks into bed rest—i.e., at 29 weeks.)

I Didn't Even Know

"During my first experience with preterm labor, my contractions just felt like mild stomach cramps. Had I not just been in a car accident, I probably would have ignored them . . . they weren't painful at all, just a little uncomfortable. When I experienced preterm labor again at 34 weeks, the contractions were again like stomach cramps. By that time, I understood what Braxton Hicks contractions were and equated my labor to that. It wasn't until I realized that they were coming three minutes apart that I recognized a need to get to the hospital. With my third pregnancy, my preterm labor began at 24 weeks. I was carrying twins and had general discomfort. I didn't realize preterm labor had started based on contractions—it wasn't until my doctor did a cervical check that she realized I was starting to dilate. The monitors

showed that I was contracting, but I really didn't feel much. As the weeks passed, my contractions were more noticeable and came in waves." ~ Jenn, Utah (even after multiple experiences with early labor, she still didn't know)

"I did not feel any contractions, and I have had preterm labor three times. They showed up during uterine monitoring, and I was treated accordingly." ~ Anonymous

"Part of my problem is that I don't feel the early contractions. I really just felt them when it was almost too late to stop anything, around the five-minute mark. I would be at my ultrasound appointment, and the doctor would see me have a contraction and ask if I felt anything, but usually I couldn't." ~ Ana, California (lost two babies at 28 weeks before she made it to 32 weeks)

"I didn't notice them with my first pregnancy until it was too late. My belly always felt hard, and I was really uncomfortable. Sometimes I felt like there was pressure in my vagina/cervix along with the tightening. With the second pregnancy, the contractions at 15–23 weeks made me feel like I always had to pee. I contracted more when I was active and busy, although I was distracted by what I was doing and usually didn't notice." ~ Carla, Canada

"In hindsight, I did notice my belly getting hard at times. I also experienced pain throughout my pregnancy and was told it was round ligament. My problem was that 1) I had been experiencing pain throughout so did not notice that this was particularly different, and 2) I had a history of kidney stones, so they thought I may have had another one." ~ Cristina, Panama

You Can Make It

"They first started in the middle of the night, and I thought it was just cramps from eating tacos. Over a few hours, they got more frequent and I wasn't going to the bathroom, so I went to the doc. By the time I got to the hospital, it was intense pain

starting in my pelvis and radiated up around my belly. With my daughter, my water broke first, and the contractions came quick and hard right after." ~ Lynn, Maine (went on to have a healthy baby girl at 36 weeks after 13 weeks of bed rest and the previous loss of twins at 22 weeks)

"In my first pregnancy, I'm not sure when the contractions started, as I didn't realize that's what they were. That pregnancy resulted in a loss at 22 weeks. In my second pregnancy, which I carried almost to term, I realized I was having contractions at 19 weeks. I had heard people say the baby can 'ball up' in your belly, so when I had that feeling in my first pregnancy, I thought nothing of it. In my second pregnancy, I felt the same thing— that there was a hard area in my belly. It wasn't the baby balling up, though—it was my uterus tightening in a contraction. As the pregnancy progressed and my uterus got bigger, I could feel the contractions more. I had the contractions off and on all day from at least 19 weeks, until I delivered at almost 37 weeks. Almost all of that time, I was taking medications to prevent preterm labor." ~ Anonymous, New York

I hope some of these words of experience will come in handy, should you need them, which I hope you won't. As you can see, the range of experiences is huge. This doesn't even come close to describing all the possible sensations you could experience, but I think you get the idea. So, listen to your body, and if something seems off, call your doc. Figuring out what's going on early is key. Good luck, girls...hang in there.

References

1. Lewis D, Pelham JJ, Done E, et al. Uterine contractions in asymptomatic pregnant women with a short cervix on ultrasound. *J Matern Fetal Neonatal Med* 2005;18(5):325–328.
2. Berghella V, Iams JD, Newman RB, et al. Frequency of uterine contractions in asymptomatic pregnant women with or without a short cervix on transvaginal ultrasound scan. *Am J Obstet Gynecol* 2004;191(4):1253–1256.
3. Herron M, Katz M, Creasy R. Evaluation of a preterm birth prevention program: preliminary report. *Obstet Gynecol* 1982;59(4):452–456.
4. Berghella V. *Preterm Birth: Prevention & Management.* West Sussex, UK. Wiley-Blackwell, 2010.

CHAPTER 6

Our Friend and Foe, Tocolytics

" *T he dreaded 'mag'—God, I HATED it! Not sure I want to go into detail on this, though. Had it three times, with each pregnancy."* ~ Klea, California

The Basics[1]

Tocolytics (from the Greek words *tokos*, meaning childbirth, and *lytic*, meaning capable of dissolving) is the official medical term for anti-contraction medications or labor depressants. They're used to halt/stop premature labor to delay the delivery of your baby, and they are given when delivery would result in a premature baby. They buy time for giving steroids, which greatly accelerates fetal lung maturity, but which take one to two days to work, or they allow for the transfer of mom to a center/hospital better able to care for her preemie baby.

The stopping of contractions is often only partial, and typically tocolytics can only be relied on to delay birth for several days. Depending on the type of tocolytic used, either the mother or the baby may require monitoring, so expect to be hospitalized—though many women are now going home with a terbutaline pump for home use to help try to control early labor.

Various types of agents are used, with varying success rates and side effects. Some medications are not specifically approved by the U.S.

Food and Drug Administration (FDA) for use in stopping uterine contractions in preterm labor; instead, these are being used for purposes other than those specified on the label.

When Tocolytics Should NOT be Used[1]

Several factors may eliminate you as a candidate from using these drugs to stop early labor, including:

✦ A baby who is older than 34 weeks. At this age, the risks from the meds outweigh the benefits, since you are at a good gestation.

✦ A baby who has intrauterine growth restriction (IUGR) or placental insufficiency.

✦ Congenital or chromosomal abnormalities that would lead to the death of the baby.

✦ Cervical dilation greater than four centimeters.

✦ The presence of chorioamnionitis or intrauterine infection.

✦ Severe pregnancy-induced hypertension, eclampsia/preeclampsia, active vaginal bleeding, placental abruption, a cardiac disease, or another condition that means there is extreme risk to both mom and baby if the pregnancy continues.

What Are the Overall Thoughts About These Drugs?

Why is this chapter titled friend or foe? Tocolytics are our friend because these drugs can help us to have healthier babies, but they can also be our foe, because as you will read throughout this chapter, there are many, many side effects when taking them. They tend be really rough on mom. Many women who are put on these drugs commonly report feeling like complete shit, but most will tell you they didn't care about that so long as it helped them carry their babies longer.

An important point to take away is that these drugs can't generally be used for long periods of time. As one article summarizes, they have "the potential to delay preterm birth for 48 hours, which is the critical period for antenatal steroid administration or to arrest an episode of preterm labor, thus delaying birth and improving neonatal outcomes." They also go on to say that the most common drug used in the U.S. to stop labor is magnesium sulfate; however, recent research has shown that oral nifedipine appears to have an equal ability to stop labor, but without as many side effects for mom. The author further recognizes that some of the side effects of these drugs can be life-threatening, so careful monitoring by doctors is mandatory.[2]

According to one author, "The use of tocolytics has proved disappointing, perhaps because inflammation rather than spontaneous uterine activity is increasingly recognized as the final common pathway." What he is saying is that inflammation, not preterm labor (early contractions), seems to be causing our babies to come too soon. He believes that the best approach to reducing preterm birth is by decreasing contagious diseases, providing improved care for diabetes, and stopping certain behaviors, like smoking and drug use during pregnancy.[3]

Another author states that, "Available tocolytics in Canada...have poor efficacy, have not been shown to increase the completion of a course of corticosteroids, are potentially associated with significant maternal/fetal side effects, and most importantly, have not been shown to improve neonatal outcomes." He goes on to say that, "Therefore, questionable efficacy and potentially serious side effects may outweigh their use."[4]

Another physician reveals, "The perfect tocolytic agent, which is completely safe for both the mother and fetus, and which will inhibit uterine contractions and stop preterm labour in every case does not exist and the search continues."[5]

Don't be completely deterred, though. On the other side, it is argued that these studies were not designed to truly look at the benefits of extending a pregnancy by 24 hours, 48 hours, or even 7 days. These studies typically use women "at relatively advanced gestational ages with predictably good outcomes." They point out that one large placebo-controlled study in particular "showed clear trends towards better survival in fetuses <28 weeks, lower rates of cerebral palsy and higher Bayley mental scores." They also cite research that shows a reduction in common premature complications.[6] So, some are saying, "Hey, they do work!"

In a survey comparing practices of Canadian obstetricians, they found that from 1997–98 to 2004, the use of tocolytics dropped slightly. The use of them for longer than 48 hours had dropped by half, from 20% to about 10%. (It can be speculated that this is due to the safety issues and known side effects from these drugs.)

There was also a shift from using magnesium sulfate to indomethacin as the most prescribed treatment to stop contractions. Also, the use of repeat doses of antenatal corticosteroids throughout pregnancy had dropped quite a bit, from 72.9% in 1997–98 to 18.7% in 2004.[7]

The best candidates for tocolysis are women who:

+ Are between 24 and 34 weeks along
+ Are less than 4 cm dilated
+ Have no other complications with their pregnancy
+ Have no signs of infection

The Common Ones (The Class of Drug)

Here, I briefly discuss each of the tocolytics typically used to stop early labor, but I spare you the boring details on how they work. Do you really care what mechanism they act upon to stop labor? Most likely not…it's way too complex for me. Should you want more information on the pathways on which each of the drugs work to stop contractions, it would be best to pick up a pharmacology book or a medical textbook.

Atosiban (Oxytocin-Receptor Antagonists)

This drug is used commonly throughout Europe, but its use is not permitted in the U.S.[8] It did not get FDA approval—the approving body of pharmaceuticals within the U.S.—cited as being due to a lack of proof in the research provided on its efficacy. In a worldwide comparison study between Atosiban versus beta-agonists (another group of tocolytic drugs), Atosiban was found to be just as effective as the others, but with fewer side effects, like cardiovascular issues, so doctors didn't have to stop using it as often.[5]

Another study, which also compared Atosiban with other drugs used to suppress preterm labor, showed that in women taking Atosiban, 78.7% of them were still pregnant after 48 hours, and 64.3% after 7 days. Atosiban reduced contractions from an average of 5.4 to 1.6 every 30 minutes. Similarly, this study concluded that Atosiban was effective and had fewer side effects related to its "lack of cardiovascular activity."[9]

Women between 23 and 33 weeks who had preterm labor were either treated with an IV of Atosiban for as long as 45 hours or a terbutaline IV for 24 hours (control group). In the Atosiban group, 2.5% of the women delivered before 48 hours, while birth occurred before 48 hours in 22.5% of the women in the control group. The average interval to delivery in the Atosiban group was 28 days, versus only 5 days in the control group. (Those extra 23 days could make a huge difference.)

Side effects were experienced by 27.5% of the women in the Atosiban group, and none had a fast heart rate or breathing issues, while 75% of the control group experienced side effects including palpitations, a fast heart rate, shortness of breath, or headaches.[10] So, based on this study, it appears that Atosiban is more effective and has fewer side effects than terbutaline.

Generally, there are fewer reported side effects for Atosiban than for any other tocolytic. The side effects are minimal and only consist of increased sensitivity and reaction of the injection site.[8] This is all great news, but if it isn't totally awesome in terms of its effectiveness, then what's the point? If only they could make a tocolytic that works without question to stop contractions until the baby is ready, with no significant side effects. I'm sure many of you who have been on these drugs would appreciate the lack of nausea/vomiting, dizziness, and heart palpitations. Disappointingly, this drug has shown not to work all that well overall.

Betamimetics[8]

A review concluded that this group of tocolytics was effective in reducing early birth within 48 hours by 37% and seemed to reduce birth within 7 days by 33%. The studies included in this review were limited, however.

Some side effects in mom are nausea, headaches, stuffy nose, nervousness, tremors, racing heart rate and palpitations, as well as chest pain, shortness of breath, irregular heartbeat, and to a lesser degree, fluid accumulation in the lungs. There are also side effects for the baby, including: fast heart rate, low blood sugar, and low blood pressure.

As one medical text concluded about this group of drugs, "Due to the significance and high frequency of side effects, we never use these medications as treatment for preterm labor." The available date is confusing/conflicting, yet, in spite of all this, these are still commonly used by many doctors.

Common Betamimetics

1. Ritodrine[8]

This drug is the only tocolytic that is approved by the Food and Drug Administration (FDA) for the treatment of preterm labor. None of the other drugs that are used to stop early labor are registered or intended for that specific use. The newer tocolytics don't have the side effects of Ritodrine; therefore, most doctors don't use this drug any longer.

2. Terbutaline (a.k.a. Terb Pump)

In a small study of women with recurrent preterm labor at less than 32 weeks, they found that a continuous dose of this medicine at home reduced preterm birth markedly. The rate of delivery before 32 weeks was 47% in women who received no tocolysis, but fell to zero in those using Terbutaline. It was found that its use not only allowed for longer "baking time" for the baby, which reduced NICU time, but also reduced the amount of time mom spent in the hospital.[11]

If there's one thing that sucks worse than bed rest, it's hospitalized bed rest. Being surrounded by your family in the comfort of your own home has a large impact on how well you can handle it. Just this factor alone, being able to take the medicine continuously while being at home, can really help you make it through this difficult time. But, be open with your doctor about discussing the possible side effects, which are many.

Indomethacin (Prostaglandin Inhibitors)

This drug is not only a tocolytic but also an anti-inflammatory. It is sometimes given to women after they receive a cerclage to prevent uterine activity (contractions).

In a study of women with cervical dilation of greater than or equal to 1 cm between 14 and 25 weeks, they found that it had no apparent benefit in extending the pregnancy or in preterm birth rates when compared to the control group who did not receive it, regardless of whether or not they'd had a cerclage.[12]

Another study found that women who took Indomethacin when they received an ultrasound-indicated cerclage had the same amount of preterm birth as those who didn't take the drug. Hence, Indomethacin was shown to have no effect on the rate of preterm birth.[13]

Yet another trial, which looked at women with short cervical lengths and no cerclage, found that the use of Indomethacin in asymptomatic women did not reduce births before 35 weeks, but did seem to reduce preterm birth at less than 24 weeks. It's interesting to note that the overall preterm birth rate at less than 35 weeks was 29.3% in those who took Indomethacin and 42.5% in those who didn't take it. (Based on the number of participants, this was found to be an insignificant difference, and they recognized that a larger study is needed to fully understand this.)[14]

When compared to a placebo, this drug reduced early births prior to 37 weeks, led to babies with a higher birth weight, and had a tendency to lessen birth of the baby within 48 hours to seven days. The side effects in mom are mostly nausea. Side effects in the baby are minimized when this tocolytic is used for 48 hours or less and before 32 weeks gestation. More recently, doctors have agreed that Indomethacin should be used for women in preterm labor before 32 weeks, as long as it is used for no more than 48 hours.[8]

Magnesium Sulfate (Myosin Light Chain Inhibitor)

This is one of the most commonly used therapies to halt preterm labor. In a large survey within the U.S., 94% of the doctors surveyed use it as their main drug to stop preterm labor.[8]

In a study that looked at the ability of magnesium sulfate to reduce cerebral palsy and death in babies who were expected to be born within 24 hours at less than 30 weeks, they found that it can improve outcomes. They also found no serious side effects.[15]

Like the last study, recent research has sought to look at possible brain-protective benefits for preterm babies when using mag. In a recent review of 19 randomized, clinical trials, they found that magnesium sulfate *does not* reduce the number of deliveries within 48 hours or seven days, or early/late preterm birth, and does not appear to improve the babies' outcomes. They confirmed that it can be used to allow time for antenatal corticosteroid administration or other suddenly occurring reasons, but treatment can be stopped once these have been satisfied. In women with recurrent preterm labor, multiple treatments shouldn't be used, although they do acknowledge that three trials did show neuroprotection benefits associated with the use of this drug.[16]

As one article puts it nicely, magnesium sulfate "is among the most commonly used pharmaceuticals in American obstetric practice. Although most clinicians are in accord regarding its value for seizure prophylaxis (*treatment*) in the setting of preeclampsia, such unanimity is not the case regarding its role in preterm labor. Credible scientific data indicate not only a lack of efficacy, but also toxicity to susceptible fetuses when magnesium sulfate is used in the high dosage found in tocolysis." They also acknowledge that "it may have both neuroprotective and toxic effects." This protective benefit appears to be at lower doses.[17]

So, why is it being used to stop early labor so often? As you've read so far, much of the data on tocolysis is unclear and confusing, so my guess would be that doctors are using this drug to stop early contractions because of vague training/understanding of tocolytics as a whole, the suspected neuroprotective benefits, the fact that its use has been "grandfathered" in because of proven effectiveness in other conditions, like preeclampsia, or because of the cost.

Side effects for mom include flushing, nausea, visual issues, and headaches. Rare issues, such as fluid in the lungs and cardiac arrest, are also possible. In the baby, as I stated before, they have found that short exposure may actually protect their brain.[8]

Since there is limited data that clearly demonstrates the benefits of this drug, as well as the side effects, many have asked for this drug to no longer be used as the primary drug to stop preterm labor.[8]

Nifedipine (Calcium Channel Blocker)

In a study that reviewed previous research in an attempt to compare Nifedipine to Atosiban, they found that Nifedipine showed a reduction in respiratory distress syndrome in babies and a non-significant delay in delivery by 48 hours above that seen with Atosiban.[18] It should be made clear that this was NOT the results of a study where X women got Nifedipine and Y women got Atosiban—i.e., it was NOT a direct comparison of these two drugs against one another. This in itself presents any number of limiting factors when making comparisons.

Another study concluded that the safety and ability of oral Nifedipine to halt preterm labor for greater than or equal to 48 hours or 7 days was comparable to Terbutaline injections to stop preterm labor. They also found that mothers receiving Nifedipine had fewer side effects.[19]

It should be noted that there are no gold-standard studies that directly compare this drug to a placebo, but "the overall data of Nifedipine as a tocolytic appears favorable." They have found fewer side effects when using this compared to several other drugs, and the need to stop treatment because of side effects is reduced by a whopping 86%. (The side effects in mom are low blood pressure, fast heart rate, flushing, and dizziness. There are no side effects for baby.)[8]

Summary on Tocolytics[8]

The whole point of using these drugs is to extend the baking time of your baby long enough to give steroids or to transfer you to a hospital better equipped to take care of you and your baby. In certain women, they can be used to delay delivery until a safer point in gestation.

Typically, tocolytics are only given for 48 hours, to allow time for the steroids to do their thing. Sometimes, especially between 24 and 28 weeks, they are used for a longer time period, even though the effectiveness of this is unproven in the research. Each additional day of gestation during this critical time increases your baby's chance of survival by 3%. The current stance as stated in *Preterm Birth: Prevention & Management* is that, "We currently never administer maintenance tocolysis, which has no scientific basis for its use."

According to this medical text, it's recommended to first use Nifedipine because of its overall safety (fewer side effects than the other drugs) and its ability to delay birth for seven days. Use of Indomethacin is also advised, but for no more than 48 hours.

Research clearly doesn't support the use of home uterine monitoring, as it has not been shown to help prevent preterm birth, nor has the use of what is called "maintenance tocolytics" (long-term treatments) after a bout of early labor has *stopped*.

What's a Girl to Think?

With all the "has not been shown to reduce preterm birth" disclaimers and talk of maternal side effects, the thought of using these medicines can be quite scary. Many women have used them, and yes, it may not have been pretty, as many have felt awful while taking them, but the reality is that lots and lots of women have used these drugs and gotten over a bout of preterm labor or a major hump in gestation with their help. Having to take any of these will not be easy, and most of the women I have talked to felt strongly that they just had to keep reminding themselves that it was what was best for their baby.

If you are having any problems or side effects, I urge you to bring up anything and everything with your doctor. It's very important to be completely honest so they can evaluate how your body is responding to a particular drug and switch if need be. Don't feel like a wimp for complaining if you are noticing something as a result of taking these meds. Trust me, it's better to speak up than to suffer the remote possibility of long-term heart effects or something else. There are so many different tocolytics available, and one could be better for you than another. Again, this is where it's best to have a good and knowledgeable doctor, one who is experienced with the use of these meds, caring for you. Hang in there, girls!

References

1. Wikipedia, http://en.wikipedia.org/wiki/Tocolytic.
2. Blumenfeld YJ, Lyell DJ. Prematurity prevention the role of acute tocolysis. *Curr Opin Obstet Gynecol* 2009;21(2):136–141.
3. Steer PJ. The epidemiology of preterm labour – Why have advances not equated to reduced incidence? *BJOG* 2006;113(Suppl. 3):1–3.
4. Smith GN. What are the realistic expectations of tocolytics? *Br J Obstet Gynaecol* 2003;110(Suppl. 20):103–106.
5. Lamont RF. The development and introduction of Anti-Oxytocic tocolytics. *Br J Obstet Gynaecol* 2003;110(Suppl. 20):108–112.
6. Fisk NM, Chan J. The case for tocolysis in threatened preterm labour. *Br J Obstet Gynaecol* 2003;110(Suppl. 20):98–102.
7. Hui D, Liu G, Kavuma E, et al. Preterm labour and birth: A survey of clinical practice regarding use of tocolytics, antenatal corticosteroids, and progesterone. *J Obstet Gynaecol Can* 2007;29(2):117–130.
8. Berghella V. *Preterm Birth: Prevention & Management.* West Sussex, UK. Wiley-Blackwell, 2010.
9. Helmer H, Brunbauer M, Rohrmeister K. Exploring the role of tractocile in everyday clinical practice. *Br J Obstet Gynaecol* 2003;110(Suppl. 20):113–115.
10. Cabar FR, Bittar RE, Gomes CM, Zugaib M. Atosiban as a tocolytic agent: A new proposal of a therapeutic approach. *Rev Bras Ginecol Obstet* 2008;30(2):87–92.
11. Morrison JC, Chauhan SP, Carroll CS Sr, et al. Continuous subcutaneous Terbutaline administration prolongs pregnancy after recurrent preterm labor. *Am J Obstet Gynecol* 2003;188:1460–1465.
12. Berghella V, Prasertcharoensuk W, Cotter A, et al. Does Indomethacin prevent preterm birth in women with cervical dilation in the second trimester? *Am J Perinatol* 2009;26(1):13–19.
13. Visintine J, Airoldi J, Berghella V. Indomethacin administration at the time of ultrasound-indicated cerclage: Is there an association with a reduction in spontaneous preterm birth? *Am J Obstet Gynecol* 2008;198(6):643 e1–3.
14. Berghella V, Rust OA, Althuisius SM. Short cervix on ultrasound: Does Indomethacin prevent preterm birth? *Am J Obstet Gynecol* 2006;195(3):809–813.
15. Crowther CA, Hiller JE, Doyle LW, et al. Effect of Magnesium Sulfate given for neuroprotection before preterm birth: A randomized controlled trial. *JAMA* 2003;290:2669–2676.
16. Mercer BM, Merlino AA. Magnesium Sulfate for preterm labor and preterm birth. *Obstet Gynecol* 2009;114(3):650–668.
17. Pryde PG, Mittendorf R. Contemporary usage of obstetric Magnesium Sulfate: indication, contraindication, and relevance of dose. *Obstet Gynecol* 2009;114(3):669–673.

18. Coomarasamy A, Knox EM, Gee H, et al. Effectiveness of Nifedipine versus Atosiban for tocolysis in preterm labour: A meta-analysis with an indirect comparison of randomized trials. *Br J Obstet Gynaecol* 2003;110:1045–1049.
19. Laohapojanart N, Soorapan S, Wacharaprechanont T, Ratanajamit C. Safety and efficacy of oral Nifedipine versus Terbutaline injection in preterm labor. *J Med Assoc Thai* 2007;90(11):2461–2469.

CHAPTER 7

To Cerclage or Not to Cerclage: That Is the Question. All About Transvaginal Cerclages

The cerclage, for those who are dealing with an incompetent cervix and the chance of a preemie, is a highly sacred piece of string, a literal lifeline. For those within the medical community, it's a source of controversy over its true effectiveness and who the right candidates are. "Do cerclages really work?" and "Which women should be getting them?" are two of the biggest and the most difficult questions to answer. I'll attempt to answer them, but I should warn you up front, there are no straight or simple answers. It's far from being as easy as, "Yes" and "You!"

The issues with cerclages are compounded by conflicting research and opinions. A cervical cerclage—i.e., a transvaginal (TV) cerclage or transvaginal cervical cerclage (TCC)—is when a piece of "string" is looped in and through the cervix to strengthen it and hold it closed. This type is much more common than a transabdominal cerclage, which is most often placed by going in through the stomach. (These are discussed in another chapter.)

I don't like the word "management," but it's often used to describe the treatment of this problem. Your doctor can't really "manage" a cervix, or even a uterus, when it's acting up and contracting when it shouldn't. They can, however, take steps to try to increase how long you'll carry your bab, or reduce your chances of delivering early.

As one paper puts it, "Management of a short cervix poses a significant dilemma for clinicians."[1] We know that placement of a cerclage is an option, as well as progesterone, and even bed rest, though they aren't sure if it really works.

It's estimated that 1% of pregnancies, or around 40,000 women in the U.S. alone, get cerclages each and every year.[2] In 2005, the rate of cerclages was 3.7 per 1,000 births, being more common in twins and higher order multiples (triplets, quads, etc.) than in singleton pregnancies.[3] (Note: research does NOT support the use of cerclages in pregnancies with multiples...keep reading.)

After my loss, I was told matter-of-factly that, "You'll just get a cerclage next time," and "Don't worry, they're *very* effective." This sounded like an easy, simple treatment to my problem; a no-brainer for my next pregnancy. It seemed I had little to worry about in any future pregnancies. Boy, was I wrong!

I had no idea how tough it would be to be pregnant and living with IC, no clue about the issues surrounding treatments, the constant worry and stress, or the specific problems we face, such as bed rest, pelvic rest, and the stresses of a potential premature delivery. I most certainly knew nothing about cerclages and the debate over the use of them, especially in situations of a questionable loss such as mine. Did infection lead to my IC and ultimately to my loss, or did IC lead to the infection?

The reality that bed rest, and lots of it, was to be a big part of my future, and the impact it would have on my life and, more importantly, my emotional stability, was never even a thought. It wasn't until I actually got pregnant again that the reality of the situation, and especially the fear, the worry, and the stress, began to surface.

I had originally intended to summarize ALL the research out there and present it for you to digest, absorb, and then draw your own conclusions, but this proved to be impossible, due to the enormous number of studies (not to mention that it would be terribly boring and hard for you to read). Instead, I have addressed a good number of the studies/opinions and tied them into the various subtopics to try to make it a bit less complicated...not an easy task with this topic.

I have relied on the use of several review articles, which did a lot of the work for me. Review articles examine, evaluate, and summarize existing research and comment on the overall "pool" of data, often including only those studies they deem up to their standards. Then they statistically analyze it all to draw their own conclusions. Basically, they research the research...go figure.

An ever-important decision you may be faced with is whether to adopt the "wait and see" approach, and so this is covered in depth—both the benefits and the negative consequences. I'm an expert on this one, because I've been there, and I'm **not** a huge fan. Many women are now blogging or posting messages seeking guidance on this issue in online communities such as Incompetent Cervix Support.[4] [Note: this is a great resource to connect with other moms who are either in the same place as you or who've been there. It was started by a mom who lost a baby due to IC that went undetected when it could've been (in her opinion), as a way to honor his memory. She has since gone on to have four cerclage babies. It was my savior during my high-risk pregnancies. To be able to get support from other moms who've been there, get to go through the experience with other women who were struggling like I was, and to share/exchange information was . . . just awesome.]

Knowledge is power, and my hope for each of you is that this will help those of you who are embarking on this journey to gain some comfort and clarity, allowing you to enjoy the reduced anxiety that comes with a solid understanding of the nature and issues surrounding this condition, specifically cerclages. Welcome to the wild and stressful world of IC.

Introduction: The People Who Discovered IC and Cerclages

This problem, whereby the baby "falls out," was recognized as far back as 1658.[5] Cerclages were first introduced by an Indian doctor named Dr. Shirodkar in 1955[6] and a couple years later by an Australian doctor named Dr. McDonald.[7] The techniques they used, with some modifications, are still in use today and are named after them.

The authors of an article directed toward OB/GYNs point out that both inventors and medical researchers agree that for a woman to be a suitable candidate for this procedure, she must have an obstetrical history that includes MULTIPLE second-trimester losses, and she must show signs of changes to her cervix in her PRESENT pregnancy.[2]

Notice the two emphasized words, "multiple" and "present." These are important themes that run through the research shaping current opinion on the use of cerclages. I, along with moms who've been through this, and even some doctors, have a hard time digesting the need for multiple losses in order to receive treatment. Many standards consider three or more losses as a prerequisite for an IC diagnosis. Do they have any idea what three losses does to a woman and her family?

The long-term emotional effects from a single loss are incomprehensible, yet I've heard of women suffering four, five, or more losses before the determination of IC was made. I can't even begin to understand how these women gathered the strength to go on, and my heart goes out to them. I barely survived the loss of one baby.

The second highlighted word is "present." Elsewhere, I've pointed out that IC isn't an all-or-nothing condition, meaning it doesn't necessarily present itself in the same manner during each pregnancy, or even at all.

Despite these problems, they're saying that before a woman can get a cerclage, she must have had multiple second-trimester losses, and her cervix should be observed to be shortening in her current pregnancy.

Regrettably, part of the problem, and the reason for current push back on the use of cerclages, is that they're commonly being placed in women for reasons other than their intended use and, by some docs, in large numbers of women, like when they're used to prevent preterm birth in women with short cervixes, as seen on a sonograph, who may not have a history consistent with IC.[8] This practice by certain doctors who see cerclages as "the answer" is contributing even further to this controversy.

Also, the rarity of this condition hinders diagnosis and treatment by some doctors, who just haven't been exposed to it. They either don't recognize early symptoms, such as changes in discharge or pressure, or they miss a red flag in the woman's history, like LEEP or other cervical procedures, DES exposure, etc.

Since there's no set test to determine whether a woman has IC, or even uniform standards to treat it, doctors' opinions and practices differ. One study sent questionnaires to 1,421 obstetricians/gynecologists in Canada to evaluate their views regarding the use of transvaginal ultrasound in determining cervical length, as well as the circumstances in which they would place a cerclage.

In certain clinical scenarios, the percentage of doctors who were unsure was high, meaning they didn't know whether they would or wouldn't place a cerclage. For example, if the length of the cervix was 1.5–2.5 cm, the gestational age of the baby was 20–23 weeks, and the woman had additional risk factors (spontaneous second-trimester miscarriage, preterm birth, early rupture of membranes, previous cervical surgery, history of DES exposure, or cerclage in a previous pregnancy), 54% would NOT place a cerclage, but of those who wouldn't consider a cerclage, an astounding 62% of them were unsure of this decision.[9] Wow, 54% would NOT place a cerclage in those circumstances. That's quite scary. (If it were me, I would demand a cerclage.)

Not until the last couple of decade have well-designed, controlled, and randomized studies looked at the effectiveness of cervical cerclages. The design and subsequent conclusions of older studies, many showing glowing successes, have subsequently come into question, casting doubt over the use of cerclages.

McDonald Versus Shirodkar

Both procedures involve inserting a string (mersilene is one of the more common materials used, or tevdek, or prolene[10]) around the cervix to "cinch" it closed. The Shirodkar technique is more invasive, requiring dissection of the bladder and rectum in order to place the stitch higher up on the cervix. One review article says this approach could lead to more complications than the McDonald technique, and placing the stitch higher, as in the Shirodkar method, hasn't been shown to provide any extra benefit. Because of this, the established effectiveness of the McDonald technique means that it's preferred by doctors over a Shirodkar cerclage.[2]

Basically, a McDonald cerclage is easier to place and take out, and it takes less time, so it's used more often. One medical text reports that analysis of the available randomized studies has shown no difference in effectiveness between the two types.[10]

One study looked at the efficacy of both types of cerclages in preventing preterm birth in women with short cervical lengths. They found no significant difference between them in preventing preterm birth before 33 weeks. (Both types of cerclage only had about a 20% early birth rate.)[11]

The labor outcomes in women who got Shirodkar cerclages, which were then removed before labor, were examined. They found a C-section rate of 18.8%, and noted that this was a higher rate than expected. They also observed a disturbing trend of uterine rupture and umbilical cord prolapse.[12]

A study looked at tightening the McDonald suture (squeezing the stitch so tight as to close off the vaginal canal completely). They used ultrasound as a guide during the preventative cerclage placement at 12–14 weeks, in order to determine why cerclages fail and to observe the shape/size of the canal before and after tightening of the stitch. They witnessed an hourglass shape after tightening in some women. Unfortunately, even though they noted this observation during the study, it was later found that this shape was likely a risk factor for preterm delivery.[13] Based on this, I would recommend asking for my cerclage to NOT be tightened all the way.

Medical Jargon: Deciphering the Language of Cerclages

Primary, secondary, tertiary, prophylactic, therapeutic, ultrasound-indicated, salvage, emergency, rescue, urgent, physical examination–indicated, elective, history-indicated, emergent . . . uhhhh, so many terms. You've watched the shows, *ER*, *House*, *Grey's Anatomy*, so it should come as no surprise that the medical establishment loves to use lots of words—lots of very confusing words.

Several researchers have suggested a standardization of the nomenclature to reduce uncertainty and confusion associated with the descriptions of cerclages. As one author suggests, naming it based on the reason why it's being placed would be beneficial and would get rid of any misunderstandings. They feel that this type of classification would oblige doctors to specify why the surgery is being suggested, be it history-indicated, ultrasound-indicated, or physical examination–indicated.[2] (I tend to use these terms throughout this book.)

Another author suggests naming the cerclage based on the various stages of prevention, defining these as primary, secondary, or tertiary transvaginal cervical cerclages. Primary refers to avoiding IC—i.e., stopping your cervix from shortening in the first place by placement of the cerclage early on. Secondary means placement after early symptoms appear, like if your cervix goes from 3 cm down to 1.5 cm. Tertiary means that the "disease" (not my word, the author's; I don't like to consider IC as a disease) has already progressed.[14]

History-Indicated/Elective/Preventative/Prophylactic/ Primary Cerclage

These terms imply that the cerclage is being placed based on risk factors alone, regardless of what is occurring during the current pregnancy.[2] (It doesn't mean you have a short cervix presently.) This type is placed early in pregnancy based on a history of risk factors, such as spontaneous second trimester loss(es) after painless dilation, a preterm birth, cervical surgeries, etc. It's usually put in around 12 to 14 weeks after the miscarriage period has passed, but sometimes it can be placed before pregnancy.[2,14] Because the cervix is still long and thick, the chance of infection is very low. A loss caused by placement of a preventative cerclage occurs in about 1 in 50 women.[14]

One study looked at research from 1994 to 2007 to determine the best time to place a history-indicated cerclage. Women were placed into two groups, one group who received cerclages at less than 14 weeks, and the other who did at 14 or more weeks. The average gestational age at placement for the first group was 12 weeks, and it was 15 weeks for the second group. They found no difference in the outcomes between the groups; 17% vs. 20% had an early baby, the length of pregnancy was 38 vs. 37 weeks, and the occurrence of preterm premature rupture of membranes was 17% vs. 18%. The best time for cerclage placement was concluded to be between 12 to 14 weeks, after testing the baby for abnormalities and chromosomal issues.[15]

The confusion/controversy with this type of cerclage is: how many losses are enough before you are considered a candidate? Also, what are the acceptable previous or current risk factors that make you eligible? Like I said, many doctors go by the standard that a woman must endure THREE second-trimester losses. I hope that in future this will change as a result of further research, a better understanding of IC, and the spread of knowledge among doctors practicing obstetrics, so that many women will hopefully be spared such trauma.

Ultrasound-Indicated/Therapeutic/Urgent/Secondary Cerclage

> *"I decided to have the septum removed. It was after this surgery that I was advised that I may be at risk for IC, but because I had carried my daughter to term, the risk was deemed VERY low. With my third baby, I was booked in for cervical length scans at 16, 20, and 24 weeks. At my 24-week scan, the cervix was seen to have shortened to 1.5 cm and was funneling, so I was given an emergency stitch. So far, I have gotten to 29 weeks and, please God, our second little miracle baby will stay safe and sound inside me for at least another six weeks."* ~ Oonagh, Dublin (had a bi-cornuate-septate uterus and got a cerclage after ultrasound showed cervical changes; technically, this is not considered an emergency cerclage.)

Often, the "wait and see" approach is used. This is when your cervix is routinely monitored using ultrasound in order to watch for any changes, shortening, or funneling that may occur. If changes are detected and you receive a cerclage at this point, one of these terms is used to describe it.

The commonly accepted cut-off when this type of cerclage is suggested is if less than 2.5 cm of cervical length is observed.[2] In women with a previous preterm birth and a length of less than 2.5 cm observed in the second trimester, a reduction of 29% in early birth before 35 weeks has been shown.[10]

Several recent studies have shown that ultrasound-indicated cerclages are equally as effective as history-indicated cerclages in high-risk women. These studies have been very important in shaping current opinion and practice regarding the placement of cerclages.

Women with a previous spontaneous loss between 14 and 24 weeks who were either given a history-indicated cerclage or managed by multiple transvaginal ultrasounds starting at 14 weeks were examined. They were given a cerclage if their length went down to less than 2.5 cm, or if they had more than 25% funneling. Of the 177 women identified, 66 got a McDonald history-indicated cerclage, and 111 were watched. Only 40 ladies (of the 111; i.e., 36%) actually ended up getting a cerclage after changes were detected. Remember, these were all high-risk women. The two groups showed virtually no difference in preterm delivery or the baby's age at delivery. (History-indicated cerclage babies were born at 34.6 ± 6.8 weeks, while ultrasound-indicated babies were born at 34.4 ± 6.8 weeks.)[16]

So, why is waiting it out to see cervical shrinkage now the preferred approach to managing IC? To those in the field, it *possibly* reduces unnecessary surgeries. Yes, there are downfalls to this approach for the women who are living it, including the enormous emotional burden, or the chance of missing the cerclage "window," which we'll talk about later, but this is a huge plus for the medical side of things.

Physical Examination–Indicated/Rescue/Emergency (or Emergent)/Salvage/Tertiary Cerclage

> *"The ER doctor gave me a choice of letting them take my baby then, or getting a room and having the baby in less than a week. Then, a wonderful doctor came and offered me the chance to save my baby."* ~ Evette, New Jersey (received a rescue cerclage between 18 and 19 weeks, and her baby was born at 28 weeks)

This is a cerclage that is placed after critical cervical changes with dilation have occurred. Sometimes the membranes, which house the baby in the amniotic sac, can be seen actually falling/protruding into the vagina. [More specifically, in medical jargon, the unruptured membranes are at or beyond the external os (opening).] The membranes must be intact—i.e., not ruptured—in order to get a rescue cerclage.

The vast majority of women (90%) who are dilated in the second trimester will deliver early if no interventions occur, and, unfortunately, a large portion of them will deliver before 28 weeks. It's mandatory that some form of treatment, like a cerclage, is considered for these ladies. The authors of one medical text state that, "Placement of a physical exam–indicated cerclage should be considered for all women with a singleton gestation and premature manually detected cervical dilation prior to 24 weeks."[10]

Placement of this type of cerclage, where cervical length is at a minimum, is a much more difficult and sensitive procedure than the other types, because there's little or no cervix left to work with, and the amniotic membranes are exposed. They found that the rate of amniotic sac rupture during surgery is between 4 and 19%, and if the membranes have dropped down into the vagina, the risk is even higher.[10] I know this goes without saying, but make sure the doctor who's going to do this surgery is experienced in placing emergency cerclages.

The techniques used to push the membranes back up in order to enable cerclage placement are reducing the amount of fluid (amnioreduction), using a Foley catheter balloon to gently push them back in, manually using a stick, which is covered with a sponge, or using gravity (the upside-down Trendelenburg position). None of these is 100% guaranteed to work.[10]

In one small study, they found that the extension of pregnancy was the same in women who had and didn't have amnioreduction.[17] In another study evaluating the effectiveness of amnioreduction, they found that it prolonged pregnancy by an average of 100 days versus 10 days for the non-reduction group. Deliveries before 32 weeks were also significantly lower in the women who underwent amnioreduction.[18] Given these conflicting results, you should talk to an EXPERIENCED doctor about your specific situation.

One study looked at the risk of amniocentesis prior to an emergency cerclage in women with a dilated cervix (1–4 cm) before 26 weeks to see if it would increase the risk of preterm delivery. They found that the amnio itself wasn't a factor for preterm birth at less than 28 weeks.[19] [An amniocentesis is the name of the procedure that is done to remove amniotic fluid or/and to test for the presence (or markers) of infection in amniotic fluid.]

I had an amnioreduction, and it was an extremely nerve-wracking experience, to say the least. The pain itself was minimal, just a quick burning pinch as the needle was pushed in, but it was scary. The size of the needle is very overwhelming, so don't look. In this situation, you're already in a state of complete shock, panic, fear, and sadness at the thought that you might lose your baby, but try to stay as calm as possible (even though it's damn near impossible).

I remember my husband having to leave the room after he saw how big the needle was, and I was so scared that I was going to lose my baby that the room seemed to whirl around me. The doctor was using ultrasound to guide the needle, and he was smiling and saying something like, "Look at your baby...here's his nose," but I just lay there and looked away from the screen, tears rolling down my cheeks. He looked at me oddly and said something like, "What's wrong? Why are you crying?" I thought, "Duh, you asshole. I don't know if my baby will even make it!" He then shook his head as he grasped the reality of the situation and looked down at me as if to say he was sorry.

I have come to the realization that our doctors are only human, and they deal with these situations in various ways too, in order to cope. It has to be hard on them to see these things. Maybe my doctor was trying to convince himself that he was in the middle of a routine sonogram in order to deal with it. I don't know.

Infection of both mother and baby is a major threat in this situation, and one of our biggest fears. Bacteria in the vagina, such as fecal bacteria that are found in poop, can invade and lead to infection, which is an extremely serious situation. The good news is, there are lots of healthy babies who've been born at good gestations, even at or near term, after the placement of an emergency cerclage.

What's terrible is that many babies are lost when dilation has progressed to this advanced stage. Dilation in itself can cause membrane rupture and the triggering of preterm labor, as well as increased risk of infection. Sometimes, when a woman's cervix is in a really bad state, there's just not enough flesh left to place a good, solid stitch.

Looking at the success rates of emergency cerclages over an eight-year period, 47% of the women had a delivery after 32 weeks, with a healthy baby at the time of discharge, while 44% of the pregnancies reached 36 weeks. In the women who had bad outcomes, most of them were due to infection (79%). The authors concluded that emergency cerclages appear beneficial.[20]

In women with Shirodkar rescue cerclages, 24% made it to term, 34% delivered between 34 and 36.9 weeks, 22% between 30 and 33.9 weeks, 10% between 24 and 29.9 weeks, and 5% before 24 weeks.[21] Almost 80% of the women birthed their babies at a good gestation of 30 weeks or later. Another study also found an 83% survival rate in women who had dilation with and without bulging of the membranes. Pregnancy was longer in those who didn't have bulging, as you would expect.[22] This is great news.

Yes, 30-weekers will be in the NICU for a while, but their chance of survival is 95%, and the majority of these babies will suffer no long-term effects. Those odds should make you feel a bit better. They're not as bad for a situation that many consider to be hopeless as I had believed. Certainly, that's what I was told: "There's really no chance of survival." So keep this in mind.

When comparing the length of additional "baby growing time" in women who had rescue cerclages versus those who opted not to get a cerclage, it was found that those with cerclages carried their babies an average of 9.1 weeks compared to only 3.3 weeks for those without.[21] That study clearly shows the benefit of a cerclage in this situation.

In women between 17 and 26 weeks who had prolapsed membranes, which is when the amniotic sac has dropped down into the vagina, who either received a cerclage and conservative management (bed rest, tocolysis, antibiotics) or were treated conservatively with no cerclage, amazingly, they found that the cerclage group averaged an extra 41 days before the birth of their babies, while, sadly, those who just had conservative management made it only three more days on average. They found that 72% of the babies in the cerclage group survived, compared to only 25% in the bed rest, tocolysis, and antibiotics group.[23]

When every day counts, these extra days in utero can be the difference between life and death, or a healthy, developed baby versus a sick baby, possibly with lifelong disabilities. Length of pregnancy is related to the health of the baby. The farther along you are, the healthier your baby, typically.

In a review of bed rest versus cerclage outcomes in women with dilation greater than 4 cm between 20 and 27 weeks, cerclages resulted in a significantly longer time to delivery than bed rest alone. The women who got cerclages also had shorter hospital stays, less use of tocolysis, and less preterm rupture of their membranes. The authors concluded that the benefit of emergency cerclages is quite clear.[24] Physical examination–indicated cerclages have been shown to prolong pregnancy. Cerclages were associated with better survival of the baby, higher birth weights, and fewer babies born before 28 weeks.[25]

In 400 low-risk women whose cervical lengths were examined at various time points to determine if emergency cerclage procedures were effective in preventing preterm deliveries at less than 34 weeks, they found a preterm birth rate of only 3.8%. Of these women, only five needed to have emergency cerclages placed between 20 and 28 weeks, and each of these ladies made it past 34 weeks. The researchers concluded that routine length measurements of short cervices and monitoring of vaginal bacteria will avoid unneeded prophylactic cerclages and increase the success of emergency cerclages when a dilated cervix is seen.[26]

Questions I have with this rationale are: Why would you place a rescue cerclage on someone who's 26 or 27 weeks along? And more importantly: Why would you prefer to wait until such a critical situation, with more risks to both mom and baby, to place a cerclage? The majority of doctors would NOT place a cerclage much beyond viability (around 24 weeks), never mind at 26 or 27 weeks. At 27 weeks, there's a good chance of a healthy baby at a hospital equipped with a level III neonatal intensive care unit (NICU) and the administration of steroids to speed up lung development.

The more common approach to treatment at the 25-, 26-, and 27-week mark is to administer tocolysis to prevent/stop contractions, antibiotics to prevent/stop infection, Trendelenburg position bed rest (where your head is lower than your feet—picture yourself lying on an inclined bench) in order to take pressure off the cervix, and steroid shots to speed up fetal lung development. Each of these is an attempt to "buy" some time. (Antenatal steroids need 48 hours in order to be completely effective. After the first shot, another shot is given 24 hours later, and 24 hours after the second shot is the window they hope to clear.) There's a lot of variation among doctors on how late into pregnancy a cerclage should be offered.

It's often not recommended to place a cerclage after 23 weeks because babies are able to survive outside the womb at this gestation. A Saudi Arabian study found that emergency cerclage outcomes were better when they were performed early in the second trimester (at or before 22 weeks) compared to later on,[27] but this is a debatable area. There's limited scientific evidence in support of a 23-week cutoff point.[2] The further along you are, the higher the chances of infection and that contractions will occur.

A gestation of 24 weeks, or even 25 weeks, with prolapsed membranes is on the borderline of whether the benefits of a cerclage out-weigh the risks. This is a situation where it's very important for you to talk with your doctors about your options, and their opinions/experi-ence on the best course of action. Demand answers to questions about what's going on. They won't have all the answers, but based on my experience, you can easily get overlooked in this critical situation. They tend to forget about the mom, so speak up if you have to. I just hope you never have to experience this scary situation.

A large study at Northwestern University Medical School in Chicago examined the data from a 20-year period to determine the fac-tors that lead to a successful emergency cerclage (success being defined as delivery at or after 28 weeks). They found that nulliparity (a woman who has not given birth), membranes prolapsed beyond the external cervical OS (low into the vagina), and a gestation of less than 22 weeks at the time of cerclage placement were all linked to babies coming before 28 weeks.[28]

A French study looked at the outcomes of women who'd received late emergency cerclages, placed after 20 weeks along, and found a sur-vival rate of 86.5%. Only 17.6% delivered before 28 weeks, and infec-tion was found in only about 15% of these women. The babies who were admitted to the NICU were followed up at one year and showed no signs of major handicaps.[29]

Other studies have shown lower survival rates, around 50%, and have determined that protruding/prolapsed membranes are a bad sign, with a higher chance of early delivery and death of the baby.[30]

Why have different survival rates been observed? There are many reasons why different outcomes have been reported, including not only the doctor's ability/experience in placing the cerclage, but also the abil-ity and experience of the hospital in caring for preemies. Technology in caring for tiny babies has come a long way in recent times, but it isn't universally available, so obviously, a better doctor or a hospital with a good NICU leads to better outcomes/healthier babies.

There's not enough research yet supporting the use of bed rest, progesterone, pessary, indomethacin, or other treatments besides a cer-clage in women who show no symptoms of preterm labor but have manually detected cervical changes in the second trimester of preg-nancy.[10] In these situations, therefore, you should be offered a cerclage.

You'll need to consult with a perinatologist, because they're experienced in this area, whereas a typical OB/GYN will most likely have never dealt with advanced IC or might only have seen it a couple times. You need to understand that this is one of the most ominous situations in all of obstetrics.

I really want to give you some hope, a glimmer of light in the darkness, should you ever encounter this, because a flicker of hope is what you'll need in what will be one of the darkest moments of your life in order to get by. To be contemplating an emergency cerclage is an extreme situation. I only wish I could say that none of you with IC will ever experience this, but I know that's not true. We can only hope that in the future, they'll find better diagnostic tools to determine who has IC before this occurs, and develop a concrete plan of treatments for women who have this condition, but the human body is extremely complex, and this is a complex puzzle to solve.

> *"I found that taking it one day at a time helped me following my rescue cerclage. I knew that every minute, hour, day was a milestone for baby. I remained mostly positive and never really acknowledged the idea that I could lose my baby."* ~ Melissa, Oregon (She was already dilated 3 cm, with membranes exposed, at the time of her cerclage procedure, and she made it.)

I was looking at the possibility of a rescue cerclage at 22 weeks. I was dilated 6 cm, and my membranes were bulging down into my vagina. At that time, I was told that we should consider terminating the pregnancy, because the chances of success were so low. I was led to believe that a cerclage was futile at this point, but the idea of aborting our baby was insane and out of the question for us... this was our boy. As I've said previously, there's always hope, even in this situation. Unfortunately, I was one of those who succumbed to infection, but many don't, and they end up leaving the hospital with babies in their arms.

Often, if you have dilation with or without bulging membranes, you'll be monitored to make sure you're not in active labor. If you're in active labor, unfortunately you're no longer a candidate for a cerclage. What they'll do in this situation is give you contraction-stopping medicines (tocolytics) to allow time for steroids to mature the baby's lungs and try to extend your baking time. If labor can be stopped, a

Tips/Expectations Should You Be Dilated in the Second Trimester[10]

1. NO, NO, NO—say no to repeated cervical checks. One gentle manual examination using a sterile speculum is all that's needed. Beyond that, you shouldn't be afraid to speak up and say no. This was the best advice I got from a nurse. Hands = bacteria = infection. Multiple checks can also increase inflammation. Reduce your chances of getting an infection/inflammation. It may seem that every doctor, nurse, resident, and med student wants to examine you, but just say, "NO!" This is your right, so use it.

2. A transvaginal length check will probably be done. Rest assured that even if you're dilated some, a length of more than 2.5 cm is a good sign.

3. You'll be hooked up to a monitor that determines and measures contractions, known as a tocodynamometer. Try to stay calm, and don't become too fixated on that damn printout, difficult as this will be.

4. This will be the worse time of your life. You'll feel the reality that the death of your baby is possible at any moment, and obviously this will weigh heavily on you and your spouse/partner and could push you right over the edge. Lean on people, keep calm, do whatever you need to do to get through each minute, hour, and day. Remind yourself often that there's hope. Healthy babies are born to moms in your situation all the time.

5. Expect to be hung upside down, in Trendelenburg position, for at least a while until a cerclage can be placed. No sitting up is allowed. Expect this to do wonders in terms of knots in your hair. Tip: put your hair back to avoid knotting and having to cut it later. (I fell prey to this.)

6. Expect to not be able to get up at all, not even to use the bathroom or to eat. It's very hard to eat while upside down, not to mention the joy of normal pregnancy heartburn, and I have no suggestions to help make this better, other than to suggest you just let go of being polite, being ladylike, feeling pretty, and being in control of yourself and your emotions. Throw all that out the window. Sometimes, you've got to poop in a bedpan, but don't worry about it; they've all dealt with this before in the hospital. For me, pooping was a major milestone when I was in the hospital, and pooping in a bed pan with a roommate was very awkward and stressful, but just let go. You deserve at least this minor comfort.

cerclage may be considered depending on the specifics of your situation. You'll also be monitored for signs of infection. An amniocentesis should be performed to ensure the absence of infection. This is a test in which they remove some of the amniotic fluid and test for the presence of bacteria or increased white blood cells, which indicate the presence of infection. (Under normal circumstances, amniotic fluid is sterile.)

Multiple Gestation–Indicated Cerclage

This is a cerclage placed solely because you're carrying multiples. In one study, they found that elective cerclages in twin pregnancies did not prolong pregnancies or reduce preterm birth,[31] and another study came to the same conclusion. In fact, they found that cerclages in twin pregnancies had a significantly higher rate of preterm delivery before 35 weeks[32]—that is, they actually harmed the pregnancies. Scary.

In a study where cerclages were placed in multiple gestations after the observation of cervices of 2.5 cm or less before 24 weeks compared to a control group who were placed on bed rest alone, they found that cerclages were not related to a reduction of preterm delivery. Women carrying twins who received cerclages delivered on average at 34.0 weeks compared with 34.4 weeks for those who didn't have cerclages. For women carrying triplets, it was 34.1 weeks for those with a cerclage and 33.0 weeks for those without. They found no difference in preterm delivery or in preterm premature rupture of membranes.[33]

In summary, be VERY hesitant if your doctor recommends a cerclage if you're pregnant with multiples. Make sure he/she is aware of the research. A cerclage in women with a short cervix carrying multiples was found to cause a more than 200% increase in preterm birth.[10] Research to support the use of cerclage in multiples just isn't there. There's no justification for preventative cerclages in multiple gestations. Instead, serial ultrasounds starting at 16 to 18 weeks is best.[34] (Though if you have a history of IC, that's a different story.)

Comparison of Outcomes from Different Types of Cerclages

The outcomes of elective (after the first trimester in women with a history of loss, high-risk women), urgent (after observation of cervical shortening), and emergent (dilation and possibly bulging membranes) cerclages are shown below.[35/36]

	Elective (History-Indicated)	Urgent (Ultrasound-Indicated)	Emergent (Physical Exam–Indicated)
Average gestational age at delivery (weeks)	35.9 **35.5**	34.2 **33.1**	29.3 **30.5**
Delivery beyond 36 weeks	73.9%	57.7%	23.5%
Death of the baby	6.8%	9.5%	43.8%
PPROM	19.3% **18%**	38.5% **40%**	64.7% **51%**
Infection (chorioamnionitis)	1.4%	18.2%	42.9%
Extension of pregnancy (weeks)	**20.2 ± 0.9**	**12.2 ± 1.5**	**8.3 ± 0.9**

Note: Results in **bold** are from the second reference. Similar results are seen in both studies, which were done a decade apart.

No Cerclage If Any of the Following Apply[2,10]:

+ Your baby has a severe anomaly.

+ Intrauterine/intra-amniotic infection is present. (Testing of your amniotic fluid via an amniocentesis to rule out infection is desirable.)

+ You have active bleeding. (If the bleeding is able to be stopped and the cause of the bleeding is determined, then a cerclage may be placed.)

+ You are experiencing active preterm labor. (Again, there's hope. If the contractions can be stopped and then controlled, a stitch can be placed. Sometimes, dilation of the cervix itself can trigger preterm labor.)

+ Your waters have broken (PPROM).

+ Your baby has died.

+ You're carrying multiple babies.

+ You have a uterine anomaly.

Some have suggested that neither a cerclage nor cervical length checks are suggested for women with a prior preterm birth or second-trimester loss if they've had a subsequent term pregnancy with no treatment, believing that the risk of another preterm birth is less than 10%. I think that even with those odds, I would at least ask for some cervical length checks in my second trimester. Just a thought.

Possible Risks From the Procedure[2,37]

+ Chorioamnionitis (infection)
+ Rupture of membranes (ROM)
+ Suture displacement
+ Bleeding
+ Contractions
+ Cervical damage

Rarer complications that can cause maternal and/or fetal death include:

+ Sepsis
+ Uterine rupture
+ Scarring of the cervix
+ Avulsion (the tearing away of the cervix)

The frequency of these complications varies widely, depending on the timing and the actual indications for the procedure. Ultrasound-indicated and emergency cerclages are related to worse outcomes due to a short cervix and exposure of the fetal membranes (amnion) to bacteria that is present in the vagina.[37] In one study that looked at almost 17,000 women who had cervical lacerations after a vaginal delivery, they concluded that cerclages were linked to an 11.5-fold increase in the incidence of cervical lacerations.[38]

Two Must Be Better Than One?

It would seem to make sense that if one cerclage may do the trick, then surely two would be better, but this isn't necessarily true. The use of a reinforcing cerclage was actually linked to significantly earlier deliveries (20.8 vs. 32.9 weeks) compared to women who did not receive a second cerclage.[39] That's terrible. Another study concluded that there was no benefit of two cerclages over one in preventing preterm delivery.[40]

One study did find that a single cerclage produced higher rates of preterm delivery before 28 weeks than a double cerclage, 29.4% vs. 5.9%, in high-risk women who'd had at least one previous loss in the second trimester. The average gestational age was 32.9 weeks for the single cerclage and 35.9 weeks for the double cerclage. Importantly, they found no significant differences in terms of survival of the baby *or* admission to the NICU.[41]

Doctors in the previous study had placed double cerclages so that one was in the lower portion of the cervix, while the other was placed in the high (upper) portion of the cervix. When the cervix was short, they dissected the bladder from the uterus in order to place the cerclages. (They took this approach as research has shown that a single cerclage placed close to the internal OS, or the inside upper portion of the cervical opening near the uterine cavity, was more effective than when placed in the middle or lower third of the cervix.)[41] It is unclear whether the difference in early birth rates was due to the double cerclage or due to the placement location of the cerclages.

As you can see, as with everything in the IC and preterm labor world, there's no 100% certainty. You should discuss this option with your doctor and decide whether it's right for you. Overall, the conclusion of experts is that a reinforcing cerclage is linked to worse outcomes. A better option is for the doctor to initially place the cerclage as high as possible, at a *minimum* of 2 cm from the external OS.[10]

What Can I Expect If I Get a Cerclage?

Depending on the circumstances, the stress level you'll experience will vary. If you're getting a history-indicated cerclage, you'll probably experience typical surgery jitters, but you can be confident that your cervix is still long and closed, so the chance of nicking your bag of waters or introducing infection is greatly reduced. At this point, you should be confident that a good stitch will be placed to hold your baby in. I'm not saying you're not going to be scared or nervous, but try to relax, confident in the knowledge that you're at a good point to get the stitch.

If shortening of your cervix has been detected, the level of stress and anxiety will increase significantly. In an emergency situation, you'll be under enormous strain, and the support of your loved ones is essential to help you make it through this. Try not to give up hope. (Note the success stories throughout this book.)

During my second pregnancy, I got an ultrasound-indicated cerclage placed at 21 weeks when my cervix measured around 1 cm. Needless to say, I was on pins and needles from the time of my ultrasound until the surgery the next day. I was a complete wreck, scared beyond anything I've ever experienced before. All I could think about was losing another baby. After they'd detected my short cervix, I was sent home and told to come back the next day for surgery. Sent home? I couldn't believe they were sending me home. For the next 16 or so hours, I refused to stand up except to use the bathroom, using my wedge pillow to tilt my uterus up in order to relieve the pressure of the baby off my cervix. I was completely freaked out, convinced that my cervix would dilate overnight and that my baby was going to fall out, just like the last time.

On the way to the hospital, I was so frightened I could've vomited. I sprawled across the back seat of the car on the way there. When I arrived at the hospital, I took up several seats in the waiting room just so I could lie down, still much too afraid to be upright. I didn't care about all the people who were staring at me.

I remember the cold of the operating room, and I prayed for my baby. Everything was a haze. I was placed on display, my legs spread as wide as they could open, in a room full of strangers. All I could do to prevent myself from screaming and suffering a breakdown was to try to visualize myself on a Caribbean beach. I tried to escape the reality of the situation in my mind.

At one point, I saw a tube sucking up my blood, so I decided that keeping my eyes closed was a better idea. I heard people chatting and talking; was I even there to them? My anestheologist was my savior. He kept checking on me and asking if I was all right, telling me we were going to be fine. Before I knew it, the procedure was done, and I was being wheeled back to outpatient recovery. The best thing about cerclages is that the procedure itself is really quick.

In my third pregnancy, I had a cerclage placed preventatively at 14 weeks. What a different experience this was from the previous time. During the drive down, and while we were waiting, we chatted and laughed, and I felt a lot less stress and anxiety. Apprehension returned when I got inside the surgical suite, because these places can have that effect on even the most seasoned, but the room felt much less tense than last time, and once again, it was over quickly. Both times, the hardest part for me was recovering from the epidural anesthesia. (I'm very sensitive to them, and they took an extremely long time to wear off.)

After the procedure, you can expect cramping and bleeding over the next couple days. The bleeding I had was period-like for two to three days, and the cramping was strong for the first couple days. Pay attention to your body. If you feel any sort of regular contractions, an increase/change in blood flow, or something just feels off, call your doctor.

I've heard some ladies say that they were put completely under during the procedure (meaning general anesthesia). I can understand why it would be preferable to be "asleep," but the favored anesthesia option is regional, where only a portion of your body is "blocked" from feeling pain. The reasoning is that due to the short procedure time, regional anesthesia is preferred because it's relatively short-lasting and safe. A spinal is typically used for pain control during cerclage procedures.[2]

When they're placing it, you're asked to sit and curl your spine (to provide space for inserting the pain med), while a nurse helps to hold you still. The needle is put into your back to first numb the area in epidurals or to give you the one-shot pain relief of spinals. It's definitely scary to get a needle in your back, but it just feels like any other shot, with a bit of extra burning. The anesthesiologist then checks the area to make sure it's sufficiently numb. In epidurals, a larger needle is then placed into your back, and a catheter (a small line) is run through the needle and secured. The catheter carries the medicine to your spine continuously, blocking the pain receptors. Typically, numbness is from the waist down, although sometimes one side will be more numb than the other.

Some doctors perform cerclages on an outpatient basis, while others prefer you to stay for observation. The circumstances will also dictate whether you'll be staying at the hospital. If it's an emergency situation, you should expect observation for a while, and you may even be kept in hospital until you deliver.

If you're having the procedure as an outpatient, you'll be allowed to go home once you've stabilized (blood pressure), contractions/baby have been monitored, you're able to move your legs around/stand, and you can pee on your own. For most women, this should only take a couple hours, but for me it was more like eight hours.

Until it wears off, your bladder will be emptied using a catheter inserted into your urethra (pee hole). This doesn't sound too comfortable, but it isn't really too bad, since you're numb. It's more embarrassing than anything else. Even though you won't feel the urge to pee, you can experience pain, almost like contractions, in your back when your bladder is full.

The only pain I experienced during this entire ordeal were strong contractions in my back, but because I'd done this before, I suspected that it was because I had to go. Boy, was I in agonizing pain. I grabbed the nurse, and sure enough, my bladder was as full as it can get. They have this scanner machine to check if you need to be "tapped" with the catheter, so speak up. Rarely will they say, "Honey, when was the last time you peed or emptied your bladder?" so don't wait until you're in tears, like I did...twice.

Some doctors only request that you rest in bed for a day or so. Generally speaking, this is the case for women who get history-indicated cerclages and show no signs of contractions or heavy bleeding after the procedure. Some doctors, however, may suggest bed rest or reduced activity for longer, perhaps even a week or more, and depending on the situation in which your cerclage was placed, your history, and your recovery from the procedure, indefinite bed rest may be prescribed.

It's important to monitor your body following the procedure for any changes in discharge, fever (both of which could be a sign of infection), continued bleeding, cramping, leaking of fluids as a possible signal of ruptured membranes, or contractions. Some cramping is normal; after all, they've been digging around in there, and a foreign material is now stitched into your insides. Sometimes, irritation of the uterus from either the procedure or the cerclage can trigger contractions, so it's important that you discuss any concerns with your doc.

Epidural Versus Spinal Anesthesia[42]

+ The injected dose is larger for an epidural than for a spinal, so more space inside the back is needed.

+ A catheter is often used in epidurals to allow for multiple/continuous doses of medicine compared with the one-shot deal of a spinal.

+ It takes 15–30 minutes for an epidural to kick in and only about 5 minutes for a spinal.

Side Effects/Risks of Spinal/Epidural Anesthesia[42]

This is only a partial list. Make sure you talk to your doctor/anesthesiologist about ALL the risks.

+ Spinal shock
+ Cardiac arrest
+ Hypothermia (This leads to shivering and is based on my experiences. I chattered and shivered uncontrollably each time but was told this was normal.)
+ Broken needle
+ Bleeding resulting in a hematoma
+ Infection
+ Spinal/epidural headache
+ Breathing difficulty if the numbness travels too high
+ Loss of sensations
+ Loss of muscle power
+ Drop in blood pressure
+ Lowered heart rate
+ Breathing issues
+ Catheter needed for urination
+ Itchiness

Failure to obtain pain relief occurs in about 5% of patients, while 15% experience partial or "patchy" pain relief, factors include:

+ Being overweight (obesity)

+ Carrying multiple babies (You guys just can't seem to get a break.)

+ A history of a previous failure

+ Cervical dilation of more than 7 cm at the time of insertion

+ The anesthesiologist using air to find the epidural space while inserting the epidural, instead of alternatives

+ People who are regular opiate users.

Should I Expect to Get Any Other Meds After Surgery?

Some doctors will administer tocolytics after the procedure to "calm" your uterus and ward off contractions. Most women with a short cervix at less than 24 weeks are having contractions when they're monitored, even though they can't feel them.[2] There's a lack of research on the use of tocolytics in this situation.

Some doctors will prescribe the use of a specific tocolytic, indomethacin, and it's been suggested that if this drug is used, it should be used for no more than 48 hours after the surgery. Many studies have been unable to show that the use of antibiotics in women with unruptured membranes prevents preterm birth. Research hasn't supported the use of antibiotics, anti-inflammatory meds, activity restriction, and tocolytics, even though they're often used after a cerclage placement.[10]

Similar ambiguity exists when it comes to the precautionary use of antibiotics after cerclage placement. Some doctors routinely use them; others don't. There are no clinical trials that have looked at the effect of antibiotics at the time of cerclage placement. Screening for and treatment of sexually transmitted diseases should be done before surgery,[2] and you'll probably be told that you can take Tylenol after the surgery to deal with the aches and the cramping.

Why Cerclages Fail

Sometimes, cerclages don't do the job they're supposed to do and don't hold the baby in until term. One study looked at 793 women who had history-indicated McDonald cerclages in an attempt to calculate the risk factors that lead to preterm delivery and cerclage failure. They determined that first pregnancy, fertility treatments, severe preeclampsia, second-trimester bleeding, premature rupture of membranes, infection (chorioamnionitis), and placental abruption lead to early babies, even with a cerclage. According to the docs I spoke to, the approximate failure rate of transvaginal cerclages is 20%.

They found that the average reduction in pregnancy length was 6.4 weeks for bleeding, 5.6 weeks for infection, 5.1 weeks for placental abruption, 3.2 weeks for premature rupture of membranes, and 2.4 weeks for severe preeclampsia. The average gestation was 38.1 weeks in women without these risk factors.[43]

What They Do Agree On: The Shorter the Cervix, the Higher the Risk of an Early Baby

Many studies have looked at the correlation between cervical length and preterm delivery. As one author noted, it's important to consider that no studies have looked at the association between cervical length and preterm delivery due specifically to an incompetent cervix.[14] There's general consensus within the medical community that the shorter your cervix, the greater the risk of an early delivery.

Berghella *et al.* reinforced this relationship in a study examining cervical lengths between 16 and 24 weeks in women who'd had a previous cone biopsy. They found that a length of less than 2.5 cm was clearly linked to birth before 35 weeks.[44] (Yes, that's the same Berghella who's a contributor to this book. You'll see lots of his studies popping up.)

Another study that checked cervical lengths every two weeks between 16 and 24 weeks in women at high risk who had a prior preterm birth before 32 weeks found that women with lengths of 3 cm or less before 22 weeks were much more likely to have micropreemies before 26 weeks than those who had 3 cm or less after 22 weeks.[45] Again, this relationship was confirmed when they found that the shorter the cervix, the higher the incidence of preterm delivery. A cervical length of less than 2.5 cm and the use of ultrasonography between 14 and 22 weeks were the best indicators of an early baby.[46]

Yet another trial found that cervical lengths of 2.5 cm or less before 20 weeks was linked to a greater risk of delivery within four weeks.[47]

A study of 469 high-risk women between 15 and 24 weeks found that a length of 2.5 cm or less during this time period was best in predicting preterm birth before the major milestones of 28, 30, 32, and 34 weeks. They also found that 2.5 cm or less of cervix between 21 and 24 weeks was an ominous sign of preterm delivery, more so than the 15- to 20-week measurements.[48] Note: all these studies were only looking at cervical length and preterm birth. They didn't consider/calculate outcomes for women with cerclages.

A study that focused strictly on twin pregnancies found that lengths of greater than 3.5 cm had only a 4% preterm delivery rate. This study did not include women with preterm labor, prophylactic cerclages, or placenta previa. These were non-IC ladies who happened to be pregnant with twins. (Twins have a higher rate of preterm delivery than do singleton pregnancies.) Twenty-three percent delivered before 35 weeks, and they found that a cervix of 3.0 cm or less and any funneling, greatly increased the risk of a premature baby.[49]

As you read through all this, remember, the takeaway message is NOT that if you have a cervix of less than 2.5 cm, you're automatically destined to deliver early. Not so. Large percentages of these women who had short cervices still carried to term. Just be aware that you're at higher risk, and act accordingly. Work with (or push) your doctor to determine the best direction for care, given that you're in this higher risk bracket. (Just so you know, my cervix measured 2.5 cm at 18 weeks and was under 1 cm from 21 weeks on, and yet I carried to term with my daughter. But, as you know, I did get a cerclage at 21 weeks.)

One interesting trial examined cervical effacement rates on a weekly basis in high-risk women, some with IC and some without, between 15 and 24 weeks. They found that IC cervices shortened at an astounding rate of 0.41 cm per week versus a rate of only 0.03 cm per week for women without IC. (The women who were found to have IC, defined as shortening to 2 cm or less before 24 weeks, received cerclages.)[50] Wow! If this doesn't prove the reality of this condition, then I don't know what will.

Cerclages: The Controversy Over Their Effectiveness

The research on cervical incompetence, cerclages, bed rest, and cervical length is endless. Even though the incidence of IC is so small, it's a very popular subject with obstetrical researchers. There are literally hundreds and hundreds of studies spanning several decades. When attempting to draw general conclusions from all these studies, a very difficult if not impossible task, you have to remember that many of them were set up differently from one another, making it hard to look at them in one collective "clump."

One study may have different inclusion criteria from another. (An example of an inclusion criterion is if one study includes women who had one or more losses, while another might only include women with two or more losses.) Some studies include hundreds of women from the general population of pregnant women, and then filter down these women based on cervical length, or on whether they receive a cerclage or not. The potential design of studies is endless.

The Cochrane Review on cerclages for preventing preterm birth isn't even published yet, even though it's been in the works since 2009. A review on cerclages and preventing pregnancy loss in women was completed back in 2002, and concluded that, "A cervical stitch (cerclage) may help prevent miscarriage due to a cervical factor, but has not been shown to benefit other women."[51] How can our doctors know what's up when there isn't even clear guidance in a Cochrane Review? (Vague reviews are common with many issues in the preterm birth world.)

The problem with saying that cerclages absolutely work is that there haven't been any fully randomized and controlled trials conducted into the placement of a cerclage in women with a history of IC (multiple painless second-trimester losses).

So, why don't they do these trials and provide an answer once and for all? Well, that's an easy one. Say you have 5,000 women with a history of painless dilation and second-trimester losses. 2,500 of them are chosen at random to get a cerclage, while the other 2,500 are assigned to the "no cerclage" group. Now, say that of those 2,500 in the "no cerclage" group, some women show changes in their cervical length, or even dilation. No matter how dire their situation, because they're in the 'no cerclage' group, they can't receive a cerclage. Is this ethical? I think not.

169

They have done studies where this design was initially adopted, but when changes were detected in women in the "no cerclage" group, the women were then given a cerclage. The outcomes of history-indicated and ultrasound-indicated cerclages were then compared, and no difference was found between the two groups. (See the sections on ultrasound-indicated cerclages and the "wait and see" approach in this chapter.)

Several studies included women with a history of second-trimester losses (i.e., high-risk women) and women who were pregnant for the first time who showed a short and/or funneled cervix on ultrasound (i.e., low-risk women). The problem, however, was that all these women were pooled together, leading to bias within the results. Studies also used past pregnancies as the control, which is a big no-no.[5] Designing the perfect, flawless, unquestionable study is extremely difficult, if not impossible.

The conclusions that can be drawn from a study are only as good as the study design itself (and, of course, the statisticians who look at the data). Potentially, a poorly designed study can get published, and the results can be taken as fact by the doctors who read them. This information then gets passed along, when it shouldn't have held much weight in the first place. How can this be, you ask? We would hope that the editors of medical journals would assess the study completely before it's published, but this isn't always so.

For the average doctor, it can be hard to judge the merits of a single study without examining the subject as a whole, and this takes a lot of time, energy, and resources. Doctors typically aren't trained researchers; they're trained to treat their patients, not determine the validity of a study. They don't have the time to read an entire study, contemplate the design, and then analyze the conclusions to then apply to their own practice. I can't stress enough how complex all this cerclage stuff is. The American College of Obstetricians and Gynecologists (ACOG) doesn't even have recommendations for low-risk women who have a short cervix,[37] and these are the experts.

We would like to think that all scientific studies publish results with solid conclusions, but we know all too well that this couldn't be further from the truth. One month we hear that X has been found to cause cancer, and then the following month we're told that this same

X can help fight cancer. This is enough to drive you crazy, and it's the same with the wonderful condition we find ourselves with…IC.

And, here's where the problem lies: most of us don't have the time or knowledge to read, understand, and comprehend all this "stuff," which is loaded with medical jargon, let alone try to apply it all to our own care. That's what we pay doctors for, right? This is where so many of us go wrong. We put all our faith in someone else. Unfortunately, as I said before, often either doctors don't have the time to keep up with all the latest research, or they have so few patients with IC that they're relatively inexperienced in dealing with it. That's why it's so important for you to educate yourself (and that's where this book comes in), so you can work *with* your doctor(s), question/discuss options, push for the pregnancy you desire (advocate for yourself), make decisions, or just know what the hell it is your doctor is talking about.

There are also problems with incorrect comparisons of studies and false/skewed interpretation of the results. It's been pointed out that three randomized trials on preventative cerclages have NOT exclusively included women with IC. Duh…that doesn't make sense. A cerclage is used to treat women with IC. The author uses this to support the argument that there isn't enough evidence to show a benefit of cerclages in women with less than three prior losses. He says that if you've had two losses, you can be a candidate for a preventative (history-indicated) cerclage, but there's less proof to support this.[2] Confusing.

There are huge differences in the reported success of cerclages. Some cite between 70 and 100% survival rates of the baby in treated pregnancies, compared to only 10 to 30% when being compared to past pregnancies.[52] This is a design flaw. It's not totally accurate to use two separate pregnancies to calculate results, since IC doesn't show itself the same way in each pregnancy.

Several studies have demonstrated the effectiveness of cerclages in extending pregnancy to term, while several other studies have shown them to be ineffective. Contradictory findings regarding cerclage effectiveness for women with short cervices have been seen for both high- and low-risk women. This is very frustrating for us and our doctors.

For example, one study published in 1984 found no differences in preterm labor, premature rupture of membranes (PROM), or infant survival in women with cerclages compared to those who didn't have them who were at medium to high risk,[53] and yet another study, published in 2008, concluded that there was a high success rate in high-risk women who got a cerclage when cervical changes were seen on ultrasound.[54]

The studies that found that cerclages are very, very effective would lead one to believe that they're a no-brainer, right? Every doctor who even suspects IC should just place a cerclage, no questions asked, right? The criticism of these studies was that they weren't necessarily placed on women with "true" IC, and women who didn't have IC were included in the study. This led to inflated results on how good cerclages were, since many of these women would've most likely carried to term anyway.

After the loss of my baby, the studies showing the undeniable benefits of cerclages were the ones that were presented to me, so I thought, "No problem; next time I get pregnant, I'll just get the cerclage and go about life as usual." I had no idea about the real impact IC would have on me, and the decisions I would have to make. I only knew that A) I would get a cerclage, and B) I would carry to term. As simple as that.

Don't let all this boggle your mind, though. Your goal is to review the information so you can then open up the lines of communication with your doctor. I can't provide all the right answers, because there are too many scenarios and circumstances, but I hope that this book can help you develop a plan of attack.

The Problem with the "Wait and See" Approach

Based on the conclusions of some large, well-designed studies, such as the Cervical Incompetence Prevention Randomized Cerclage Trial (CIPRAT),[55] many doctors are now confident that an ultrasound-indicated cerclage is just as effective as a history-indicated cerclage and is the best course of action. To them, this reduces the amount of unnecessary cerclages and the potential risks associated with surgery—the thought being, why fix it if it isn't broken? First, let's see if it (the cervix) acts up, and if it does, only then will we do the procedure. One study suggested that out of 100 women who got cerclages, only one really needed it.[14]

It's not always clear in women who suffered a prior preterm birth or loss that it was definitely caused by cervical weakness. Often, it's not easy to determine whether IC was at work or whether it was due to other factors, like preterm labor or an underlying infection. In these cases, doctors recommend close monitoring of your cervix, often in conjunction with reduced activity (and pelvic rest), as well as progesterone shots to decrease your risk of premature delivery again.

The majority of women (60%) who are considered high risk, meaning they had a previous preterm birth or spontaneous delivery, will have a good length until after 24 weeks and therefore will not need *any* interventions.[10] On the *clinical* side, these are important arguments for the "wait and see" approach. If all those women were given a history-indicated cerclage, then 60% of them would not have needed it.

The CIPRAT trial[55] concluded that bed rest, along with an ultrasound-indicated cerclage if a length of less than 2.5 cm prior to 27 weeks is observed, reduces preterm birth. The women were not on bed rest for the entire study. After they had experienced shortening of their cervices, they were randomized into two groups: 1) get a cerclage and then be on bed rest, or 2) bed rest only.

Another study concluded that placing a cerclage only when indicated (upon observation of a cervix of 2.5 cm or less), as opposed to preventatively, will reduce the number of cerclages and improve the baby's outcome.[56] Again, it was confirmed that surveillance of cervical length in high-risk women and placement of a cerclage only if needed seems to reduce cerclage rates "without compromising pregnancy outcomes." They acknowledged the need for a large, multi-centered randomized study to confirm this,[57] and at the time of this writing, more research is needed into both low-risk and high-risk women who develop a short cervix in the second trimester.

The medical text *Preterm Birth: Prevention & Management* states that "expectant management with serial cervical examinations starting at 16–18 weeks"[10] should be done to keep an eye on whether that cervix of yours is behaving.

A study that had quite different findings from the CIPRAT trial was the CIRCLE trial. This was also a good study—well-designed, like the CIPRAT study. They found that women randomized into the ultrasound-indicated group were much more likely to receive a cerclage (32% vs. 19%) and progesterone (39% vs. 25%) than those in the history-indicated cerclage group. Interestingly, they found that the number of babies born between 24 and 34 weeks was only 15% in both groups.[58]

According to this study, there's no benefit in cervical-length checks to determine ultrasound-indicated cerclages over placement of a history-indicated cerclage; indeed, it appears to lead to more unnecessary cerclages. Yikes…this goes against the whole rationale behind the "wait and see" approach.

An article titled *Ultrasound Adds No Value to Cervical Cerclage Decision Making* addresses this last study. Originally, when designing their study, the doctors from St. Thomas' Hospital, King's College, London, U.K. believed they would find the opposite of what they actually observed. They went in thinking that the long-established approach of history-indicated cerclages (or preventative cerclages) was actually leading to unnecessary procedures.

One of the authors of this article who conducted the study in question, Dr. Andrew H. Shennan, spoke about how difficult it was to even get other doctors to participate, since they preferred history-indicated cerclages and firmly believed in their effectiveness.

His overall conclusion after his research was that "these data do not suggest any benefit in replacing historical indications for suture placement with ultrasound surveillance in all women with a history of preterm birth. Do not assume interventions are good without proper evaluation. There is little evidence ultrasound scanning–indicated sutures are beneficial."[59]

In examining the figures from the table presented earlier in this chapter, you can see that the women who got history-indicated (or elective) cerclages had longer gestations and fewer preemie babies. The infection rate was almost 18 times higher in the women who got ultrasound-indicated (or urgent) cerclages, and they had double the amount of PPROM. Hey, I'm no expert, but that concerns me. (The authors did acknowledge this in the conclusions. The purpose of these studies was to compare outcomes of the types of cerclage, not to evaluate the "wait and see" approach.)

With this approach, you're "watched" with serial transvaginal ultrasounds. The problem with that is that there's no set timeframe or protocol for when ultrasounds should be performed. Should it be every week, every two weeks, or once a month? If you do decide on this approach with your doctor, it's beneficial to have an ultrasound every week during the high-risk period of about 16–23 weeks, then one every two weeks until 28 weeks. Unfortunately, this may not always be possible if you live a long way from a center, and in my experience, docs usually prefer ultrasounds every two weeks. I simply demanded checks more often, especially during rough periods when I needed reassurance that my cervix was fine.

Another problem with this approach is in the measurements themselves. Many technicians are untrained in how to perform an accurate cervical measurement. Why? Because many rarely, if ever, have to perform one. Therefore, this type of measurement can have great variability among technicians. It takes a trained eye to choose the correct spot to measure from. (On the ultrasound, the end of the cervix is just a faint line, slightly darker than the surrounding tissue. See the chapter on transvaginal ultrasonography for more information.)

When weighing the benefits of the "wait and see" approach it's best to consider both your ability to get regular ultrasound cervical-length checks and the center's experience with performing length measurements.

During my second pregnancy, my group of doctors felt this was the best approach based on the circumstances of my loss. Originally, before I was pregnant, I was told I would get a cerclage early, which just messed with my head. Now I had to make a decision about whether I would follow my doctor's advice. I looked at the studies, I posted on the boards, and we very hesitantly agreed to go this route. I lost many nights of sleep contemplating this, and on each and every visit, my measurements were a source of extreme stress.

In a single session during the early weeks, my cervix could measure 2.1 cm, 2.5 cm, and 3.0 cm. What did this mean, exactly? I didn't know. Each time, I prayed that my length would jump up to a safe 4 cm or even stay at around 3 cm (it never did.) I got to the point that after they "connected the dots" and the measurement became visible on the screen, I would immediately begin to cry, believing that I was destined to lose my baby again.

Another concern with this approach is that a cervix can change over a few hours, so do the math...two weeks between measurements... changes within hours...It doesn't always add up. As I said previously, the shorter your cervix is (especially if dilation is present), the greater the chance of infection.

Obviously, you can tell that as a woman who has lived through the added stress that this approach brought, I'm not a big fan. I do recognize that every woman is different, and every pregnancy is different. In my case, it was determined that I did have "true" IC, so after suffering, and I mean suffering—the stress, complete bed rest, and then an ultrasound-indicated cerclage when my cervix shrank to less than 1 cm, I wished I'd just gotten the damn preventative cerclage in the first place. I survived two pregnancies after my loss, and yes, I know a cervix behaves differently each time, but the pregnancy I had with a preventive cerclage, though not easy, was a walk in the park compared to waiting it out. For a start, there was no bed rest. Enough said.

As with anything having to do with preterm birth, how are we supposed to know this without actually going through it? My main concern with the "wait and see" approach is the extra emotional stress it places on a woman and her family, as well as the added risks in waiting when your cervix misbehaves. Every day, you feel like you're dangling on a string that could break at any time, 100 feet up in the air, over pavement littered with shards of glass containing venom. You spend your days on pins and needles, thinking the worst.

So you don't drive yourself crazy should you and your doctor decide on this approach, it's extremely important to let go and try to relax—just go with the flow as best you can. You need to take it day by day, measurement by measurement, and NOT let your imagination take over. Reduce your activity, follow your doctor's orders, and try to lead as normal a life as possible. Don't worry about the what-ifs; you only need to deal with them if they happen. The emotional side of this situation, and the effect it can have on your entire life, is an area that I wish more doctors would take into account and address when pushing for this approach. If you have any doubts about why your doctor wants to wait, get another opinion. (Seriously!)

When to Remove The Stitch

Most doctors will remove the cerclage at 36 to 37 weeks, because it's extremely important to have it removed PRIOR to the start of labor. Real labor causes contractions that result in cervical changes, while false labor (i.e., Braxton Hicks) doesn't. Contractions could actually tear your cervix, causing even further damage, if the cerclage is still in place. When contractions occur, they pull on your uterine muscles, which in turn pull at the cervix to dilate it. If there's a string tying it closed, well, you get the picture. Ouch!

One study actually found the opposite, concluding that you can leave Shirodkar cerclages in place until labor, because they didn't see any increased risk of cervical dystocia, cervical laceration, or uterine rupture.[60] In my opinion, I'd rather just get it taken out at term.

If you start to see a change in your contractions; if they become stronger, longer, in a pattern, even period-like pains; or you experience a dull backache or an increase in mucus (this could be your mucous plug coming loose, signaling a change in your cervix) while your stitch is still in, make sure you call your doctor.

One study looked at the time from removal of the stitch to delivery and found that the average time from removal to delivery was 14 days. Only 11% of women actually delivered within 48 hours, although those who'd had ultrasound-indicated cerclages were more likely to deliver within 48 hours.[61] Prior to actually going through this experience twice, I thought that as soon as it came out, I would have the baby, but both times I walked around dilated for two weeks.

In some cases, it can be decided, between the woman and her doctor, to leave the stitch in and perform a C-section. This is typically the case for transabdominal cerclages, as these are more difficult to place and more invasive than a transvaginal cerclage. If you're being pushed to get a C-section for a transvaginal cerclage in order to leave it in place, you need to understand that you do have options.

If you've had C-sections in the past, there may be the opportunity for a VBAC (Vaginal Birth After a C-section) although lots of doctors aren't trained in these, and still more are hesitant to even assist in these deliveries for fear of lawsuits. There's research available showing the relative safety of VBACs, but this is a whole other issue.

Many women choose a scheduled C-section for convenience. They've had a stressful pregnancy, and they want one less thing to worry about. If this is your situation, I urge you to really think about this decision before you go ahead and to read the chapter on this elsewhere in this book. There's no right or wrong here; just don't short-change yourself on what is probably a once (or maybe twice, or thrice) in a lifetime experience. You deserve to have the birth experience you've always dreamed of. Maybe it's fear that drives you, which is understandable, but read up. There are some great books out there that can help you overcome the fear of giving birth. (That and you should make yourself aware of all the risks associated with C-sections.)

What to Expect During Removal

One fear for most of us is the pain/discomfort of the actual removal. In reality, the pain isn't completely unbearable. Yes, it does hurt, but just for a brief time while they root around inside looking for the string. (One time, my string was embedded, so they really had to dig. It hurt but was definitely manageable.)

There's some blood involved, and so I recommend that those husbands who have weaker stomachs stay up by your head. You'll experience period-like bleeding for a few days or so, and there's also cramping and often contractions involved. Overall, based on my experiences and discussions with other women, the removal of the cerclage is not traumatic. At this point, you've already made it past the hard stuff: fear of the actual placement, fear of losing the baby after the procedure, dread of a premature delivery, a sick baby, and the overall anxiety from a high-risk pregnancy, so this is a piece of cake. Hey, you've nearly made it!

Both times when I had my cerclage removed, I assumed I would go straight into labor. With my daughter, I popped open to 6 cm, which in turn triggered contractions. I was told to stick around the area, since we lived quite a distance away, so we went out to dinner, excited that I would be returning to the hospital soon. As dinner went on, however, the contractions moved further apart, and then stopped all together, so we finished eating and went home. Not quite the dramatic scenario I'd envisioned. I walked around 6 cm dilated for another two weeks prior to my water finally breaking.

With my second son, I practically had a nervous breakdown on the day my cerclage was removed for fear that I wasn't ready to have the baby yet. I cried in the hours leading up to it and during the one-hour ride to the hospital. I wasn't scared of the actual removal, because I knew what that was like. I just had this fear of having a newborn again. Oh, the joy of pregnancy hormones.

This time, I dilated 3 cm, still a good start (this was most likely because I'd had a preventative cerclage placed when my cervix was still closed and long), but again, I went two weeks, despite many false labor episodes, an attempt at castor-oil induction, several sex-capades, which weren't that great, even after not getting laid in eight months, and a little walking (I was feeling lazy), until I was eventually induced. So, we fight to keep them in, and then sometimes we fight to get them out. (Note: often scar tissue develops around the cerclage, so there's a "barrier" to dilate past, which can be a bit difficult.)

Some doctors insist on a quick in-office procedure, while others prefer to remove it in the hospital. Often, pain meds aren't needed for a McDonald stitch, but a Shirodkar is more difficult to remove, and I've even heard of some doctors giving their patients a spinal to eliminate any pain. My advice is to talk to your doctor about your options. If they prefer the hospital/pain-relief route, discuss it to find out why. My feeling is that this is a quick and relatively easy procedure, so why draw it out? This will only add to your anxiety if it's done in the hospital setting. Obviously, though, there are certain circumstances that would dictate this as the preferred path.

Full Steam Ahead

So, your stitch is out, and you haven't dropped the little munchkin on the floor of the doctor's office. Now what? Go home and enjoy being a normal, pregnant woman. Really, by this stage in your pregnancy, you can enjoy being a normal, albeit extremely large and uncomfortable, possibly slightly crabby, pregnant lady. There's not much time, though, because baby will be here soon, so don't waste a single minute. Soak it all in.

At this point, most doctors feel that it's safe to have sex again, unless your water has broken. You may not be feeling too sexually energized, but unfortunately for us, our husbands have been deprived for several months, so you may have to "take one for the team."

In a study of women who'd had Shirodkar cerclages, the average time from removal to delivery was 9.4 days (± 8.8 days).[62] Based on this, you won't likely pop the baby out immediately, but there are the lucky—or maybe unlucky, depending on your point of view—few who do deliver immediately.

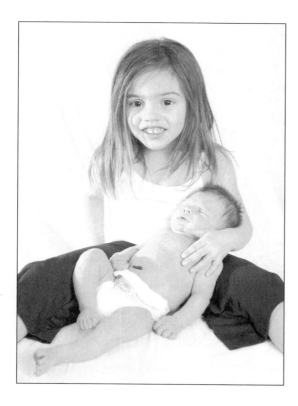

My two cerclage babies. (Madison at almost 4 years old, Drew at 5 days old.) *Photo by: Anthony Ziccardi Studios (www.aziccardi.com)*

References

1. Sinno A, Usta IM, Nassar AH. A short cervical length in pregnancy: management options. *Am J Perinatol* 2009;26(10):761–770.
2. Berghella, V, Seibel-Seamon J. Contemporary use of cervical cerclage. *Clin Obstet Gynecol* 2007;50(2):468–477.
3. Menacker F, Martin JA. Expanded health data from the new birth certificate, 2005. *Natl Vital Stat Rep* 2008;56(13):1–24.
4. Incompetent Cervix Support Forum, http://ic.hobh.org/forums/.
5. Fox NS, Chervenak FA. Cervical cerclage: a review of the evidence. *Obstet Gynecol Surv* 2007;63(1):58–65.
6. Shirodkar VN. A new method of operative treatment for habitual abortions in the second trimester of pregnancy. *Antiseptic* 1955;52:299–300.
7. McDonald IA. Suture of the cervix for inevitable miscarriage. *J Obstet Gynecol* 1957;64:346–350.
8. Romero R, Espinoza J, Erez O, Hassan S. The role of cervical cerclage in obstetric practice: can the patient who could benefit from this procedure be identified? *A J Obstet and Gynecol* 2006;194(1):1–9.
9. Pramod R, Okun N, McKay D, et al. Cerclage for the short cervix demonstrated by transvaginal ultrasound: current practice and opinion. *J Obstet Gynaecol Can* 2004;26(6):564–570.
10. Berghella V. *Preterm Birth: Prevention & Management*. West Sussex, UK. Wiley-Blackwell, 2010.

11. Odibo AO, Berghella V, To MS, et al. Shirodkar versus McDonald cerclage for the prevention of preterm birth in women with short cervical length. *Am J Perinatol* 2007;24(1):55–60.

12. Fox NS, Rebarber A, Bender S, Saltzman DH. Labor outcomes after Shirodkar cerclage. *J Reprod Med* 2009;54(6):361–365.

13. Hershkovitz R, Burstein E, Pinku A. Tightening McDonald cerclage suture under sonographic guidance. *Ultrasound Obstet Gynecol* 2008;31(2):194–197.

14. Althuisius S, Dekker G. Controversies regarding cervical incompetence, short cervix, and the need for cerclage. *Clin Perinatol* 2004;31(4):695–720.

15. Suhag A, Seligman NS, Bianchi I, Berghella V. What is the optimal gestational age for history-indicated cerclage placement? *Am J Perinatol* 2010;27(6):469–474.

16. Berghella V, Haas S, Chervoneva I, Hyslop T. Patients with prior second-trimester loss: prophylactic cerclage or serial transvaginal sonograms? *Am J Obstet Gynecol* 2002;187(3):747–751.

17. Makino Y, Makino I, Tsujioka H, Kawarabayashi T. Amnioreduction in patients with bulging prolapsed membranes out of the cervix and vaginal orifice in cervical cerclage. *J Perinat Med* 2004;32(2):140–148.

18. Locatelli A, Vergani P, Bellini P, et al. Amnioreduction in emergency cerclage with prolapsed membranes: comparison of two methods for reducing the membranes. *Am J Perinatol* 1999;16(2):73–77.

19. Airoldi J, Pereira L, Cotter A, et al. Amniocentesis prior to physical exam-indicated cerclage in women with midtrimester cervical dilation: results from the expectant management compared to physical exam-indicated cerclage international cohort study. *Am J Perinatol* 2009;26(1):63–68.

20. Gupta M, Emary K, Impey L. Emergency cervical cerclage: predictors of success. *J. Matern Neonatal Med* 2010;23(7):670–674.

21. Ventolini G, Genrich TJ, Roth J, Neiger R. Pregnancy outcome after placement of 'rescue' Shirodkar cerclage. *J Perinatol* 2009;29(4):276–279.

22. Debby A, Sadan O, Glezerman M, Golan A. Favorable outcome following emergency second trimester cerclage. *Int J Gynaecol Obstet* 2007;96(1):16–19.

23. Stupin JH, David M, Siedentopf JP, et al. Emergency cerclage versus bed rest for amniotic sac prolapse before 27 gestational weeks. A retrospective, comparative study of 161 women. *Eur J Obstet Gnecol Reprod Biol* 2008;139(1):32–37.

24. Olatunbosun OA, al-Nuaim L, Turnell RW. Emergency cerclage compared with bed rest for advanced cervical dilation in pregnancy. *Int Surg* 1995;80(2):170–174.

25. Pereira L, Cotter A, Gomez R, et al. Expectant management compared with physical examination-indicated cerclage (EM-PEC) in selected women with a dilated cervix at 14(0/7)–25(6/7) weeks: results from EM-PEC international cohort study. *Am J Obstet Gynecol.* 2007;197(5):483 e1–8.

26. Caliskan E, Cakiroglu Y, Dundar D, et al. Integrating cervical length measurement into routine antenatal screening and only emergency cerclage when indicated. *Clin Exp Obstet Gynecol* 2009;36(1):40–45.

27. Eskandar MA, Sobande AA, Damole IO, Bahar AM. Emergency cervical cerclage. Does the gestational age make a difference? *Saudi Med J* 2004;25(8):1028–1031.

28. Terkildsen MF, Parilla BV, Kumar P, Grobman WA. Factors associated with success of emergent second-trimester cerclage. *Obstet Gynecol* 2003;101(3):565–569.

29. Benifla JL, Goffinet F, Darai E, et al. Emergency cervical cerclage after 20 weeks' gestation: a retrospective study of 6 years' practice in 34 Cases. *Fetal Diagn Ther* 1997;12(5):274–278.

30. Lipitz S, Libshitz, Oelsner G, et al. Outcome of second-trimester, emergency cervical cerclage in patients with no history of cervical incompetence. *Am J Perinatol* 1996;13(7):419–422.
31. Eskandar M, Shafiq H, Almushait MA, et al. Cervical cerclage for prevention of preterm birth in women with twin pregnancy. *Int J Gynaecol Obstet* 2007;99(2):110–112.
32. Berghella V, Odibo AO, To MS, et al. Cerclage for short cervix on ultrasonography: meta-analysis of trials using individual patient-level data. *Obstet Gynecol* 2005;106(1):181–189.
33. Roman AS, Rebarber A, Pereira L, et al. The efficacy of sonographically indicated cerclage in multiple gestations. *J Ultrasound Med* 2005;24(6):763–768.
34. Parilla BV, Haney El, MacGregor SN. The prevalence and timing of cervical cerclage placement in multiple gestations. *Int J Gynaecol Obstet* 2003;80(2):123–127.
35. Nelson L, Dola T, Tran T, et al. Pregnancy outcomes following placement of elective, urgent and emergent cerclage. *J Matern Fetal Neonatal Med* 2009;22(3):269–273.
36. Kurup M, Goldkrand JW. Cervical incompetence: elective, emergent, or urgent cerclage. *Am J Obstet Gynecol* 1999;181(2):240–246.
37. National Guideline Clearinghouse, www.guideline.gov, American College of Obstetricians and Gynecologists (ACOG), Cervical Insufficiency, 2003 Nov 9 (ACOG practice bulletin; no 48) (reaffirmed 2008, updated Feb 9, 2010).
38. Parikh R, Brotzman S, Anasti JN. Cervical lacerations: some surprising facts. *Am J Obstet Gynecol* 2007;196(5): e17–18.
39. Baxter JK, Airoldi J, Berghella V. Short cervical length after history-indicated cerclage: is a reinforcing cerclage beneficial? *Am J Obstet Gynecol* 2005;193(3 pt 2):1204–1207.
40. Woensdregt K, Norwitz ER, Cackovic M, et al. Effect of 2 stitches vs 1 stitch on the prevention of preterm birth in women with singleton pregnancies who undergo cervical cerclage. *Am J Obstet Gynecol* 2008;198(4):396 e1–7.
41. Tsai YL, Lin YH, Chong KM, et al. Effectiveness of double cerclage in women with at least one previous pregnancy loss in the second trimester: a randomized controlled trial. *J Obstet Gynaecol* 2009;35(4):666–671.
42. Wikipedia, http://en.wikipedia.org/wiki/Spinal_anaesthesia.
43. Sheiner E, Bashiri A, Shoham-Vardi I, et al. Preterm deliveries among women with McDonald cerclage performed due to cervical incompetence. *Fetal Diagn Ther* 2004;19(4):361–365.
44. Berghella V, Pereira L, Gariepy A, et al. Prior cone biopsy: prediction of preterm birth by cervical ultrasound. *Am J Obstet Gynecol* 2004;191:1393–1397.
45. Owen J, Yost N, Berghella V, et al. Can shortened midtrimester cervical length predict very early spontaneous preterm birth? *Am J Obstet Gynecol* 2004;191:298–303.
46. Berghella V, Tolosa JE, Kuhlman K, et al. Cervical ultrasonography compared with manual examination as a predictor of preterm delivery. *Am J Obstet Gynecol* 1997;177:723–730.
47. Andrews WW, Copper R, Hauth JC, et al. Second-trimester cervical ultrasound: associations with increased risk for recurrent early spontaneous delivery. *Obstet Gynecol* 2000;95:222–226.
48. Guzman ER, Walters C, Ananth CV, et al. A comparison of sonographic cervical parameters in predicting spontaneous preterm birth in high-risk singleton gestations. *Ultrasound Obstet Gynecol* 2001;18:204–210.

49. Yang JH, Kuhlman K, Daly S, Berghella V. Prediction of preterm birth by second trimester cervical sonography in twin pregnancies. *Ultrasound Obstet Gynecol* 2000;15(4):288–291.

50. Guzman ER, Mellon C, Vintzileos AM, et al. Longitudinal assessment of endocervical canal length between 15 and 24 weeks' gestation in women at risk for pregnancy loss or preterm birth. *Obstet Gynecol* 1998;92:31–37.

51. Drakeley AJ, Roberts D, Alfirevic Z. Cervical stitch (cerclage) for preventing pregnancy loss in women. *Cochrane Database of Systematic Reviews* 2003, Issue 1. Art No: CD003253. (Last assessed as up-to-date Sept 7, 2002.)

52. Althuisius SM, Dekker GA, vanGeijn HP. Cervical incompetence: a reappraisal of an obstetric controversy. *Obstet Gynecol Surv* 2002;57(6):377–387.

53. Lazar P, Gueguen S, Dreyfus J, et al. Multicentred controlled trial of cervical cerclage in women at moderate risk of preterm delivery. *Nr J Obstet Gynecol* 1984;91:731–735.

54. Shamshad MY, Jehanzaib M. Evaluation of cervical cerclage for sonographically incompetent cervix in at high risk patients. *J Ayub Med Coll Abbottabad* 2008;20(2):31–34.

55. Althuisius SM, Dekker GA, Hummel P, et al. Final results of the cervical incompetence prevention randomized cerclage trial (CIPRACT): therapeutic cerclage with bed rest versus bed rest alone. *Am J Obstet Gynecol* 2001;185(5):1106–1112.

56. Higgins SP, Kornman LH, Bell RJ, Brennecke SP. Cervical surveillance as an alternative to elective cervical cerclage for pregnancy management of suspected cervical incompetence. *Aust N Z J Obstet Gynaecol* 2004;44(3):228–232.

57. Groom KM, Bennett PR, Golara M, et al. Elective cervical cerclage versus serial ultrasound surveillance of cervical length in a population at high risk for preterm delivery. *Eur J Obstet Gynecol Reprod Biol* 2004;112(2):158–161.

58. Simcox R, Speed PT, Bennett P, et al. A randomized controlled trial of cervical scanning vs history to determine cerclage in women at high risk of preterm birth (CIRCLE trail). *Am J Obstet Gynecol* 2009;200(6):623 e1–6.

59. Boggs W. Ultrasound Adds No Value to Cervical Cerclage Decision Making. Reuters Health (Imaging Economics), 6/30/2009.

60. Abdelhak YE, Aronov R, Roque H, Young BK. Management of cervical cerclage at term: remove the suture in labor? *J Perinat Med* 2000;28(6):453–457.

61. Bisulli M, Suhag A, Arvon R, et al. Interval to spontaneous delivery after elective removal of cerclage. *Am J Obstet Gynecol* 2009;201(2):163 e1–4.

62. Fox NS, Rebarber A, Bender S, Saltzman DH. Labor outcomes after Shirodkar cerclage. *J Reprod Med* 2009;54(6):361–365.

CHAPTER 8

Transvaginal Ultrasonography: The Only Allowable Penetration for the Lady on Pelvic Rest

dvances in ultrasound technology over the last decade have brought transvaginal ultrasonography (TVU) to the forefront of aiding the management and treatment of suspected IC pregnancies, and most importantly, for the prediction of preterm birth. This has become the major weapon in the medical world's arsenal for use in determining cervical length to assess the chances of your baby coming early. It is the most reliable and the best technique, far exceeding determinations made using fingers or external abdominal ultrasound.

TVU of the cervix allows our providers to more accurately identify those women who are considered more likely to deliver before term. Compared to vaginal examinations—you know, the old finger stuck inside to measure trick—this is much more consistent and reproducible, and also has less variability among the people whose job it is to determine cervical length/dilation.

It also allows for observation of the entire birth canal, not just what can be felt when you go in "blindly" using your fingers for measurements within the exterior vaginal portion only. The historically used manual examination looks at the position, thinning, softness, and of course dilation of the cervix. Each of these is dependent on the observer's interpretation.

A real benefit is the ability to watch the cervix in "real time." TVU allows for the observation of the progress of effacement (thinning) from the internal to the external opening. This effacement is able to be seen even when the cervix is closed (undilated), which can't be detected using the "finger" technique. I've heard that during ultrasounds, a technician/doctor has actually observed the cervix opening up on the inside (funneling) and seen the bulging of the amniotic sac into the cervical canal, sending up an early warning sign. This is a signal that, "Hey, something's up here."

Imagine if we didn't have transvaginal ultrasonography. This sort of thing wouldn't be detected as clearly or as early in the process. Maybe it wouldn't be caught until a much worse situation developed, like dilation or even complete prolapse—i.e., where the membranes have dropped into the vaginal canal.

The knowledge of funneling, dilation, and/or length changes with contractions is important in figuring out if we are really in preterm labor. It also helps our doctors to make decisions about how to proceed with care to help us carry our babies closer to term, even if some of our options are not 100% clear and supported by research. I'd rather them try to do something than nothing.

According to Dr. Ana Monteagudo, in an article titled *Worth a Thousand Words: The Ultrasound Advantage*, ultrasound is especially important, superior to finger examinations, because you are able to see the upper half of the cervix [i.e., the portion just above the internal OS (opening)].

Her belief is that this is an important region for detecting the initial or development of labor. As she states, "Effacement and shortening of the cervix start here but may go undetected by digital palpation regardless of the examiner's experience."[1]

I think it's important to note that transabdominal ultrasonography, the kind we normally think of, where the probe is rubbed across the stomach in order to obtain images, has been shown to result in the (false) appearance of a longer cervix.[2] Transabdominal ultrasound requires a full bladder in order to optimally and accurately visualize the cervix. An overfull bladder can incorrectly provide a longer cervical length measurement.[1]

Although the use of TVU in women with symptoms of preterm labor has been demonstrated in several studies, the exact clinical applications and limitations are not yet fully known. Particularly in question is the routine use in low-risk women.

This "tool" can become your best friend or your worst enemy. The numbers it spits out can be the source of either great happiness or intense dread and fear. The most important thing for you to remember is that it is ONLY another tool. The numbers—i.e., the length of your cervix—DO NOT dictate with exact precision how your pregnancy will turn out.

Case-in-point: during my second pregnancy, I was mid-second trimester when I underwent a transvaginal ultrasound. At this point it wasn't my first time at the rodeo, so I was familiar with watching the technician mark the ends of my cervix and then calculate the length of my cervix end to end. My measurement would then be projected on the screen.

A couple weeks before this visit, my cervix had been measured, and it was seen to be decreasing. (I believe the average was 2.5 cm at that time.) At this visit, I immediately saw the numbers 0.9 cm and 1.2 cm and freaked. I was hysterical and started crying, sure that within moments my baby would fall out.

The technician looked at me, put her hand on my shoulder, and said something like, "Honey these are only numbers, and they don't mean anything. You can still have a healthy, full-term baby. You need to stop looking at that screen." Boy, was she right. Her words to me at that moment meant more than she will ever know.

At that time, it didn't immediately cause me to relax or feel that everything was going to end well. Those almost weekly length checks, even after my cerclage, were extremely stressful and emotional for me. As soon as I walked into that room, I would begin to sweat, my heart rate would increase and I would fight back tears, for I was certain I was going to lose another baby. I just kept trying to remind myself of what that nurse had said to me. Oh, I made it to term, even though they didn't think my stitch would hold, or that I would make it to even 28 weeks. They don't know for sure, and so it *can* happen.

At a later visit, at around 23 weeks (after my stitch placement), when there was pretty much no measurement since my cervix was right up to my stitch, the nurse tried to joke when she looked at the screen, saying, "Wow, you could drive a bus through that funneling." I know from experience that we tend to live and die each visit based on our lengths. A good measurement means a happy day, while a short one or any changes is a bad one. Needless to say, I didn't think her joke was very funny, though she meant well.

This is the downside, from the woman's perspective. Always remember . . . just a TOOL. I cannot stress that enough. It is not our lifeline, even though we believe it is.

Who Should Get Cervical-Length Ultrasounds?

Although it is used extensively, there are no standards for treatments at various measurements, set techniques, or accepted intervals at which exams should be performed. In 2004, the American College of Radiology recommended that each obstetric ultrasound exam in the second trimester should include an assessment of the cervix and lower uterine segment to look for a short cervix (less than 30 mm) or funneling.[3]

On the other hand, the American College of Obstetricians and Gynecologists DOES NOT recommend the routine use of length measurements, due to the lack of proven treatments or intervention approaches. They do acknowledge that cervical-length information could help in predicting the risk of preterm delivery, especially the strong negative predictive value.[3] (This means that they are near certain that if your cervix is long, you WILL NOT deliver early; however, they're not confident that if you have a short cervix you will deliver early.)

There is little evidence to support routine screening of cervical lengths in low-risk women. (Many doctors are now pushing for a length check around 20 weeks in **all** women and treatment with progesterone if a short cervix is seen.) In high-risk women, those with a history of prior preterm birth or those who are carrying more than one baby, knowledge of cervical length can be useful for bringing peace of mind,[4] much like another tool that is covered later, fetal fibronectin testing. High-risk women should have serial cervical-length screenings between around 15/16 to 24 weeks. Serial checks, though expensive, are better than a one-time check of your length.

It has been shown that most women who deliver early tend to have a cervix of less than 2.5 cm at an average gestation of 19 weeks, typically between 16 and 24 weeks, and not at an earlier gestation. A length check earlier than 16 weeks is usually only done in women who have had a large proportion of their cervix removed. Early on, your cervix is usually a normal length, and a measurement before 14 weeks is not accurate at this lower gestation.[3]

Suggested TVU Screening Scenario[3]

+ One check at around 18–22 weeks in low-risk women, which is when most would get their typical growth scan anyway.

+ For high-risk women—e.g., those with a prior preterm birth— two checks, one at 14–18 weeks and another at 18–22 weeks.

+ For extremely high-risk women—i.e., those of you who've had a second-trimester loss or a very early spontaneous preterm birth—TVUs are recommended every two weeks from 14 weeks until 24 weeks.

Causes of an Early Short Cervix[3]

+ Weakness of your cervix, which can just happen for no apparent reason, or an incompetent cervix, which can be caused by any number of reasons, as discussed in the earlier chapter on IC.

+ Infection or inflammation: what is unknown and unclear is whether these actually cause your cervix to shorten or if they happen because of your cervix shortening; the old chicken-or-the-egg argument. Great, just what you need, right? (The shorter your length, the more chance you have of getting an infection. That risk is really quite low, at only 1–2% when your length is less than 2.5 cm in the second trimester. Since the risk is so low, an amnio to rule out infection prior to an ultrasound-indicated cerclage is not necessary.)

✦ The presence of contractions, silent or not. The chicken-and-egg argument applies here, too. Did having contractions shorten your cervix, or did your cervix shortening actually trigger your body to have contractions? (Many women with a short cervix are having contractions that they don't even feel.)

✦ A unicornuate uterus (a type of uterine malformation).

✦ Carrying multiple babies. Women carrying twins tend to have shorter cervices starting at 20 weeks. Making use of cervical length to predict a preterm baby is quite a challenge for those of you having more than one baby.

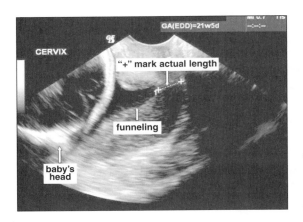

TVU 1: A short and funneling cervix at 21 weeks and 5 days. *Picture courtesy of Dr. Laughlin Dawes.*

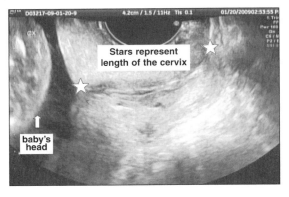

TVU 2: A nice, long, closed cervix at 17 weeks. *Picture courtesy of Dr. Vincenzo Berghella.*

I would like to throw in a word of caution here from the viewpoint of women who have dealt with this. I've heard from many women that their cervices had literally shrunk overnight, which put their pregnancies at great jeopardy. Because of this, they were unable to get cerclages, since they had no cervix left to stitch. They were susceptible to infections due to the loss of this barrier, and their risk of membrane rupture increased dramatically.

Please, please, talk with your doctors and discuss ALL the benefits and risks before making a decision in your particular case. If you choose to wait and watch for changes, don't wait until it's too late. Work with your doctors to optimize observation of shortening, even if this means more ultrasounds and measurements. In one of the stories submitted, a short cervix was noticed on a Friday, but the doctors wanted to wait until Monday, which was probably more convenient, to put in the mother's stitch. By that time, it was too late, and she was unable to get a cerclage. In the end, she lost her baby.

Don't be afraid to speak up—and even be a bitch if need be—if your doctor dismisses another length check after initial changes are observed. There's nothing wrong with demanding a TVU; I've done it several times myself. I could care less about being the office pain when my baby's life is at stake.

Short Cervix Equals a Preemie Baby—or Does It?

What is a short cervix? It's generally considered to be a cervix that measures less than 2.5 cm. Funneling can also be observed and can contribute to a short cervix. This is when there's ballooning of the membranes into the dilated internal portion of the cervix (called the "internal OS," or opening), but it has a closed outer portion (called the "external OS," or opening). Factors such as a short cervical length, uterine anomalies, previous cervical surgery, being pregnant with more than one baby, or positive fetal fibronectin results are all linked to an early delivery.[5]

The research is clear: the shorter your cervical length, the greater the chance of preterm labor.[6] A short cervical length of less than 2.5 cm at 16–18 weeks in high-risk women leads to preterm delivery in 75% of these women.[7] The shorter your length and the earlier it's seen, the higher the risk of your baby coming early.[3]

A study of 2,258 women looking at the ability of length measurements in those with a history of spontaneous preterm birth, uterine anomalies, or cervical surgical procedures who were asymptomatic to predict spontaneous preterm birth found that length does predict an early baby.[8] Again, the shorter your cervix, the higher the *chance* of a preterm birth. You need to understand, however, that they did not find, and are not saying, that if you have a short cervix, you WILL deliver early.

They also studied whether cervical length can predict early birth in women who'd had multiple previous induced abortions. (Multiple abortions are a risk factor for IC.) They found the overall occurrence of premature delivery to be 21.5%, about double the average, with a 47% incidence in those who also had a short cervix. They concluded that women with multiple previous abortions who have a cervix of less than 2.5 cm have a 3.3-fold greater chance of a spontaneous early baby.[9]

One trial, which looked at the progression of cervical shortening of over 1,000 women who had a previous early birth at between 17 and 34 weeks, found that women who had their baby at less than 24 weeks were more likely to have cervical shortening in subsequent pregnancies. They also tended to shorten more, and earlier, than women who'd had a later preterm delivery at 24–33 weeks.[10]

This is saying that if your loss occurred at 19 weeks, you're more likely to have shortening earlier in gestation than someone who had a preterm delivery at 28 weeks.

Even with tocolysis and bed rest, shortening to less than 2.5 cm before 31 weeks is a risk factor not only for preterm delivery, but also for preterm labor and sudden delivery.[11] Let me repeat this…you are not guaranteed a preemie, you are simply at a higher risk than someone who has a long cervix.

Early birth before 26 weeks is more likely than a later preterm birth (26–34 weeks) in women who have a cervix less than 2.9 cm. Thirty-seven percent of women whose cervix was less than 2.5 cm had their baby before 26 weeks, and 19% had a later preterm delivery. (Still, only a 56% risk of a preemie even with that short of a cervix.) For those women whose cervix was at 2.5–2.9cm, the figures fell to only 6% and 3%, respectively. Women with a cervical length of 3.0 cm or more had an early delivery rate of only 1% and a later preterm delivery rate of 9%.[3,12]

Another study determined that neither the timing of a prior preterm birth nor the number of prior preterm births was auseful factor in determining risk when cervical length was less than 2.5 cm in the current pregnancy.[13] However, the research is split here, so let's face it: they don't know for sure.

Could abnormal vaginal bacteria be linked to shorter cervical length and preterm birth? It seems to be a possibility. They found that the presence of aerobic vaginitis, or *Mycoplasma hominis*, is related to a shorter cervix.[14]

They also found that a really short length of less than 1.5 cm before 24 weeks carries a 50% chance of having your baby before 32 weeks. So, should you see a low number on that ultrasound machine, tell yourself, "I still have a 50% chance to carry my baby to a good or even great gestation."

All this information is worth keeping in the back of your mind. For me, I knew, based on my first pregnancy, that the shit hit the fan at around 21 weeks, when I was hospitalized. This was the point at which I tended to lose length, and it was also the case in my second pregnancy. During that pregnancy, before I even got a cerclage, we kept this in mind, and I was even more careful at this point not to do too much.

The research isn't clear on what exactly comes into play with this observation, or phenomenon. Is it contractions, is it infection, or is it a weak cervix? Many women with a cervix of 2 or 1 cm or even less, myself included, have gone on to have healthy full-term babies. (I had a whopping 8 lb 14 oz one at that.) Was carrying my baby to term easy or fun. Absolutely, positively...NO! It was hell, but it was well worth it. True, this is not always the case, and sometimes we suffer terrible losses.

The Benefits and Disadvantages of TVU

In the past, practices used, and some still use, manual examination techniques only. This technique has a high degree of variability, being solely reliant on the individual performing the exam. Yes, it's fine for determining a rough length or for dilation at term for labor and delivery reasons, but it should not be used routinely for cervical-length assessment in mid-pregnancy, because if they see something, it's too late. The cervix actually starts to shrink and dilate from the inside out.[2] If your doctor can feel changes by doing a manual examination, then ripening, softening, and dilation have already progressed quite a long way.

Many doctors say that 14 weeks is the point of differentiation, where you can actually visualize the start and endpoint of the cervix clearly, but there doesn't appear to be a consensus. Any earlier than this and your cervix isn't well defined, and an accurate measurement isn't really possible. If you're in the "wait and see" scenario, when a prior loss wasn't clearly IC related and was possibly caused by another problem, such as premature labor or infection, this 14- to 16-week check serves as a baseline measurement.

The average mid-pregnancy cervical length is around 3.6 to 4 cm. This is not to say that if your cervix is 3.2 cm, you have a problem. Research has found that a cervical length of 2.5 cm is in the 10th percentile for risk of preterm delivery.[6,15] Many ladies who do deliver early have a length of less than 2.5 cm between 16 and 22 weeks.[16]

An issue with TVU is taking the actual measurement, because there's a lot of variability among technicians. On the same day, on the same machine, I've experienced a range of different measurements from two technicians. Like much in the health field, this is far from an exact science.

Unless you are at a high-risk practice or a practice associated with a bigger hospital, chances are the technician may have never performed a TVU or has only done a handful of them. Length measurements are not all that common, so I recommend finding a center that is experienced in performing pregnancy ultrasounds outside the normal 18- to 20- week growth checks. At the very least, go there until you are in the safe zone.

According to Dr. Vincenzo Berghella, a man who has dedicated his life to researching and helping families dealing with preterm birth, this technique for measurement of the cervix "is an effective screening test for the prevention of preterm birth (PTB)…it is safe for and acceptable by >99% of women; it recognizes an early asymptomatic phase that precedes PTB by many weeks…is predictive of PTB in all populations studied so far; and, perhaps more importantly, it has been shown that 'early' treatment is effective in prevention." He goes on to say that the known preventions for high-risk gals are ultrasound-indicated cerclages and vaginal progesterone.[17]

The phenomenon that he discusses—whereby the symptoms of preterm birth, namely shortening of the cervix, even if it is "silent," precede the actual birth by weeks—is key to current understanding and treatments to prevent early birth.

In one study, the ethics of which made me queasy, they found that knowledge of cervical length and fetal fibronectin results were tied to a shorter evaluation time in triage, and with less early babies (13% vs. 36%) in women who had preterm labor.[18] Basically, in this study they randomized women into two groups: 1) where their length and FFN results were determined and shared, and 2) where they were unknown. Researchers found that it took longer for the women in the unknown group to get care, and they had their babies earlier and more often. The takeaway: cervical length check and FFN results...good. Post them on your forehead...just kidding. If your docs and nurses know your cervix is on the short side and you have a positive FFN, you should get seen, stat. You need to keep in mind that within any healthcare system, it helps to be knowledgeable and proactive.

Sometimes we aren't so lucky. We don't always get a two-week heads-up. The cervix is dynamic and, therefore, is always changing. For some women, their cervix had literally shrunk over a day or two, so keep this in mind when discussing options with your doctor.

The first time you looked on as they measured your cervix, you were probably like, "Huh, what the hell are they even looking at?" They basically look for two somewhat darker lines, more like smudges, in a mass of gray haze and connect the two points to get the measurement. [They're actually measuring from the internal to the external cervical openings (OS).] This is no easy task if you've never done it before. It takes a trained eye to lock into the true points in order to get an accurate measurement. Another possible downside is if you have a tough cervix to measure. So, though it is just another tool, it's potentially a very good one.

There is also the issue of differences in opinion regarding the best procedure. Does the bladder have to be full? Or freshly emptied? (Luckily, I never had to have a full bladder at any of the three practices I went to, as I would've peed on the table.) Do you apply fundal pressure (the fundus is the top of the uterus) to mimic contractions to induce shortening? If so, how much pressure? How do we know that all technicians and doctors are applying the same amount of pressure? Do they take 1 measurement, or an average of 3, or maybe even 10 measurements? How long should the cervix be observed for changes? Here again is where the research and common practice varies greatly.

One study suggested the optimum timeframe for observing the cervix in order to best detect changes is 10 minutes.[19] The basis of this belief is that if changes are detected during that period, they are better able to predict the risk of early delivery based on the shortest observed length. Now really, how many technicians/doctors will take that extra time to sit and watch just to make sure? Unfortunately, with the basic premise of healthcare being that time is money, I suspect not too many. If they get one, or even three, measurements right away, I don't think many feel it's necessary to take those extra minutes just to wait and see.

Common practice is to take at least three measurements and use the shortest—i.e., worst-case-scenario—measurement. One trial found that when an established set of guidelines was followed, the average difference in length was only 1.24 mm, or 0.124 cm.[20] Unfortunately, a large portion of practices performing ultrasounds are not trained in these "standards," and the extent of actual standards being used is questionable. So, if you have a problematic history of any sort, research your options, including doctors AND ultrasound facilities.

The greatest benefit of TVUs is that the doctor can use this information to detect cervical changes and to determine a course of action if changes are seen (e.g., place a stitch, prescribe P17, or even recommend bed rest, even though this is not supported by the research). The bad thing is that your cervix is dynamic and constantly changing, so your doc can't foresee if changes will occur. It can be at 2.5 cm one day and 3 cm the next. Did it grow or stretch? Maybe, or is the difference due to any one of the many factors I mentioned previously. Alternatively, one day your cervix can be long and closed, and then the next day short and open. This is why it is important to have a full plan with your doctor for checks, and not just rely on one random cervical check.

In a well-respected review of the data on this topic titled "Cervical Assessment by Ultrasound and Prevention of Preterm Delivery" (a Cochrane Review), they sought to determine whether TVU was effective in preventing preterm births based solely on knowing cervical length. They identified a total of five studies that fit their criteria, which included 507 women.

Their goal was to determine whether knowing a woman had a short cervix led to better "antenatal management" or, simply, better care during her pregnancy. They only looked at randomized controlled trials, which, as you'll recall, are the gold standard in research.

They found that knowing the cervical length did not provide a *substantial* reduction in preterm birth at less than 37 weeks (22.3% versus 34.7%, which was termed a "non-significant decrease"). They did, however, find that delivery generally occurred at a later gestational age when the length was known compared to when it was unknown. Interestingly, they found that in women with preterm premature rupture of membranes (PPROM), there was no difference in infection rates between women who had length checks and those who didn't.

The overall conclusion was that there was currently not enough evidence to support routine screening of cervical length in both asymptomatic and symptomatic pregnant women, since there was no link to reducing preterm birth. In conclusion, they stated the need for further research and also stressed the importance of determining a protocol on how to treat women based on cervical-length results.[21]

I guess I would rather know, although for the woman who knows, it's a double-edged sword. If you know your cervix is short, it adds an enormous amount of anxiety and means taking more caution as the "baby carrier." "No, I will not lift that basket," or, "I think I'll relax with my feet up for the rest of the day," and maybe, "Honey, I think you're going to have to be in charge of dinner, laundry, garbage, cleaning...sorry, I have a short cervix." (Hey, really, at what other times in our lives do we have the chance to let go of our "womanly duties?")

The Dreaded Funneling

Funneling is something else we live in fear of and fixate on—maybe even unnecessarily so, as the use of funneling to predict early delivery is not recommended. The good news is its presence has been shown to add no extra risk of an early birth in most women.[22,3] The most impor-

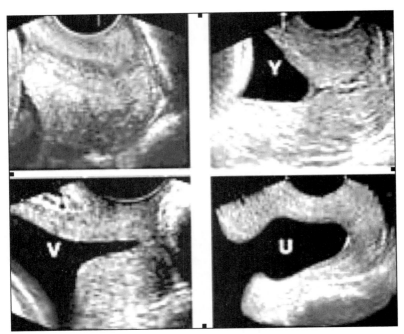

TVU 3: Examples of cervical funneling. *Picture reference: Imaging Consult (a website of Elsevier Health).*

tant factor in determining your risk is your actual cervical length, not the presence or absence of a funnel. (If there is a funnel, though, most likely your cervix is on the shorter side.) Between 25 and 33% of high-risk women and 10% of low-risk women funnel.[3]

Most of the time, funneling does not extend the entire length of the cervix to the exterior portion. Also, there are different types of funneling, from the less severe T-shaped funnel, to a not-so-good Y-shaped opening, worsening to a V-shaped funnel, and finally the serious scenario of a U-shaped funnel.

Now for the bad news. Some researchers have suggested that the very presence of funneling is a significant risk factor for preterm labor. One study found that the women in the non-funneling group carried longer than the women in the funneling group, 36.2 ± 4.6 weeks versus 33.8 ± 5.4 weeks.[23]

Again, the conflicting findings. Unfortunately, that wasn't the only study that found funneling to be a risk factor. Another study found that funneling was linked to early birth before 35 weeks,[24] so the extent of risk presented by a funnel is still under debate.

In a study that looked at the progression of funneling in the second trimester in high-risk women to determine whether it increased the probability of an early birth, they found that of the 183 women in the study, 33% had funneling in at least one of the scans. These women tended to deliver earlier than those without funneling (31.7 ± 7.9 weeks vs. 36.9 ± 4.4 weeks). They also noted that in the women with funneling, those women who went from a "T"-(no funneling) to a "V"- to a "U"-shaped funnel were linked to an earlier delivery than those who had "V"-shaped funneling, which was linked to delivery at term. But—yes, I said "but"—they found that in women with less than 2.5 cm of cervix, both those who had funneling and those who didn't had similar gestational ages at birth.

Overall, they concluded that there is much variability with funneling and a substantial association with earlier delivery. On the other hand, if you already have a shortened cervix, funneling does not really increase your risk.[25]

In yet another study of women who had cervices of 2.5 cm or less, the no-funnel group had considerably fewer readmissions for preterm labor (43.2% vs. 67.1%), chorioamnionitis (2.4% vs. 23.2%), abruption (1.2% vs. 13.4%), premature rupture of membranes (6.1% vs. 23.4%), and cerclage placement (23.2% vs. 43%). The no-funnel group delivered later, so they had healthier babies. They found no link to the baby's outcome based on how big or wide the funnel was. Therefore, they concluded that funneling is best measured by presence or absence only.[26]

In women with funneling observed at an average of 21.4 weeks, preterm delivery occurred in 42% of those women. They found that funneling greater than or equal to 40% and a short cervix was linked to early delivery. The preterm delivery rates were 17% for funneling of less than 25%, 29% for funneling at 25–50%, and 79% for those who had more than 50% funneling.[27]

I suspect your eyes went straight to that 79%, and you said, "Oh shit!" Now, let's examine the reality of that number. That 79% includes not only women who delivered at 25 weeks but also those who delivered at 28 weeks, 30 weeks, and 32 weeks. You get the picture. Of course, none of us wants to deliver even a week before term, but the reality is, if you deliver a baby at 28 weeks or beyond, you can rest assured, provided you have the right care, that your baby's chances of being healthy are really good.

Many women who had funneling went on to have healthy full-term babies. Girls (and everyone in their families who may read this), STAY POSITIVE AND HOPEFUL. Even if you have funneling and a short cervix. Many have sat in the same seat you're in and made it.

What's It Really Like?

I'm not going to lie and say that it's just a step below the pleasure of your vibrator. After all, you're there at a stressful time, in a foreign and cold environment, naked from the waist down in front of strangers. The good news is, it's not *that* bad. The diameter is only about an inch or so, and we know you're not a virgin, or you wouldn't be in this position, so the insertion part doesn't hurt.

Look, sorry to those of you whom I might have offended, but I had to use some humor here. I vividly remember each and every one of these visits during the pregnancy following my loss as being an emotional marathon. With each visit, there was the bad news about my loss of length and comments like, "We're just going to aim to get you to 28 weeks at this point," which left me devastated.

Try not to get completely overwhelmed and discouraged. I dreaded going to each appointment, for fear of bad news, but it doesn't have to be that way. If I knew then what I know now and what I'm setting out for you, it wouldn't have been as bad.

I prefer to put the probe in myself. This tends to be less awkward for all of us and feels less violating to me. Believe it or not, the technician or doctor really doesn't want to violate you either (and they're generally nice enough to lube it up for you for easy maneuvering).

It really doesn't have to go in too far, just a couple inches. When the technician or doctor takes over is when it can cause anywhere from no pain, to slight discomfort, to all-out "Holy shit, stop that!" pain (although the latter only happened to me once or twice). The "touch" of the person performing the ultrasound and the location of your uterus/cervix determines how easy it will be for you. For me, it was often quick and painless, while at other times, when it was difficult to see my cervix and the probe had to be twisted to the side, it really hurt.

Often, if you have a tilted cervix, it can make for more difficult measurements. My advice is that if it gets to be too much, and long, deep breaths aren't getting you through it, simply ask them to give you a break. Sometimes this break is just enough for you to recover your bearings and get yourself together.

TVU in a Nutshell

+ Go pee to empty your bladder.

+ They'll put a condom on the probe.

+ The probe will be inserted, either by you or by the tech. Tell them if you would rather do it yourself. It doesn't have to go in too far.

+ The tech/doc will move the probe around until a clear image is obtained, avoiding extra pressure, as this can make the cervix appear falsely longer.

+ The length should be measured at least three times over at least three minutes, to allow time for observing a funnel if one is present, measuring from the external to the internal OS (openings). (Length is defined as the closed portion of your endocervical canal.) The shortest measurement will be considered the appropriate one to use. A normal/good length is 2.5 cm or more.

+ Fundal pressure, or pressure on the top of the uterus, may be applied to see if any changes occur, such as funneling or shortening of your cervix.

The Typical Cervical Length[28]

One study looked at 1,061 "normal" women with "normal" pregnancies from 20 to 34 weeks and found that cervical length normally shortens throughout pregnancy. (In this study the percentage of preterm births before 37 weeks within this low-risk population was 11%, consistent with the overall rate.)

They found the following for cervical lengths:

Percentile	23 Weeks Gestation	28 Weeks Gestation	34 Weeks Gestation
5% i.e. the low-end length, a minority	2.0 cm	1.7 cm	1.0 cm
50% i.e. the average length, the majority	3.6 cm	3.3 cm	2.9 cm
95% i.e. the high-end length, a minority	4.7 cm	4.3 cm	4.3 cm

So, what does this mean? The majority of women (remember, these were low-risk women) will have a cervical length of around 3.5 cm between 23 and 28 weeks. (Most of us with IC or preterm labor can only dream of seeing those numbers on the screen.) They found that during this period, very few women will have lengths in the mid-4 cm range, i.e., the high end, and very few will measure around 2 cm—i.e., the low end. Note that after 30 weeks, shortening of the cervix is common in many women, even those who go on to carry to full term.[3]

In another study that looked at cervical lengths in the South African population, the average length at 23 weeks was 3.37 cm, and they only found a length of 1.5 cm or less in 3.3% of the ladies. The women who had shorter lengths tended to have a history of miscarriage or of preterm delivery, to be under 20 years old, or to have an abnormal BMI (body mass index). They found no significant differences in cervical lengths between black women and white or colored women.[29]

More good news, though: in low-risk women, most of those who have a cervix shorter than 2.5 cm at 24 weeks go on to have their babies after 35 weeks. In high-risk women with a prior preterm birth or second-trimester loss, a short length is a good predictor of an early birth.[3]

Not only is your length important in attempting to predict your risk of an early delivery, but so are several other factors, such as how far along you are when the measurement is taken, whether you are high or low risk, how many babies you're carrying, FFN results, whether or not you're having contractions, and whether or not you have an infection.[3]

Is There a Need for Measurements After a Cerclage?

Many doctors will dispute the value of routine TVU measurements after a cerclage, including my doctor in my third pregnancy, when I got a preventative cerclage after the first trimester. His point was that we would expect to see my cervix shrink—after all, I had IC—and that the stitch was there to do its job. I was to pay attention to any changes that would suggest issues, such as spotting, changes in discharge, and cramping/contractions. This was reassuring, I guess, so I thought I was OK with that, until I panicked at around 16/17 weeks and asked for a measurement.

As a woman who has lost a baby, I can easily say that yes, I needed measurements, even after my cerclage. There was probably no medical necessity for them, but mentally, they made a world of difference to me. Without them, my anxiety level would've risen a hundredfold, and I would have had many more sleepless nights.

At that 16/17-week visit, to see for myself that my cervix was long and closed, and the stitch was in there nice and tight, was an awesomely reassuring feeling. (I also pushed for—more like demanded—another measurement late in my second trimester to ease my mind.)

Cervical length typically increases after a cerclage. This was true for me after I had an early preventative cerclage placed, and my cervix measured in at around 3 cm. This was by far the longest length I'd ever seen.

One study looked at ultrasound-indicated cerclages and cervical lengths. They found that length had drastically decreased, from an average of 4.2 cm to 2.1 cm, when the cerclages were placed. After the cerclages, the average length increased to 3.4 cm at 22 weeks.[30]

They also studied the frequency of preemie babies in women who got cerclages after the observation of shortening. These women were grouped based on the length of cervix below their cerclage. Women who had lengths of 1.8 cm or more tended to have fewer preterm deliveries at less than 35 weeks (4%) than those with shorter lengths

(33%).[31] Note: only 33% of the women with cerclages and short lengths actually had their babies early.

Other researchers found that the length of cervix below the cerclage in women who received one after experiencing cervical shortening to less than 2.5 cm or funneling was not connected to how long they carried their baby. They analyzed the ratio of length to cerclage versus total cervical length and the gestational age of the baby when born and found no differences. This is good news, but the research is split here, too. The average cervical length below the cerclage was 1.8 ± 0.6 cm, while the total length after cerclage placement rose to 3.6 ± 0.9 cm after.[32]

Another study looked at the value of cervical-length measurements after a cerclage in predicting preterm delivery. In comparing the lengths before cerclage placement, two weeks after placement, and before delivery in women who delivered before term and those who went to term, they found NO DIFFERENCE between the women who went to term and those who delivered early at any of these time points.

Fifty-six percent of these women had no cervical length at 26.7 ± 4.4 weeks, and of these, 50% delivered early due to preterm premature rupture of membranes (PPROM) and infection (chorioamnionitis). They concluded that lack of cervical length is associated with preterm delivery, infection, and PPROM.[33] It has been shown that the body prepares for delivery by shortening the cervix after 30 weeks.[34]

Conclusion: it isn't recommended that you undergo routine length measurements after a cerclage, because your length generally increases after a cerclage. If they do find that your length has decreased, there are no further treatments they can provide (other than to prepare for an early baby by giving steroids to speed up lung development). As I mentioned previously, a reinforcing cerclage has not been shown to help and can actually do more harm.[3]

If, on the other hand, you're freaking out and need a bit of reassurance to get by, by all means go ahead and push for one. I did…several times (and I did sleep better at night because of them). Oh, and for the record, when I had my cerclage, my doc told me not to worry if I was down to the stitch. I was funneled to my stitch for many, many weeks with my daughter, and she ended up being induced at 38 weeks after my water broke.

Table 2. Predicted Probability of Preterm Delivery Before Week 35, by Cervical Length (mm) and Time of Measurement (Week of Pregnancy)

Cervical Length (mm)	Week of Pregnancy													
	15	16	17	18	19	20	21	22	23	24	25	26	27	28
0	69.8	68.7	67.5	66.3	65.2	64.0	62.7	61.5	60.2	59.0	57.7	56.4	55.1	53.8
5	62.5	61.3	60.0	58.7	57.5	56.2	54.9	53.6	52.2	50.9	49.6	48.3	47.0	45.7
10	54.6	53.3	52.0	50.7	49.4	48.1	46.7	45.4	44.1	42.8	41.6	40.3	39.0	37.8
15	46.5	45.2	43.9	42.6	41.3	40.1	38.8	37.6	36.3	35.1	33.9	32.8	31.6	30.5
20	38.6	37.3	36.1	34.9	33.7	32.5	31.4	30.3	29.2	28.1	27.0	26.0	25.0	24.0
25	31.2	30.1	29.0	27.9	26.9	25.8	24.8	23.9	22.9	22.0	21.1	20.3	19.4	18.6
30	24.7	23.7	22.8	21.8	21.0	20.1	19.3	18.5	17.7	16.9	16.2	15.5	14.8	14.2
35	19.1	18.3	17.5	16.8	16.1	15.4	14.7	14.1	13.4	12.8	12.2	11.7	11.2	10.6
40	14.6	13.9	13.3	12.7	12.1	11.6	11.1	10.6	10.1	9.6	9.2	8.7	8.3	7.9
45	11.0	10.5	10.0	9.6	9.1	8.7	8.3	7.9	7.5	7.2	6.8	6.5	6.2	5.9
50	8.2	7.8	7.4	7.1	6.7	6.4	6.1	5.8	5.5	5.2	5.0	4.7	4.5	4.3
55	6.0	5.7	5.5	5.2	4.9	4.7	4.5	4.3	4.0	3.8	3.7	3.5	3.3	3.1
60	4.4	4.2	4.0	3.8	3.6	3.4	3.3	3.1	3.0	2.8	2.7	2.5	2.4	2.3

Figure 8-1. *Chart reproduced with permission[35]*

Even with no cervix at 15 weeks, you still have a 30% chance of your baby being born after 35 weeks.

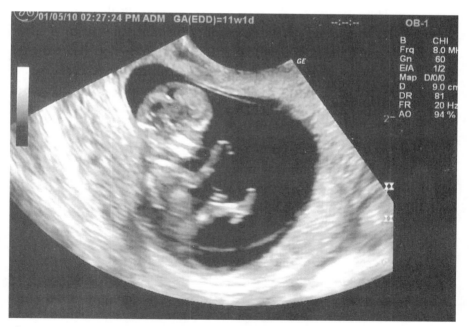

Figure 8-2. This is a 'typical' ultrasound, the type we're used to, much nicer than a boring length check. (This is actually my nephew. Isn't he cute?)

Key Takeaways[3]

+ Serial transvaginal ultrasonography cervical-length checks for all women with a prior spontaneous preterm birth are suggested. (More than 60% of these pregnancies will be normal and will require NO intervention to deliver full term.)

+ Short cervix ≠ preemie baby. Even with a short cervix, you can still make it to term and have a healthy baby.

+ A length of less than 2.5 cm is best for predicting an early birth. The earlier a short length is seen, the higher the risk of having your baby early.

+ A cervix shorter than 2.5 cm (high-risk gals) upon vaginal ultrasound = get a cerclage. (Unless you have symptoms that exclude you from being a candidate, including known infection, preterm premature rupture of membranes, or active preterm labor.) The reduction in preterm birth following a cerclage is almost 30%.

+ Carrying multiples ≠ cerclage. In fact, cerclages have been shown to do harm in women carrying multiples. However, if you have a history of IC and happen to be carrying more than one baby, that's a different scenario, and you should discuss this option with your doc.

+ Cervical length of greater than 3.0 cm at 24 weeks = low risk of an early delivery, despite your previous history. (There's only a 1% chance of delivery at less than 26 weeks and a 9% chance of having your baby before 35 weeks.)

+ Normal cervical length (2.5 cm or more) + funneling ≠ a higher chance of a preemie.

+ Low-risk women (no history of an early birth or loss) + short cervix between 16 and 24 weeks ≠ a benefit from an ultrasound-indicated cerclage. A benefit has not been shown in the research. Note: this doesn't mean for sure that a cerclage in this instance won't work, just that it hasn't been proven in research trials. You may be one of those women whose problem was caught the first time a round. Good for you.

References

1. Monteagudo A. Worth a thousand words: the ultrasound advantage www.obgyn.net/us/cotm/0002/Monteagudo.htm. 1998.
2. Hill LM. Cervical length in preterm labor prediction. Institute for Advanced Medical Education Reviewed 6/6/09. https://iame.com/online/cervlength/cervlength.html.
3. Berghella V. *Preterm Birth: Prevention & Management.* West Sussex, UK. Wiley-Blackwell, 2010.
4. Doyle NM, Monga M. Role of ultrasound in screening patients at risk for preterm delivery. *Obstet Gynecol Clin North Am* 2004;31(1):125–139.
5. Chao AS, Chao A, Hsieh PC. Ultrasound assessment of cervical length in pregnancy. *Taiwan J Obstet Gynecol* 2008;47(3):291–295.
6. Iams JD, Goldenberg RL, Meis PJ, et al. The length of the cervix and the risk of spontaneous premature delivery. *N Engl J Med* 1996;334:567–572.
7. Owen J, Yost N, Berghella V, et al. Mid-trimester endovaginal sonography in women at high risk for spontaneous preterm birth. *JAMA* 2001;286:1340–1348.
8. Crane JM, Hutchens D. Transvaginal sonographic measurement of cervical length to predict preterm birth in asymptomatic women at increased risk: a systematic review. *Ultrasound Obstet Gynecol* 2008;31(5):579–587.
9. Visintine J, Berghella V, Henning D, Baxter J. Cervical length for prediction of preterm birth in women with multiple prior induced abortions. *Ultrasound Obstet Gynecol* 2008;31(2):198–200.
10. Szychowsi JM, Owen J, Hankins G, et al. Timing of mid-trimester cervical length shortening in high-risk women. *Ultrasound Obstet Gynecol* 2009;33(1):70–75.
11. Yoshizato T, Obama H, Nojiri T, et al. Clinical significance of cervical length shortening before 31 weeks' gestation assessed by longitudinal observation using transvaginal ultrasonography. *J Obstet Gynaecol Res* 2008;34(5):805–811.
12. Owen J, Yost N, Berghella V, et al. Can shortened midtrimester cervical length predict very early spontaneous preterm birth? *Am J Obstet Gynecol* 2004;191(1):298–303.
13. Yost NP, Owen J, Berghella V, et al. Number and gestational age of prior preterm births does not modify the predictive value of a short cervix. *Am J Obstet Gynecol* 2004;191(1):241–246.
14. Donders GG, Van Calsteren C, Bellen G, et al. Association between abnormal vaginal flora and cervical length as risk factors for preterm birth. *Ultrasound Obstet Gynecol* 2010, Jan 26 (Epub ahead of print).
15. Anderson HF, Nugent CE, Wanty SO, et al. Prediction of risk for preterm delivery by ultrasonographic measurement of cervical length. *Am J Obstet Gynecol* 1990;163:859–867.
16. Berghella V, Tallucci M, Desai A. Does transvaginal sonographic measurement of cervical length before 14 weeks predict preterm delivery in high-risk pregnancies? *Ultrasound Obstet Gynecol* 2003;21:140–144.
17. Berghella V. Novel developments on cervical length screening and progesterone for preventing preterm birth. *BJOG* 2009;116(2):182–187.
18. Ness A, Visintine J, Ricci E, Berghella V. Does knowledge of cervical length and fetal fibronectin affect management of women with threatened preterm labor? A randomized trail. *Am J Obstet Gynecol* 2007;197(4):426 e1–7.

19. Kurtzman JT, Jenkins SM, Brewster WR. Dynamic cervical changes during real-time ultrasound: prospective characterization and comparison in patients with and without symptoms of preterm labor. *Ultrasound Obstet Gynecol* 2004;23:574–578.
20. Burger M, Weber-Rossler TW, Willmann M. Measurement of the pregnant cervix by transvaginal sonography: an interobserver study and new standards to improve the interobserver variability. *Ultrasound Obstet Gynecol* 1997;9(3):188–193.
21. Berghella V, Baxter JK, Hendrix NW. Cervical assessment by ultrasound for preventing preterm delivery. *Cochrane Database Systematic Reviews* 2009, Issue 3. Art. No.: CD007235. (Last assessed as up-to-date: February 21, 2009.)
22. Owen J, Yost N, Berghella V, et al. Can shortened mid-trimester cervical length predict very early spontaneous preterm birth? *Am J Obstet Gynecol* 2004;191:298–303.
23. Rust OA, Atlas RO, Kimmel S, et al. Does the presence of a funnel increase the risk of adverse perinatal outcome in a patient with a short cervix? *Am J Obstet Gynecol* 2005;192:1060–1066.
24. Berghella V, Pereira L, Gariepy A, et al. Prior cone biopsy: prediction of preterm birth by cervical ultrasound. *Am J Obstet Gynecol* 2004;191:1393–1397.
25. Berghella V, Owen J, MacPherson C, et al. Natural history of cervical funneling in women at high risk for spontaneous preterm birth. *Obstet Gynecol* 2007;109(4):863–869.
26. Rust OA, Atlas RO, Kimmel S, et al. Does the presence of a funnel increase the risk of adverse perinatal outcome in a patient with a short cervix? *Am J Obstet Gynecol* 2005;192(4):1060–1066.
27. Berghella V, Kuhlman K, Weiner S, et al. Cervical funneling: sonographic criteria predictive of preterm delivery. *Ultrasound Obstet Gynecol* 1997;10(3):161–166.
28. Silva SV, Damiao R, Fonseca EB, et al. Reference ranges for cervical length by transvaginal scan in singleton pregnancies. *J Matern Fetal Neonatal Med* 2010;23(5):379–382.
29. Erasmus I, Nicolaou E, Van Gelderen CJ, Nicolaides KH. Cervical length at 23 weeks' gestation—relation to demographic characteristics and previous obstetric history in South African women. *S Afr Med J* 2005;95(9):691–695.
30. Althuisius SM, Dekker GA, Van Geijn HP, Hummel P. The effect of therapeutic McDonald cerclage on cervical length as assessed by transvaginal ultrasonography. *Am J Obstet Gynecol* 1999;180(2 pt 1):366–369.
31. Scheib S, Visintine JF, Miroshnichenko G, et al. Is cerclage height associated with the incidence of preterm birth in women with an ultrasound-indicated cerclage? *Am J Obstet Gynecol* 2009;200(5): e12–15.
32. Rust OA, Atlas RO, Meyn J, et al. Does cerclage location influence perinatal outcome? *Am J Obstet Gynecol* 2003;189(6):1688–1691.
33. Hedriana HL, Lanouette JM, Haesslein HC, McLean LK. Is there value for serial ultrasonographic assessment of cervical length after a cerclage? *Am J Obstet Gynecol* 2008;198(6):705 e1–6.
34. Heath VCF, Southall TR, Souka AP, et al. Cervical length at 23 weeks of gestation: prediction of spontaneous preterm delivery. *Ultrasound Obstet Gynecol* 1998;12:312–317.
35. Berghella V, Roman A, Daskalakis C et al. Gestational age at cervical length measurement and incidence of preterm birth. *Obstet Gynecol* 2007;110(2 pt 1):311–317.

CHAPTER 9

When Transvaginal Cerclages Fail, There's Still Hope of Beating IC: The Transabdominal Cerclage

"**M**y TVC failed. I did everything I was supposed to do, and it still didn't work. The TVC works for some women. It may help and buy you some time, but you must have a very diligent MD and lots of luck on your side. I think women are fooled into thinking this procedure has such a high success rate—at least I was. I am scheduled for a TAC next week. Yay! I fully trust this doctor and am excited to have a normal pregnancy." ~ Melissa, Louisiana

A transabdominal cerclage (TAC) is another type of cerclage used to strengthen the cervix to help a woman with IC carry her pregnancy to term. It's different from a tranvaginal cerclage in that it is often placed by going in through the stomach. Typically, these cerclages are placed either before pregnancy, ideally, or early on. This procedure is performed much less often than a transvaginal cerclage and is more invasive/complex, so fewer doctors are trained in doing these. So don't give up; you just may have to do a bit of research and traveling to find a qualified doc.

Candidates for a TAC[1]

1. Those who've had a failed history-indicated cerclage and/or very early premature birth (less than 33 weeks), even with a cerclage.

2. Those who are lacking enough cervical tissue to place a history-indicated cerclage (this could be due to LEEP, cone biopsy, or other cervical surgeries).

It's important to note that a history-indicated cerclage failure is specified in order to receive a transabdominal cerclage. This means that if you had an emergency cerclage placed when you were dilated 3 cm and it failed, you wouldn't necessarily need a TAC the next time you were pregnant. You would most likely get a cerclage early—i.e., between 12 and 14 weeks—the next time around, so a history-indicated cerclage, when your cervix is still long and closed, or be followed using the "wait and see" approach and have an ultrasound-indicated cerclage should your cervix start to misbehave. Technically you would not become a candidate for a TAC unless this cerclage failed as well. Most doctors aren't trained on this procedure, so do your research. Don't give up! (Hint: Ask around on the boards for recommendations.)

How Well Do They Work?

Forty-five women with one or more previous second-trimester deliveries who had a pre-pregnancy TAC were followed for eight years through 50 subsequent pregnancies. The survival rate of the babies was 100%. Yes, that's right, 100%! Now that's awesome. C-sections were performed in 97% of those pregnancies at about 37 weeks.[2]

Another study followed 11 women in New Zealand with a history of failed vaginal cerclages and recurrent miscarriages who received pre-pregnancy laparoscopic cerclages. Of the 10 women who got pregnant after the cerclages, all 10 had babies via C-section in the third trimester[3]—more evidence of the undeniable success of TACs.

And here's some more. One study looked at women who had a TAC placed during pregnancy. The gestation at placement was 13 weeks, and of the 75 women who had one or more failed transvaginal cerclages, the average gestation at delivery was 36 weeks (only three women delivered at or before 24 weeks) with a 96% survival rate.[4]

In a review of women who received TACs between 1978 and 2004, they found that the overall success rate was 93% with the cerclage compared to only an 18% survival of the baby in their previous pregnancies in the 88 women and 96 pregnancies identified. Delivery beyond 37 weeks occurred in 70% of TAC pregnancies.[5] These same rates were also found in a French study, a 93% survival rate with a TAC versus 17% without.[6]

Risks with a TAC

This procedure carries the same risks as a cervical cerclage—i.e., rupture of membranes and infection (chorioamnionitis)—as well as the very rare occurrence of uterine rupture and septicemia. There's a longer recovery period after this procedure than after a cervical cerclage, especially with the laparotomy technique, where larger cuts in the abdomen are used to insert the stitch. This is considered more of a "major operation." (Placing the TAC prior to pregnancy avoids the first two risks.)

There is an additional risk with this procedure, namely hemorrhaging from the uterine veins during placement.[7] I also found a paper describing other possible complications when they go in through the vagina to do this procedure. These range from major to minor and include bladder lacerations, cervical tears, hematoma, and temporary urinary retention with pelvic pain.[8]

A new technique, involving what is termed a "laparoscopic" approach, has been developed in the last couple years. This method is less invasive, because they don't need to cut open the stomach to place the cerclage. One paper looked to evaluate this less invasive laparoscopic transabdominal cervico-isthmic cerclage. (Cervico-isthmic is just one of several types of TAC, but I won't bore you with the details of these.) They found that it is easy to perform, with an average time to place of 45 minutes, and it increases the number of term deliveries and successful outcomes in women with failed cervical cerclages and cervical defects. In this study, 93% of the women had previous losses/preterm delivery, and 42.9% had previous failed McDonald cerclages (a type of transvaginal cerclage).[9]

A study of 67 women who received laparoscopic cervico-isthmic cerclages (about half were during pregnancy) found that 89% of the babies survived, with an average gestation of 35.8 ± 2.9 weeks. They concluded that this approach is comparable to traditional laparotomy.[10] Another study also concluded that laparoscopic cerclage "is a safe and effective alternative to laparotomy for the placement of abdominal cerclage."[11]

Two limitations of the laparoscopic method are the lack of depth perception during the procedure—because there is only two-dimensional depth, as opposed to "real-life" 3D (like when they cut you open and are actually able to see everything with their own eyes)—and a restricted ability to move around freely (because of the smaller cuts they maneuver within).[12]

They even looked at the use of a robot to assist with placement of a laparoscopic cerclage in a 12-week pregnant lady with no vaginal portion to her cervix, and she delivered a healthy term baby.[12,13] Miracles happen! Even though this lady basically had no cervix, she was able to have a healthy full-term baby with the help of a TAC.

You probably noticed that all these studies only include small numbers of women. There are no 1,000-plus women studies when it comes to TACs. This procedure is very rare within the world of obstetrics. Hopefully, the expertise and knowledge of their success will spread.

Different Approaches: Go in Through the Stomach or the Vagina?

One study looked to compare the outcomes using these two approaches—the more common transabdominal (through the stomach), and the lesser used transvaginal (through the crotch)—and found that both groups had much better outcomes after cerclages, with survival rates of around 70%, up from 27% and 12%, respectively, prior to the cerclage.

The transvaginal approach had a much shorter surgical time, at an average of 33 minutes versus 69 minutes, required a shorter hospital stay, involved less risk, and was less invasive.[14]

In another study that looked at the outcomes from going in through the vagina, they found that in all 56 pregnancies, the babies made it. The preterm birth rate was 32%, with births at less than 30 weeks in 21% of the ladies.[8]

C-Section Only

Most all of the women who receive TACs have C-sections. In order for you to have a vaginal birth, they would have to knock you out, go back in there, and remove the cerclage. This is much harder than the procedure for removing a transvaginal cerclage. It would mean another major operation, with all the usual risks involved, and then you would be all cut up and trying to deal with labor and pushing out your kid. Not so good. For me, this is a situation when a C-section is truly justified. For some of you this is a small price to pay for a healthy baby, but for others, the reality of having to have a C-section is something you must consider and come to terms with. Typically, the stitch is left in place for any future pregnancies. (According to Dr. Arthur Haney, an expert on IC and TACs, that aside from being able to birth vaginally, women with TACs have NORMAL pregnancies. Complete with sex, lifting, social life, and NO bed rest. Hmmm. Something to think about.)

Do I Get Another Vaginal Cerclage and Hope for the Best, or Get a TAC?

There are a lot of things to consider when making this decision. One is the reason for your failed cerclage. Was it because it was placed in an emergency situation? In that case, you may be better off with a cerclage placed high in the cervix, before changes happen, at 12–14 weeks. A preventative—i.e., history-indicated—cerclage may be the best choice for you the next time around. (Or maybe consider a TAC.)

Was your cervix too short to begin with to get a really good "knot" in there? Is this due to previous surgeries or to other deformities in your cervix? In this case, it's time to go doctor shopping to find a doctor who has experience performing this type of cerclage. When I said it can be hard in some areas to find a doctor experienced in transvaginal cerclages, it may be damn near impossible to find a doctor with experience in TACs. Don't give up, though. It may be a real pain in the butt, and you may have to travel, but go for it.

A resource providing support and other information about TAC is called Abbyloopers, at www.abbyloopers.org. This is a nonprofit organization whose goal is to educate and support women with IC, specifically those with or seeking a TAC. At the time of writing, it provides a limited physician-referral service. This may be a good place to start your search.[15] (Most Obs and some perinatologists don't even know about them.)

You also need to consider the added risks involved with a TAC. It's more invasive, requires more time in hospital, and has a longer recovery period. However, the upside is the very high success rate, even higher than for typical transvaginal cerclages.

In a study comparing the outcomes in women who had failed transvaginal cerclages and who then got either another transvaginal cerclage (40 women) or a transabdominal cerclage (117 women), they found that the chance of death/delivery before 24 weeks was 6% after a transabdominal cerclage and 12.5% after a transvaginal cerclage. The rate of serious postoperative complications was 3.4% after transabdominal cerclage and zero after tranvaginal cerclage.[16]

In another study that looked at the same thing, they found that preterm delivery prior to 33–35 weeks was more prevalent in the transvaginal cerclage group (42%) than the transabdominal group (18%). The average length of pregnancy was 36.3 ± 4.1 weeks in the transabdominal group and 32.8 ± 8.6 weeks in the transvaginal group. Premature rupture of membranes was also less frequent in the transabdominal group, at 8% vs. 29%.[17]

With all that said, and because this is my book and I can write what I want, if it were me, and I had a failed vaginal cerclage, I would go for the transabdominal cerclage. I would take that 3% risk for about a 93% survival rate. I know what it is like to lose a baby, and I would do anything in my power to NEVER experience that again. I would rather risk hemorrhaging than go through that again…for sure.

However, my situation may be different to yours in that 1) I live in an area where I only have to travel for 1.5 to 2 hours tops to find a doctor who specializes in this, and 2) I have the means to do it (good insurance, a job, a solid support system, etc.). I realize that not every-one is in this position, and so only you can make the decision of what is best for you.

Knock on wood, I have been blessed in that I have had two trans-vaginal cerclages to date that have not failed on me (even though there were times when I was sure they were coming loose). I am so sorry for all you ladies who have not been as fortunate as I have, and it's to you that I dedicate this chapter, to give you hope. Don't give up on your dream of a healthy baby. TACs work!

> *"Before losing my precious babies, I had no idea what a monster IC was. I was blissfully ignorant during my first pregnancy, until that fateful day in L&D when I was told my cervix was already 6 cm dilated and my membranes were bulging. The innocence of pregnancy was lost for me from that day on. One year later, I thought I would beat IC, only to be defeated once again when my TVC failed. I now pray that my TAC will keep holding and I will be able to bring my miracle home."*
> ~ Fawzia, Canada (At the time of writing she was 29 weeks pregnant after the loss of babies at 20 weeks and 21 weeks. You go, girl!)

References

1. Berghella V, Seibel-Seamon J. Contemporary use of cervical cerclage. *Clinical Obstetrics and Gynecology, Current Controversies in Obstetrics: What is an Obstetrician to Do?* 2007;50(2):468–477.
2. Thuesen LL, Diness BR, Langhoff-Roos J. Pre-pregnancy transabdominal cerclage. *Acta Obstet Gynecol Scand* 2009;88(4):483–486.
3. Liddell HS, Lo C. Laparoscopic cervical cerclage: a series in women with a history of second trimester miscarriage. *J Minim Invasive Gynecol* 2008;15(3):342–345.
4. Debbs RH, De La Vega GA, Pearson S, et al. Transabdominal cerclage after comprehensive evaluation of women with previous unsuccessful transvaginal cerclage. *Am J Obstet Gynecol* 2007;197(3):317 e1–4.
5. Fick AL, Caughey AB, Parer JT. Transabdominal cerclage: can we predict who fails? *J Matern Fetal Neonatal Med* 2007;20(1):63–67.
6. Gesson-Paute A, Berrebi A, Parant O. Transabdominal cervico-isthmic cerclage in the management of cervical incompetence in high risk women. *J Gynecol Obstet Biol Reprod (Paris)* 2007;36(1):30–35.
7. National Guideline Clearinghouse, www.guideline.gov, Cervical Insufficiency, 12/3/07.

8. Katz M, Abrahams C. Transvaginal placement of cervicoisthmic cerclage: report on pregnancy outcome. *Am J Obstet Gynecol* 2005;192(6):1989–1992.
9. Nicolet G, Cohen M, Begue L, et al. Laparoscopic cervico-isthmic cerclage evaluation. *Gynecol Obstet Fertil* 2009;37(4):294–299.
10. Whittle WL, Singh SS, Allen L, et al. Laparoscopic cervico-isthmic cerclage: surgical technique and obstetric outcomes. *Am J Obstet Gynecol* 2009;201(4):364 e1–7.
11. Carter JF, Soper DE, Goetzl LM, Van Dorsten JP. Abdominal cerclage for the treatment of recurrent cervical insufficiency: laparoscopy or laparotomy? *Am J Obstet Gynecol* 2009;201(1):111 e1–4.
12. Wolfe L, DePasquale S, Adair CD, et al. Robotic-assisted laparoscopic placement of transabdominal cerclage during pregnancy. *Am J Perinatol* 2008;25(10):653–655.
13. Fechner AJ, Alvarez M, Smith DH, Al-Khan A. Robotic-assisted laparoscopic cerclage in a pregnant patient. *Am J Obstet Gynecol* 2009;200(2):e10–11.
14. Witt MU, Joy SD, Clark J, et al. Cervicoisthmic cerclage: transabdominal vs transvaginal approach. *Am J Obstet Gynecol* 2009;201(1):105e1–4.
15. Abbyloopers, http://www.abbyloopers.org/.
16. Zaveri V, Aghajafari F, Amankwah K, Hannah M. Abdominal versus vaginal cerclage after a failed transvaginal cerclage: a systematic review. *Am J Obstet Gynecol* 2002;187(4):868–872.
17. Davis G, Berghella V, Talucci M, Wapner RJ. Patients with a prior failed transvaginal cerclage: a comparison of obstetric outcomes with either transabdominal or transvaginal cerclage. *Am J Obstet Gynecol* 2000;183(4):836–839.

CHAPTER 10

Summary of Treatment
Options for a Short Cervix

In recommendations released by the National Guideline Clearinghouse on cervical insufficiency in 2007 to aid doctors in making
decisions about care, to provide a review of the current evidence,
and to offer management standards, they included the following guidelines: serial ultrasounds to assess cervical length in **low-risk** women are
unnecessary and should not be done regularly, serial ultrasound measurements starting at between 16 and 20 weeks (or later) should be
considered in women with risk factors, an elective cerclage should be
contemplated in women who have had THREE or more unexplained
second-trimester losses or preterm deliveries, and finally, women who
were exposed to diethylstilbestrol in utero (DES daughters) can be
evaluated for IC. (Notice the weak wording they use throughout.
These don't seem like guidelines to me; they seem more like cautious
suggestions. How are these supposed to help doctors if they only
loosely propose certain practices?)

For the recommendations based on doctor's consensus and expert
opinion, they state: 1) To evaluate a woman with cervical shortening
or funneling, a detailed ultrasonographic evaluation of the baby should
be performed to rule out anomalies, as well as other evaluations to rule
out labor and infection (chorioamnionitis), and 2) in light of advances

in neonatal care (NICUs are now better able to care for preemies) and the risk to mother and baby associated with a cerclage, this procedure should be restricted to pregnancies before viability is reached (typically around 23 or 24 weeks).[1]

A survey of maternal-fetal specialists in the U.S. was conducted to determine what their practice was in reference to history-indicated cerclages, since there is little research to support treatment with this specific type of cerclage. In a scenario where a woman had painlessly and spontaneously lost her baby at 19 weeks, 75% would advise one at 12–14 weeks in her next pregnancy, 21% would agree to it if it was requested by the patient, and only 4% would not recommend a cerclage in this scenario. Eighty-nine percent felt there was little or no risk to doing a history-indicated cerclage.[2]

According to a review of the research on short cervices, there is not enough research to support the use of indomethacin (a tocolytic), pessaries (an alternate to cerclages), and/or bed rest for those of us who have a short cervix.[3]

If you've had a previous loss or an early birth, discuss the option of a history-indicated (a.k.a. preventative) cerclage with your doctor to see if maybe you would be a good candidate for one. I had one second-trimester loss at almost 23 weeks, reluctantly went with the wait-and-see approach, ultimately got a cerclage at 21 weeks when my cervix shortened to about 1 cm in my second pregnancy, then had a history-indicated cerclage placed with my third pregnancy. I was fortunate in that I didn't have to endure multiple losses or preemies in order to get an early cerclage. I knew the risks of the cerclage procedure and made an informed decision to try it.

Another Treatment Option for a Short Cervix: The Pessary

When I first read about these, they were totally new to me. These are medical devices, think diaphragm-like, that are placed in the vagina, like a dome, to cover the cervical opening. I had never heard of this, nor was it ever mentioned in the course of my experiences with IC. I'm not sure how popular these are in the U.S., because much of the

What to Expect During Your Next Pregnancy After a Loss or Early Birth

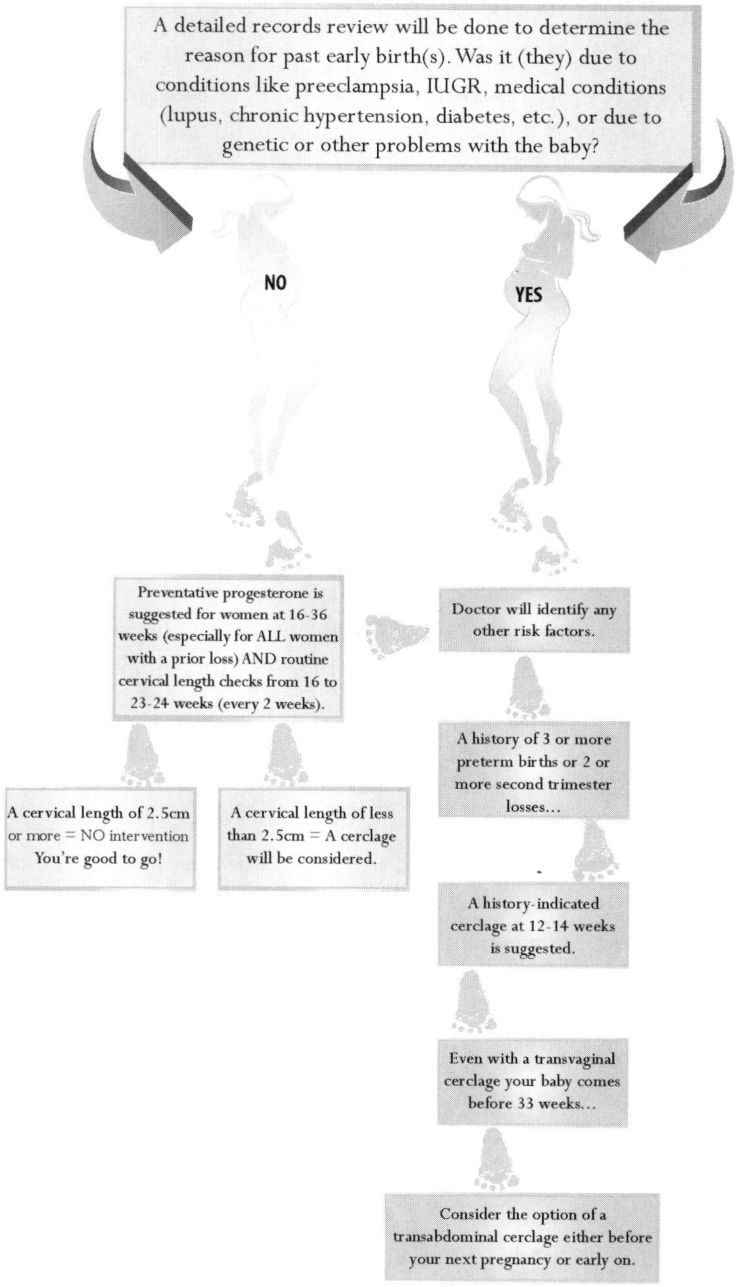

A detailed records review will be done to determine the reason for past early birth(s). Was it (they) due to conditions like preeclampsia, IUGR, medical conditions (lupus, chronic hypertension, diabetes, etc.), or due to genetic or other problems with the baby?

NO

YES

Preventative progesterone is suggested for women at 16-36 weeks (especially for ALL women with a prior loss) AND routine cervical length checks from 16 to 23-24 weeks (every 2 weeks).

Doctor will identify any other risk factors.

A history of 3 or more preterm births or 2 or more second trimester losses...

A cervical length of 2.5cm or more = NO intervention You're good to go!

A cervical length of less than 2.5cm = A cerclage will be considered.

A history-indicated cerclage at 12-14 weeks is suggested.

Even with a transvaginal cerclage your baby comes before 33 weeks...

Consider the option of a transabdominal cerclage either before your next pregnancy or early on.

Figure 10-1. The chart is adapted from the well-respected clinicians' reference book, *Preterm Birth: Prevention and Management.*[3]

research seems to come out of Europe. The benefit of these is that they're noninvasive—i.e., they're not surgically placed—so it's a less traumatic procedure, and generally doesn't require anesthesia.

Vaginal pessaries have been found to be helpful in women who are at high risk of preterm delivery since around the time cerclages were developed, and they don't carry many of the risks presented by cerclages. As the authors of one review article state, these should be used as an alternative to cerclages when women aren't candidates, or in addition to cerclages in some women (to provide additional reinforcement).[4] (The reduced surgical risk argument doesn't hold up here when they suggest both a cerclage and a pessary.)

In one nonrandomized study that looked at the use of Arabin pessaries in women with a cervical length of 1.5–3.0 cm prior to 28 weeks, about 2% delivered before 29 weeks and 83% delivered after 37 weeks. (Women who had a length of less than 1.5 cm got a cerclage.) Treatment with a pessary was effective in these women.[5]

A 2006 study concluded that "Pessary may be useful in the management of cervical incompetence. Whether it can be a noninvasive alternative to surgical cerclage merits further investigation." In this small study, they used pessaries in those who showed progressive shortening of their cervices to 2.5 cm or less before 30 weeks. The average gestation at birth was 34 weeks, and 45% of the babies were born at less than 34 weeks. It was noted that all of the women complained about increased vaginal discharge. (No other complications were observed.)[6]

Another study of 73 women using a Herbich cervical pessary found an overall early birth rate of about 36%; 89% of women delivered after 33 weeks. They concluded that this is "a safe and effective method of treatment for cervical incompetence."[7]

One study compared cerclages with pessaries in women at between 22 and 27 weeks who showed shortening. Cerclage extended the pregnancy by 13.4 weeks, while the pessary extended it by 12.1 weeks. The authors concluded that they were both "equally effective methods of prolongation of pregnancy."[8]

According to *Preterm Birth: Prevention & Management*, since randomized and controlled trials on the use of a pessary compared to no pessary are yet to be conducted, they're not recommended for use in women with a short cervix. The studies that are currently available have several design flaws and limitations, and so they conclude that, "At this time, pessaries should not be offered as first-line therapy for women with cervical insufficiency."[3]

In summary, should you not qualify as a candidate for a cerclage, for any of various reasons, such as the lack of a cervix, talk to your doctor about the option of a pessary. (Note: This choice would be at the very bottom of my list.)

Discussion

It's important to remember why they recommend minimizing preventative cerclages in women. There are some risks associated with this procedure, as discussed in the chapter on cerclages. Further, it hasn't been clearly proven that they reduce early birth in many women, most likely because cerclages are being placed for reasons other than IC. Not only does this approach avoid unnecessary risks, but it also avoids unnecessary surgery in those women who do not have IC. After all, true IC is quite rare. Talk with your doctor about your options and assess whether they're familiar with the latest research. If not, you know what to do. Move on.

References

1. National Guideline Clearinghouse, www.guideline.gov, Cervical Insufficiency.
2. Fox NS, Gelber SE, Kalish RB, Chasen ST. History-indicated cerclage: practice patterns of maternal-fetal medicine specialists in the USA. *J Perinat Med* 2008;36(6):513–517.
3. Berghella V. *Preterm Birth: Prevention & Management*. West Sussex, UK. Wiley-Blackwell, 2010.
4. Patro-Malysza J, Leszczynska-Gorzelak B, Marciniak B, et al. The use of pessaries in the treatment of incompetent cervix. *Ginekol Pol* 2009;80(1):54–58.
5. Sieroszewski P, Jasiński A, Perenc M, et al. The Arabin pessary for the treatment of threatened mid-trimester miscarriage or premature labour and miscarriage: a case Series. *J Matern Fetal Neonatal Med* 2009;22(6):469–472.

6. Acharya G, Eschler B, Grønberg M, et al. Noninvasive cerclage for the management of cervical incompetence: a prospective study. *Arch Gynecol Obstet* 2006;273(5):283–287.
7. Grzonka DT, Kaźmierczak W, Cholewa D, Radzioch J. Herbich cervical pessary-method of therapy for cervical incompetence and prophylaxis of prematurity. *Wiad Lek* 2004;57(suppl 1):105–107.
8. Antczak-Judycka A, Sawicki W, Spiewankiewicz B, et al. Comparison of cerclage and cerclage pessary in the treatment of pregnant women with incompetent cervix and threatened preterm delivery. *Ginekol Pol* 2003;74(10):1029–1036.

CHAPTER 11

Dealing with a High-Risk Pregnancy Really Sucks!

"*P*rematurity and multiple births are a world you never know exists, unless life takes you there.*"* ~ Nicole, Pennsylvania (With her first child, her preterm labor started at a shocking eight weeks. Can you believe that? The baby was born at 25 weeks. She then went on to carry twins to 37 weeks, having preterm labor from 28 weeks on. Yes girls, it can be done.)

"Even though it seems that this point in time will last forever, it is only a small hurdle for a lifetime of joy with that little miracle in your life." ~ Janna, Ohio

"Keep the faith and be strong; that's the key to making it through the downs in your pregnancy. I pray for the best, ladies." ~ Ambrel, Texas (After the devastating loss of her baby girl at 24 weeks, who lived for three days, she endured "STRICT hospital bed rest" from 19 weeks until 34 weeks. That's a long time to be in the hospital on bed rest. She delivered a healthy boy at exactly 37 weeks.)

"Today is a day you have never seen before and will never see again; let's get through it." ~ Jakaila (location unknown)

"No matter how down you feel, just remember the beautiful miracle you will have in the end." ~ Diane, Georgia

"Some days are easier than others. You have to keep your chin up and pray for a positive outcome; otherwise, you will drive yourself crazy, and that isn't good for anybody." ~ Genny, Alabama

"Hang in there. It may seem like FOREVER. But in the grand scheme of things, a few weeks or even months is over before you know it. Also, it's okay to feel overwhelmed, scared, sad, and just plain 'over it.' That doesn't make you a bad mom; it means your human and are having these feelings. Try to embrace them and get a snack!" ~ Erika, Nebraska

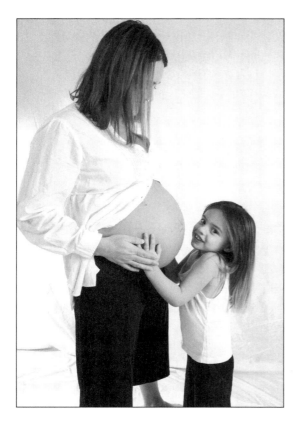

Though a pregnancy far from normal, with this one I really tried to enjoy it. (Hey I'm no Demi Moore, but I even went for those shots too.) Relief that I made it to this point, happy to be vertical and enjoying my body. I advise each of you to consider this if you can. *Photo by: Anthony Ziccardi Studios (www.aziccardi.com).*

"Every day is a blessing with your little one. We are blessed to live in a time where technology gives us the opportunity to diagnose, treat, and research further our situations. Even though technology is grand, our ultimate strength comes from within. Draw strength from whatever you believe in... God, family, your spouse. No matter the outcome, you are a strong woman."
~ Telisia Marie, Arizona (four weeks in on bed rest and up to 10 more expected at the time of writing this)

"I had to take it hour by hour, minute by minute. I couldn't handle taking it 'one day at a time.' For me, it was 'one breath at a time.'" ~ Erin, Florida

Help! I've Turned Into a Psycho, Raving Bitch

As if it isn't bad enough that you have the normal crazies of pregnancy, now you have that extra bit that comes from being in a constant state of fear and worry. I may have been a bit of a psycho, raving bitch during my pregnancies, especially when I was carrying my daughter, and I must say, I'm not ashamed to admit it. Really, can you blame me (or us) for behaving like this?

I would also like to say that we have every right to be complete bitches and have our asses kissed every second of every day during this time. Does anyone else really have any idea of what it's like to spend months in bed, or get poked and prodded more times than a junkie, or live with the fact that, at any time, the very life of the precious little being who is growing inside us could actually be taken away? No, they don't. They may try to understand, even our partners, but can they really?

No one can completely understand unless they've been through this nightmare themselves. While our partners, friends, and family get to leave for work every day, can go out with friends, and are able to do normal things like grocery shopping or even simply washing dishes, we spend every second of the day living with the reality that we can't do those things. We're stuck there feeling those kicks and wondering if we will ever get to hold this baby in our arms, or have the gift of him or her looking back up at us. It's a question that is continually circling through our minds. The stress of dealing with a difficult pregnancy is really indescribable; no words can accurately capture the intensity of what you are feeling and going through. I've been through it, so I know. It's just an awful experience, but one that leads to a beautiful gift like nothing you've *ever* felt before.

So, the reality is this: 1) having a high-risk pregnancy sucks; 2) having a high-risk pregnancy and being on bed rest really, really sucks; and 3) having a high-risk pregnancy after losing a baby is beyond sucking and can best be described as really, really shitty, emotionally stressful, and downright torturous. It brings about feelings of fear, anxiety, desperation, sadness, depression, loneliness, dependence, and any number of other bad feelings. Trust me, you may not think so while you're going through it, but you *will* survive and you *will* be normal again… one day. (Although your definition of normal may have shifted a little by that time.)

Even though I said earlier that it should be a right to behave badly as a result of our situation, to be a total bitch during our pregnancies, it isn't that easy. In reality, we can't act that way on a regular basis, nor should we want to. You really should try not to be a crazy, psycho, at least not on a regular basis. I mean, do you want to scare everyone away? Your support system will need, and deserve, a break from time to time to deal with it all, and we need to find ways to control our behavior, or else we'll drive everyone who is around us (and helping us) away. It's also possible to be so miserable during this entire experience that you miss the opportunity to derive any joy from your pregnancy. That's a big no-no.

This should be every high-risk woman's goal. Let me say it again: it should be one of our prime objectives to try to enjoy as many moments of our pregnancy as we can, since we're robbed of so much just by the very fact of being pregnant. Make sense? It should. You only gyp yourself if you fail to find any joy during this time.

On that note, don't worry if the occasional bout of bitchiness overcomes you. Also, I would like to suggest that if your rants are falling on deaf ears, it may not be a bad idea to sign up for a buddy support system on www.sidelines.org. Sidelines National High Risk Pregnancy Support Network pairs high-risk women with other women who have been through similar situations. If you're experiencing it, chances are they have the perfect match for you.

It can be very helpful to talk with someone on a regular basis. (You can have phone or email support, however you choose.) Not only does releasing your fears, concerns, and feelings to someone who understands help you emotionally, it can do wonders in helping you to survive this experience.

There are also other forums and boards aimed at supporting women during a high-risk pregnancy. Do a search and see if you can find the right one for you. I have been involved in the Incompetent Cervix forum, www.ic.hobh.org/forums. This is one of the largest support groups of its kind, with over 1,300 members from around the world. It's a great resource and a great way to connect with other women who have either been in your shoes or are walking in them right now. It was started and is run by a wonderful woman who knows all about the stresses and ultimate joys of high-risk pregnancies, who now has four cerclage kids and an angel in her heart. The loss of her baby, Tanner, due to IC was such a devastating experience that she started this forum as a way to honor her son and help others. (Thank you, Danah.) If you have IC or even preterm labor, you should check it out.

My only advice is to try to not get too wrapped up in these boards. There are women who experience and then post negative outcomes, stories of losses and other horrors, that can be quite overwhelming. Reading others losses and bad outcomes while you are in the midst of your own stressful pregnancy is not recommended. People by nature tend to be more inclined to tell the bad stuff than the good. When you get too wrapped up in reading all the stuff that could happen or has happened to others, you can start to stress that it will now happen to you, so don't spend all night reading the "Angels" section, please. (Hey, I've done it, so take my advice and learn from my mistakes.)

"Patience is key. Keep your eyes on the end result. Count down the days to your due date." ~ Angela, Michigan (Lost twins at 20 weeks due to premature labor and a boy at 23½ weeks due to PPROM. At the time of writing, she is pregnant, just got a preventive cerclage, and is thinking positively.)

STRESS! Need I Say More?

If there's one thing there's no shortage of during a high-risk pregnancy, it's stress. We have the effects of stress racing through our veins all day and all night. We think, breathe, and dream the what-ifs, and can't seem to beat off the negative thoughts of things going wrong. There's no doubt that this will be one of the most—if not *the* most—stressful experiences of your life, and this stress isn't exactly temporary or fleeting. It won't necessarily end quickly, like certain other stresses in your life, such as an upcoming presentation. This intense and heightened level of stress can stretch out for many months.

The effects of chronic stress have been studied, and it has been found that support from the baby's father helped to reduce the chances of a preterm birth. Chronic stress, low confidence for a normal birth, and fearing for the baby's health increases the risk of an early birth. Moderate-to-high stress, with no support, followed by fearing for the baby's health, carried the highest risk.[1]

If that isn't the kicker—not only are we at high risk for preterm delivery for any number of reasons, but now our fear and stress over it all can also cause us to have our babies early. We just can't seem to win. So, what can you do? Sit back, take several deep breaths, and relax. Tell yourself, "Everything's going to be okay." Now do this several times a day. They say that if you tell yourself something often enough, your brain will eventually catch on and believe it. Hey, we've got to try something, right? We need to try to find ways to reduce this stress and to find some enjoyment, even in the midst of this nerve-wracking time.

This can be as simple as a two-hour escape with a good comedy movie, or lunch with a friend to catch up on the local gossip, even if that means they need to bring lunch to your house and you need to eat while lying down. How about any number of mindless but entertaining diversions? My guilty pleasure is celebrity gossip magazines. (Sorry, celebrities. Look, I know it's not true, but it is entertaining to those of us living rather mundane lives. Money, sex, fashion...can you blame us?) It's sad but true; there's nothing like blowing an hour browsing through *OK* or *In Touch* magazine.

There are many ways you can find to reduce, even just a little bit, the stress and anxiety you're feeling—foot rubs from your cabana boy . . . wait, I'm still on the gossip-magazine thing. Seriously, though, ask your spouse for a back or foot rub. Enjoy some of your favorite take out and watch a good movie. Remind yourself of some of the research in this book. More often than not, the numbers are on your side.

Basically, just figure out things that will work for you. I found that long showers did wonders for me. Yes, I had to lie on the floor while I was taking one, but they really helped me to relax and get my thoughts together when I was ready to snap and freak out. This gave me time to regroup. If you can escape into a book or a hobby, like knitting or scrapbooking, go for it. I know it's easier said than done, but you've got to do it. Do it for yourself, do it for your sanity, and do it for the health and welfare of your baby.

Truth be told, I cried just about every day, living in a constant state of fear during my entire pregnancy with my daughter. I not only worried whether she would make it, I also worried what the long-term effects would be on her—if she even got here—from all the stress and anxiety I'd felt during this time. Would she be a colicky, unhappy baby? Would she turn out to be an anxious child? Would she be normal, or was I screwing her up for life? Extreme, I know, but I'm sure many of you have wondered the same things about your babies.

Just so you know, she's a normal kid. Yes, she's a very—and I mean *very*—emotional kid, and I often wonder if that personality trait goes back to her time in the womb. I believe they call those children "highly sensitive." Yup, that's her. But I love that she still gets upset over the death of our dog, which happened over a year ago. She recently cried and told me she didn't think Molson had enough food in heaven. When I told her he got to eat anything he wanted, including steak, she then cried hysterically and said that she didn't think he had a nice place to poop. Can you believe that? So stop worrying so much; my kid's fine, and yours probably will be, too.

Even though I don't have any cold, hard research on personality and stress, I do know that stress is not good for you or your baby, so you should try to minimize it as much as you can. Asking lots of questions about what's going on in your body, what to expect, your options, and just generally being knowledgeable can help to reduce some of the anxiety you're feeling, although I know it's impossible, realistically, to get rid of it all. Anyone who says otherwise has never been in our position.

> *"This is an emotional roller coaster. Some days I want to cry, other days I pray. Still there are days I want to scream. And there are times I want to do all three at once. I refuse to hope anymore. After losing two previous pregnancies I have "pregnancy goals." At 24 weeks, I will call my son by name. At 30 weeks, I will order his furniture. At 32 weeks, I will let my friends plan the baby shower they want to give me. I am just too afraid to hope to hold him one day, after losing two babies and knowing the risks with carrying him. Worse, I am ashamed of my fear because it proves my faith is weaker than I once believed."* ~ Jennifer, Louisiana (She experienced two early losses at less than 12 weeks and has a very short cervix, which makes her unable to get a cerclage.)

> *"My worst fear ever occurred—my placenta was tearing away. Placenta abruption. I felt completely lost, worried, and scared about my health and my baby. Noticing every little movement, or lack thereof, and constantly checking the bed sheet and toiletries for blood/blood clots became my routine. Any slight blood, and my heart would sink and race. I kept with my MD's advice, along with my hubby and strong family to support me, and after numerous scares, I feel that I have defeated all odds by carrying my boy to 34 weeks. There is not a day that goes by that I am not very grateful for the wonderful care and support. Just because you're defined as "high risk" doesn't mean you stop living, it just means you're more delicate than before."* ~ Laura, Canada (I couldn't have said it better.)

> *"My husband and I lost our little girl, Mollie, at 23½ weeks in 1994. It was a life-changing moment/time in our lives. We realized that life can change so quickly. We cherish the small amount of time that we had with her. Once we became pregnant*

with our son, Keegan, we lived each day with anticipation of week 23½. Thankfully, we made it, and Keegan made it as well. He came on time and was healthy. We were soooo thankful for all of the wonderful care that we got from our doctors and nurses, and the support that we got from family, friends, and Sidelines. Having Mollie made us totally appreciate having our son and the time that we have with him, and the time that we had with his sister." ~ Megan, Michigan (spent six and a half months on bed rest to have her healthy boy)

"Going through another pregnancy after you have experienced a loss takes a huge leap of faith and can be very scary. When you add a high-risk situation into the mix, emotions are at an all-time high. Every kick and hiccup brings reassurance, but that is countered by the fear that every 'abnormal' twinge or pain brings. It's hard to stay upbeat and positive. Days on bed rest can be long and depressing. Having the help of family members and a supportive doctor were imperative to my ability to keep my spirits up. I kept reminding myself that I was doing all I could to maintain my pregnancy for as long as I could, and the rest was up to God. Now that I'm on this side of the fence, with three healthy and energetic children, I long for someone to tell me to stay in bed and do nothing for even just one day. I wish I could have had that perspective during my days on bed rest." ~ Jenn, Utah

"You can get through this. You will survive." ~ Jessica, Colorado (This positivity is coming from someone who had five losses, one each at 5 and 6 weeks, two at 16 weeks, and another at 21 weeks. She now has a healthy two-year-old girl.)

"A complicated pregnancy is one of the most agonizing things one will go through in their life. Take one day at a time, and don't think about how far you are from your due date. Instead, think about when your next appointment is and what you are going to do between now and then to help that baby grow." ~ Autumn, Oregon

"Remember to try and find some inner peace, and find ways to mitigate the stress. Follow your doctor's advice—it's a big investment in your child(ren), but totally worth it." ~ Angela, California (spent 12 weeks on hospital bed rest to birth her twins at 34 weeks)

When asked for words of advice... *"I'm having a hard time finding words of wisdom for myself. I'm still at the depressed stage."* ~ Daniela, Brazil (Experienced several losses. At the time of writing, she's 10 weeks, 3 weeks into bed rest, and looking at a long road ahead. Her words are something anyone who is experiencing this can relate to.)

Relationship Troubles and High-Risk Pregnancy

We all know that stress in your life can lead to problems on the home front. Unfortunately, a high-risk pregnancy is no exception. This is a time in your life when you really need the love and support of your loved ones. Unfortunately, all the stress, fear, anxiety, and even depression over the current situation—or from a previous loss—can put distance between you and your family, especially your partner.

For lots of women, this is supposed to be a time of the ultimate connection with your partner, or so I've been told—total support, comfort, closeness, and bonding. For many, though, this couldn't be further from the truth. The stress of this experience, and the fact that both of you are dealing with it in different ways, can strain your relationship. You may feel isolated from being on bed rest all day, while he may feel stressed from having to take care of you and the extra household duties, and may even feel the need to let off some steam in order to cope. Combine all that with the fact that many high-risk women are not allowed to have sex, and your blissful existence may suddenly come to an end.

After my loss, my husband and I dealt with the death of our son in very different ways. He went out and drank, partied it up, and generally enjoyed socializing in an effort to forget about it, while I preferred to sit at home sulking and analyzing each and every detail. This caused many, many issues, not to mention loud screaming matches and tears, within our marriage.

Fast forward to my next pregnancy, a high-risk one where even more problems came to the surface to wreak havoc. During my long stretch of bed rest, my husband had to do everything around the house. He was commuting, working, and then had to come home and take care of me and all the household duties. I, on the other hand, was so lonely all day as I sat and watched the clock, waiting for him to come home so I would have someone to talk to.

He felt stressed and would say that he just wanted to go out for a few hours and forget about everything, which in turn led to me feeling completely abandoned. He felt that he had the weight of the world on his shoulders, and that he should be able to go and do the things that twenty-somethings did, like going out with his friends. Meanwhile, I felt like I was the one shouldering all the weight. After all, I was the one who was pregnant and on bed rest, not him.

At that time, I would get so fired up that he would even dare think about going out. I'd been home alone all day on bed rest with no means of escape. How dare he think it was okay. How dare he even consider going out. After all, I was the one who was *literally* carrying the entire burden. Back then, it never occurred to me to put myself in his shoes and understand where he was coming from.

There was a point in time when I was so upset by these antics that I went and stayed with my parents for a period of time. Yes, while I was on complete bed rest, I went and stayed with my parents. This was not a good situation to be in, on bed rest and having severe marital troubles. From speaking with other women, I've found that this scenario isn't all that uncommon. The stresses of a difficult pregnancy can have a very bad effect on your marriage and relationships. The key is to understand that this is common and deal with it through open communication, understanding, and possibly even marriage counselors. Don't be like me; throwing a glass at someone is never good.

You will find during your pregnancy that life goes on and people move on, regardless of the fact that you may be stuck in bed. People's lives are busy, and calling you or stopping by every day just isn't on their mind or possible. You need to understand this and try not to become resentful. If you're one of the lucky ones who has full support, all day every day, meals brought to you and visits on a regular basis, be thankful for your amazing circle of friends and family.

If, on the other hand, you find you're not getting the support you need, I suggest just putting it directly out there. Tell people what you need. Don't hold back, and don't be ashamed. You could say to your partner, "Hey, I would really appreciate it if you could come straight home from work. Please try to understand that I've been alone all day on bed rest, and it's really hard for me. I really look forward to the time when you come home, so I can have someone to talk to and escape some of the stresses of this pregnancy." Tell your friends how alone you're feeling; they honestly just might not realize it.

It wouldn't hurt to occasionally give your partner a free pass to do something he always used to enjoy doing, whether it's a hobby like biking, or just a night out with the guys. I know it's hard, but try to understand that he's having trouble with this too, albeit differently.

You could also explain to your family and friends how hard it is to be on bed rest, and how hard it is on your partner to be handling everything. Sometimes you'll find that all you need to do is ask, and you shall receive. "Hey, do you mind stopping by for an hour and helping to vacuum a bit?" or "I'd love it if you could just stop by sometime and we could have lunch together. It's been really difficult on me to be alone all the time." (The guilt-trip approach may work well, too.) Honestly, though, most people just don't understand what it's really like unless you tell them.

I really wish I'd taken my own advice when I was going through it, but I didn't, and my relationship with my husband suffered (although I still believe that he was a bit selfish in his actions). I felt very isolated and lonely, and we rarely, if ever, got any help around the house or with meals. It was a very rough time for both of us, an experience I would not wish upon my worst enemy.

If things get very bad, you should consider speaking to a counselor to try to sort things out. I know, I know; a counselor is so cliché, but what else is there to do at that point? If the situation with your partner is really bad, and you have somewhere you can stay for a while, consider taking time out. Sometimes, this doesn't do much more than put even more stress on a situation that's already overloaded, but other times, it may help by giving each of you a new perspective. Just hang in there.

Remember my tips:

+ Ask and you shall receive. People aren't mind readers, and unless they've been through it themselves, they can't even begin to understand what you're going through and what you need.

+ Hand out the occasional free pass. Let hubby off the hook once in a while to do a normal activity, so he can escape the stress of taking care of you/baby and all the household duties.

+ Understand that people aren't out to get you, that they don't generally suck, that they didn't forget about you, and that it doesn't mean you don't matter to them. They just don't understand. They have busy lives that must go on while you're lying there watching the seconds tick by. Though time slows WAY down for you, it doesn't for them. It's okay for you to make the effort to call them. (See the first tip.)

+ If things at home get very bad, seek the help of an experienced counselor. It might not be a bad idea to work out some of these issues before the baby comes.

+ This experience changes who you are as a person and can force changes to any relationship. If a friend/spouse/family member really just flakes on you and isn't there to support you even after you've communicated your needs to him or her, it may be time to set that person free. You don't need them. F-em.

Losses

Even though you're working toward preventing a big loss—that of your child—in a high-risk pregnancy, there are many other smaller losses that can take place—some rather subtly, and others more drastically.

Loss of Freedom

With a high-risk pregnancy comes a loss of freedom for many of us. This includes the loss of freedom to do even the simplest of activities, including being able to use the bathroom, walk around, make your own meals, lift anything, and go out and do things. And of course, there's the loss of privacy (if you're in the hospital).

You don't realize how good it is to be able to do the simplest of things until they're taken away from you. The simple pleasure of taking a shower without having to worry about whether you went over the allotted time…gone. The joy of popping out to grab a bite to eat if you feel like it…gone. Being able to go to work and be part of society…gone.

While you sacrifice and lose a lot, however, you're doing all this to gain something that's priceless—your baby. It may sound cheesy, but I really mean it when I say that it's all worthwhile. It pays off in the end.

As I write, I just kissed my baby girl, who is now five, before she ran outside to play with her friends, and I looked at her when I kissed her and thought to myself how worthwhile it all was. Seriously, I still think about all I went through to get her here nearly every day. I never thought, when I was going through that terrible chapter in my life, that it would be so plainly obvious later, that it would all be worth it—all the heartache, pain, suffering, loneliness, anger, angst, depression, and fear. It was all so worth it that if I knew I had to do it all again to have another child, I wouldn't hesitate.

What's most important is for you to keep it all in perspective. The loss of freedom is only temporary, and in the pie chart of your life, this period of time is but a very small sliver. Remind yourself of this daily to help get you by. You can and will do this!

> *"I constantly had to tell myself that these sacrifices I was making, these physical hardships to maintain a healthy pregnancy and birth, were just one small, infinitesimal slice of my life—a tiny sacrifice in comparison to an entire full life with a new child, new family, and new hope."* ~ Jessica (Location unknown)

Loss of Self

It's easy to lose your sense of self during a high-risk pregnancy, because you can become redefined as a person. It's no longer, "Hi, I'm Kelly, the scientist who likes to go out dancing." Instead, you can come to see yourself as your condition: "Hi, I'm on bed rest, and I can't even get my own food to eat. I'm now dependent on others to do everything for me." You can't let this become the new definition of you.

Even though you can no longer work or take part in any of the athletic hobbies you enjoyed prior to pregnancy, you are still *you*. Don't forget that, either. Yes, you have been derailed, but this is also temporary. Once you get your feet back on the ground, and you're up and running, you can go back to being you. Then, you'll just have to learn to adapt to life with a baby in tow. (That's another whole book in itself.)

Part of losing your sense of self is totally giving yourself over to the job of growing this baby and doing everything you possibly can to bring your baby into the world healthy. You are no longer doing everything just for yourself, but also for the tiny being growing inside of you. The key here is to do both. Come to an understanding with yourself that you're not only the ultimate baking machine, but you're also still you, and you can still enjoy "you" things. Granted, these may be limited if you're on bed rest or reduced activity, but with a little creativity and adaptation, you can hold on to your essential you-ness.

Loss of Womanhood

On top of everything else, many of you may feel a sense of sadness over the loss of feeling, well, like a hot piece-of-ass. Your body is changing, and with this can come a sense of unattractiveness, a loss of all those womanly pheromones. You're probably not allowed to engage in any sort of penetration, so NO sex, and you're worried about the well-being of your baby at every moment, so needless to say, you're far from feeling like the sex goddess you once were.

For some women who relished their femininity prior to pregnancy, this can be a dramatic change. Carrying a baby forces many to feel less like the young, desirable woman they were pre-pregnancy. Now mix that with the demands of a tough pregnancy, a lack of sex, and feelings of extreme stress, and you can see how easily your womanhood can get buried.

Those of you who couldn't have cared less about this sort of stuff before may not find this quite so bothersome, but I have to admit, this was a weird change for me. I submersed myself completely, 150% into mommyhood. It took a long time to get back to my former self, which was really now a modified version that I came to accept in time.

If you're concerned about this, and it's an issue for you, you can beat it. Even though you may not be able to have sex, there are other ways to be intimate with your partner. Buy yourself some sexy lingerie and strut yourself, big belly and all (not literally, of course, if you're on bed rest). Put on some music that makes you feel sexy, get your hair done, or read a hot romance novel. There's nothing wrong with wanting to feel good about yourself, even when you're with child. (I am obsessed with the pregnant belly and think it is soo beautiful. Work it, girls!)

Guilt, Guilt, and More GUILT

So many years after my loss and my high-risk pregnancies, I still feel the guilt over many things I did and things I thought—lots and lots of guilt.

I've never admitted this to anyone before, but while I was in the hospital, after I found out I couldn't get a cerclage because of an infection, I wanted them to just hurry up and give me the induction drugs so I could just get this over with. I wanted, for my own selfish reasons, to hurry up and deliver my son, who would not survive, in order to be done with the whole ordeal. To this day, I feel guilty about that.

In a high-risk pregnancy, there are so many places for guilt to weasel its way in. There were times when I was on bed rest and having a very difficult day when I would get up and pace around. I couldn't help myself. I felt like I was going to crawl out of my skin if I lay down for a moment more. I felt I had to get up in order to not snap completely. In the very far corners of my mind, I even questioned whether having another loss right then and there would be easier than being pregnant for what would seem like the rest of my life.

Today, it's easy for me to say it was all worth it, but back then, living it was a very different story. After getting pregnant again, I thought of backing out. What was I thinking? What had I done? Though it was only a brief thought, I still thought it. I felt so much guilt for everything I thought, and for everything I did. If only I'd done this or that. I felt guilty for having a body that couldn't carry a baby like most women.

Guilt is a terrible thing to have to experience when you're in the midst of a difficult pregnancy or after a loss, but you need to know that it's normal; you're not crazy for having these thoughts. Think them and then blow them away. You're being totally unfair to yourself when you beat yourself up like that, so stop doing it. Move on past the guilt.

> *"Listen and trust yourself. If you feel that something isn't quite right, see your doctor immediately. I sometimes question whether if I'd gone in a day earlier in my first pregnancy, the preterm labor could have been stopped, and my twins would be alive today."* ~ Brianna, Wisconsin

> *"I would just like to say, don't chance it. If you are unsure about traveling, having sex, or anything that might stimulate preterm labor or cervical changes, don't do it. You will blame yourself for the rest of your life if something bad happens. I had my first child at 27 weeks and still analyze everything I could have done wrong, but when my second child was born at 29 weeks, I knew I had done everything in my power to keep him safe, and that his early birth was not my fault."* ~ Sara, Ohio (both kids are with her today)

Listen to Your Body

Your body is an extraordinary thing. If you learn to listen to it and understand how it tries to tell you things, you'll be amazed. There's a certain intuition that pregnant women seem to have. They can know things about what's going on with their body and their baby, sometimes better than their doctors know, even with modern technology. Trust your body to tell you if/when something is wrong. If you have a dread in the pit of your stomach about something, don't ignore it. Even if you have any slight misgivings or doubts, don't let them go unchecked. They may turn out to be nothing, but as the saying goes, "It's better to be safe than sorry."

> *"If you are worried, call the doctor. Don't feel like a pain or that you are calling too much."* ~ Jenn, New York

"My contractions started low, much lighter than menstrual cramps. They would radiate up and out. This was the OPPO-SITE of what the doctors said would happen. Also, my contractions could be in just sections of my uterus, not the whole uterus. The doctors said only Braxton Hicks did that…they were wrong. If I hadn't followed my intuition and gone to the ER, I would've lost my twins at 21 weeks. I spent 54 days in labor on strict hospital bed rest, and my twins are alive and healthy today because I listened to my body." ~ Nicole, North Carolina (Spent nine weeks in labor contracting every 3 to 12 minutes, had a positive FFN at 21 weeks, was 5 cm dilated and effaced at 21 weeks…and she made it)

"They were not like labor contractions. My regular OB didn't even pick them up because they put the monitor up high on my belly. Well, at 20 weeks your uterus is not above your belly button. Everyone kept telling me I was not in labor. But I kept feeling short, very mild cramps, every four or five minutes. I felt like no one believed me. When I saw the Peri the next day, he said I was in labor." ~ Jennifer, Oregon

Fear of…Well, Everything

Fear, just like pretty much everything else, comes in all shapes, sizes, colors, and varieties. For example, you may experience any number of the following:

1. Fear of being vertical, which leads to…
2. Fear of your baby falling out
3. Fear of going to the bathroom
4. Fear of exerting yourself at all…for fear of triggering contractions
5. Fear of not eating enough healthy foods in order to help your baby grow
6. Fear of any movement, including using the bathroom, that can trigger bleeding or pressure on your cervix

7. Fear of any sort of emotional stress, which could lead to contractions or high blood pressure

8. Fear of missing some signal from your body that something is wrong

9. Fear that your baby has died inside you

10. Fear of your water breaking early

11. Fear of having a seizure

12. Fear of dying

13. Fear of brain damage or developmental issues in your baby

14. Fear that this is never going to end

Obviously, this list can go on endlessly. The first three were some of the main fears I had because of an incompetent cervix. Some of the others on this list might be more specific to those of you who suffer from preterm labor, IUGR, preeclampsia, etc. You get the picture.

Though some of these fears would seem irrational to other people, to us, they're not. I mean seriously, how many women are actually scared that their baby will fall out of their vagina, and yet this is exactly what happened to me. Or how many women fear that every wet spot in their panties is a leak in their amniotic sac? Not many there, either. Sorry gals, fear is something we high-risk mamas have to live with during our pregnancies.

We have to make sure we get a grip on this, because fear is stress. We need to minimize this for our own health, as well as for that of our baby. Stress and fear elicit an inborn response in our bodies, in which chemicals are released and our body responds by tensing up and increasing our heart rate, among other things. All of this repeated over time is no good.

So, what are we to do? We can talk with our doctors about any fears we have in relation to the pregnancy. They may be able to offer some hope or alleviate our fears, even if only a little. Similarly, talking about your fears with your family and friends may help to diminish or weaken them a little bit, although in reality, I'm not sure how well this works most of the time. There's also the old standby of the power of positive thinking, which works extremely well for some people. I've said it before: tell yourself repeatedly, "We are going to be all right," and, "My baby is going to be fine."

But my favorite, although often the hardest, way to alleviate fear was the use of distractions. This is kind of hard to do if you're on bed rest, alone all day, but distracting yourself with things such as hobbies, tasks like organizing pictures or recipes, or being busy with other children can all help you to avoid obsessing over your fears and worries. Try to engross yourself in something, even if it's just TV.

When I was pregnant with my second son, it was amazing how many fewer freak-out episodes I had compared to my pregnancy with my daughter. I was so preoccupied with everything else, especially my three-year-old, that I had much less time to worry and obsess over what could happen. I think the pregnancy right after one with a bad outcome, such as a preemie or a loss, is inherently going to be harder than one following a good outcome. Just knowing that you *can* have a healthy baby does wonders for the psyche.

The Snapping Point—It's Okay to Vent

In every high-risk pregnancy, there will come a time when you think you just can't do it anymore. You may wonder what in the hell you were thinking. You may question why you even wanted a baby, or how you could've thought you could handle this. Your resolve will be tested to the limit, but don't let yourself be pushed over the cliff of sanity.

"There are up and down days. Sometimes I was really sad, but I felt like I couldn't be, because my loved ones couldn't handle it. I had a friend who let me be however I needed to be. It is important to be positive, but sometimes I just needed to cry, and she helped me to see that was okay, too. That was very helpful. Along with that, though, I had to learn to discipline my mind. I was very tempted to blame myself for my water breaking. My husband and doctor were very firm with me that I needed to take those thoughts captive, or I could end up in a deep hole. I know this is very clichéd, but taking it all one day—no, one hour—at a time was so important. When you know that a

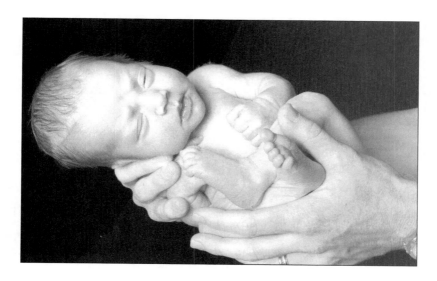

LONG *bed rest is the only hope for your child, which can be very overwhelming, it's important to see each day as a victory and an accomplishment."* ~ Linda, Missouri

Trust Me, It's ALL Worth It

"It will all be worth it once you are able to hold your baby or babies." ~ Kathleen, New York

"Often you feel so alone going through a high-risk pregnancy, and as though you will never get to see your precious little baby. But there is hope, and you are not alone. When you hold that little gift in your arms, it is all so worth it." ~ Natalie, California

"I try to keep as positive as I can, even when I'm faced with a time of uncertainty. I look at this pregnancy as a time to reflect on how I can be a better parent. It's given me time to rest and has given my family a new appreciation for all I do for everyone. I also have an amazing support system. I don't think I could do this without my friends." ~ Alison, California

Avoid Telling Yourself "I Will Not Get Attached"

Some of us try this natural protection thing where we feel we can shield ourselves from possible heartbreak by attempting to not get too attached to our babies. This line of thinking tries to tell us that if our baby dies, we will not get as hurt, but it doesn't work.

If you've found yourself falling into this pattern of thought, consider this: it's said that babies in the womb can sense the attitudes or emotions of the mother (due to the adrenaline and hormones that are released into the system with stress, fear, and other strong emotions). If you're trying to keep yourself distant from your baby because you don't want to get hurt, your baby can probably sense that in your emotions. The happier you are, and the more love you give to your baby—even when it's in the womb—the better off your child will be. Studies have proven that babies develop better when their mothers are happier.[2] (They also behave better if you experienced less stress during pregnancy.) Love your baby.

> *"One thing that I always did was talk to my babies all the time. I knew that they could die, and if they did I had to know that I was the best mom that I could be to them for however long they would be with me. This is really difficult, because if you've already lost a baby, the common-sense part of your brain says don't get too attached; it will hurt less if the worst happens. But for me (in order to stay sane), I had to give all my heart to my babies for as long as I could."* ~ Ana, California (had two losses at 28 weeks, until she eventually had a baby at 32 weeks)

> *"Giving yourself to your baby is something that happens early on in pregnancy. When I had complications very early on that continued throughout my pregnancy, I felt like I had to build a much stronger 'protective bond' with my baby."* ~ Carol, Ohio (suffered from placental abruption and preterm labor)

Possible Reconnection with Your Spirituality or an Affirmation of Your Faith

As you can tell, I'm not exactly a "holy roller," sweet-and-innocent kind of gal. I can say, though, that my experiences have brought me closer to an inner faith. I may not be a churchgoer or be overtly religious, but I can honestly say that my experiences have given me reason to have faith in and extreme gratitude to a higher power. I often say a prayer of thanks for my two blessings and ask God to watch over them and keep them healthy and safe, as well as to take care of my angel.

This is not something I ever thought I'd do, and it's something no one has known (until now) that I do. I'm not saying you have to be religious or anything of that sort. I'm saying that it's okay if you are, or if you have found religion as a way to help you get through this. Either way, it's an entirely personal decision, and pregnancy will have a different impact on each individual. No matter where you stand as far as religion or spirituality is concerned, pregnancy—whether it results in a good outcome or not—will probably have some kind of effect on your outlook or philosophy on life.

> *"I had three miscarriages before I finally had a baby. I told myself this is a gift and miracle from God. I am so thankful that he gave me one. After five years he blessed us again with another boy, who is now four months. I just prayed hard every night for a safe delivery, and God granted our prayers."*
> ~ Blanche, Arizona (She was very grateful for her cerclage baby and had another one on the way at the time of writing.)

> *"This is my first pregnancy where I have had to experience this, and yes it very hard, but I continue to think positively and pray."* ~ Natalie, Arizona

Makes You a Better Parent

This may sound a bit self-serving, but I really do believe that going through a difficult pregnancy makes you a better parent. Experiencing the death of a baby further heightens your awareness of the miracle of life. You gain that extra appreciation for the life you have created, of the precious gift of your baby, and of how lucky you are to have your children, knowing that there was the very real possibility of never getting to experience parenthood. You are less likely to take your kids for granted as a result.

The same holds true for those who decide to adopt their children after a loss or losses or because they are unable to have more kids.

Obviously, this is how I feel, and it's just my opinion, but I've heard from other women that they feel the same way.

The Best Advice of All...

"Remember, this difficult time in your life is only a snapshot in time. You can get through it...so many of us have."
~ Lisa, Florida

"STAY POSITIVE!" ~ Leslie, Florida

References

1. Ghosh JK, Wilhelm MH, Dunkel-Schetter C, et al. Paternal support and preterm birth, and the moderation of effects of chronic stress: A study in Los Angeles County mothers. *Arch Womens Ment Health* 2010;13(4):327–338.
2. A Mother's Emotions Affect Her Unborn Child, by James Goodlatte, http://www.naturalbabypros.com/mother%E2%80%99s-emotions-affect-her-unborn-child

CHAPTER 12

The Nuances of a High-Risk Pregnancy: Discharge, Pelvic Rest...Oh, the Delight!

Warning: To some, this chapter will seem like it's chock full of TMI (too much information). Don't skip it...girls, we all have to deal with this.

Oh, the Wonderful Delight of...Discharge

Yes, all pregnant women have some form of discharge during most, or portions, of their pregnancies. I'm guessing your doctors aren't going to go into detail about the fluids falling out of your body at each office visit or about what discharge is and the amount and texture you can expect. Nor are your girlfriends, who've already had children, going to say, "So, how are you feeling, and how's your discharge today?" I'll say it again; it's very important to keep a mental check on the "status" of your discharge at all times.

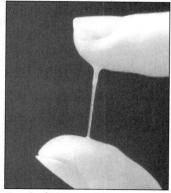

Cervical mucus. *Photo courtesy of Wikipedia.*

Changes can often be an early signal or indicator that something's up (although not always, so don't panic).

245

With my first pregnancy, I vividly remember being at work one day and noticing a lot more mucousy discharge after using the bathroom. Every time I peed, I saw a "string" of glob hanging. Being my first pregnancy, I didn't pay too much attention. I just thought, "Uh, this is what I have to expect when I'm prego. Yuck!"

The next day was a snowy day, which I just spent lounging on the couch. That night, my husband and I had sex, being the good wife that I am (hah). Afterwards, I noticed even more discharge. It was very "boogery," with a greenish tinge, but I still didn't give it much thought.

The next morning, a Saturday, I was reading *What to Expect When You're Expecting* and saw a passage in the preterm labor section that said something like, "Mucous discharge can be a sign of preterm labor."

I thought, "Oh, I guess I should call my midwife just to let her know." I called her, and she told me she would meet me at the hospital to check me while she was doing rounds. My husband and I really didn't think too much of it, so I moseyed into the shower, did my hair/makeup, and made my way to the hospital. As soon as I was in the stirrups and she peeked inside, I knew it was serious. Her face dropped, and she excused herself from the room.

I had been losing my mucous plug for several days. At that time, I didn't know we even had a mucous plug, never mind that this plug would fall out when our cervix began to thin and dilate. Located in a small corner, at the very back of my brain, is the thought that if only I'd realized this sooner, there's a chance my son would be alive today. Hindsight can be very damaging, but you can't beat yourself up over these things.

Many women experience an overall increase in discharge after the placement of a cerclage. The cerclage itself can cause irritation, which is compensated for by the body via the production of excess discharge. Not only do we have to go through the hassle of getting a string tied around our cervix, we also have to walk around with a soggy bottom because of it. Well, isn't that a kicker.

Don't fret, though; like anything to do with the human body, this is not an absolute. With my first cerclage I had tons of discharge, pretty much all day, every day, and especially after every bathroom trip. With my son, I had virtually no discharge until after the removal of my cer- clage, when I lost my mucous plug. I still was on a vigil, though, checking for changes throughout my entire pregnancy, ready to call my doctor upon the slightest change.

As most of the pregnancy books point out, if your discharge is green, brownish, or foul-smelling, call your doctor immediately, as this could be an indication of an infection. If you notice a slight blood-tinged discharge, called bloody show, call your doctor, as this could be a sign of cervical changes.

The takeaways for all you ladies are: 1) Pay attention to your discharge on a routine basis; 2) realize that what may have been normal for you in a previous pregnancy may not be the case this time around (i.e., normal for you last time could have been a lot of egg-white-like discharge, while this time you may have only spotty and thin discharge; every pregnancy is different); 3) if you do notice a change in the amount, color, or consistency, talk to your doctor about it; and 4) listen to and know your body.

Dealing with Hormones and a High-Risk Pregnancy Is One Nasty Combo

We all know that our hormones run rampant when we're pregnant. This is completely normal and part of the natural order of life. Now multiply those hormones, known as the "bitch hormones" of pregnancy, with the stresses of a high-risk pregnancy, and you get the picture…a recipe for disaster.

Honey, it's a rough ride. Hopefully, you've got not only a good, solid support system, but also a patient and understanding one. Don't be too hard on yourself. It's okay to let off some steam when you need to…just try not to become the exorcist, for your sake and that of your family and friends.

The Joy of Pelvic Rest: How to Cope

"Pelvic rest" makes it sound so mundane, so easy, simple, and effortless, but that's the term that's always used, so get used to it. The reality is—and you've heard it before—we're all sexual beings (our men more so than us, probably). Ladies, let's face up to the reality here: a high-risk pregnancy, more often than not, means NO sex. For many of us, this means for at least seven or maybe even eight months if you include the recommended post-delivery period abstinence of six weeks. Sure, there can be a small window of a week or two for some of us after the stitch is removed, or when we make it to term, but by that point, we're so huge and ready to burst that sex will be the last thing on our minds.

Chances are the lack of sex will have some sort of an impact on your life, anywhere from a minor annoyance to a major frustration. The odds are, if you have a husband/boyfriend or even a wife/girlfriend [lesbian lovers shouldn't be overlooked here, although I suspect it isn't as hard on them (no pun intended) as it would be on a guy, for obvious reasons], it will have a stronger impact on them than it will on you. What's important is for you to maintain intimacy with your partner, even if you can't experience vaginal intercourse.

In the following section, I discuss my experiences with pelvic rest and touch on some of the issues other women have discussed with me. First, a disclaimer: for any suggestions or scenarios I discuss, talk to your doctor first. Every situation, uterus, and cervix is different.

If you know about your condition prior to your pregnancy, you're somewhat better equipped to prepare yourself. Who am I kidding? Are you ever really prepared for a high-risk pregnancy and all the "things" that come with it? I guess you could treat your body like a gas tank and get your fill before pregnancy, although I think it would empty rather quickly when the going got tough. All the sex you had five months ago will be long forgotten.

Just so you know, I'm not some hot and horny little wifey. Maybe in my husband's dreams, but I'd like to think I'm just an average girl, one who has needs at times but often times could just as easily choose sleep over sex. He, on the other hand, like the vast majority of men, I suspect, needs it more than I have the energy to give it up. There were definitely a few points during my pregnancy when I was more excitable than normal, though; that whole wanting what you can't have thing.

It's natural for your partner—especially if you've had a prior bad outcome—to not even want to look at you too long in that way, so as to avoid engaging in any sort of sexual activity for fear of damaging your parts or hurting the baby. This often happens even before you hit the "no sex" point in your pregnancy. And, some men are simply turned off by the thought of their woman being with child, even if she's never had a loss or a pregnancy issue. My only advice is to try to not take it personally. Is that even possible? Turn to your girlfriends, so they can tell you how hot, sexy, and beautiful you are. (Your best girlfriend will do this, even if you look and feel like shit. She knows better than to be totally truthful with you when your hormones are raging.) Try to think, "Oh, how sweet, he doesn't want to hurt the baby."

For those men who've endured either a loss or a difficult pregnancy, their fear is understandable. These guys know too much. They understand the workings of a reproductive system gone wrong, while most men don't even hear the words cervix, amniotic membranes, or contractions until Lamaze classes. This was definitely the case with my husband. He was so freaked out that he didn't really want to have sex with me at all during my second, and especially my third, pregnancy, even early on when we were "allowed." To him, it wasn't worth the perceived risk. (Believe me, he was no saint about it, either; he had no problem complaining about it.)

For "normal" pregnancies, sex is not an issue. Women are encouraged to remain sexually active throughout. Pregnancy hormones can have wondrous effects on the female body and psyche. Many women have points in their pregnancy when they are totally repulsed by sex. This is totally normal, and can be due to fatigue, nausea, and sickness, our own unhappiness with our bodies, discomfort, etc. On the other hand, some women become hypersexual, craving sex all the time. This response seems to be less openly discussed in the media than the other, but it too is completely natural and normal. For a large number of women, sex during pregnancy is more exciting and leads to more sensitivity, both for the man, since your vaginal canal is "swollen," and for the woman. Countless women have had better and even more orgasms while pregnant. Unluckily for us, we'll never know what that's like…bummer.

Typically, most doctors allow vaginal intercourse through the first trimester for many of us. Preterm labor is less likely to start in the first trimester, so you may be free to play, but bleeding of any sort is a no-no for sex.

Unfortunately, for the approximately 50% of pregnant women who suffer from morning sickness and the 100% of us who suffer from extreme fatigue during this trimester, sex is the furthest thing from our minds. The time when we can have sex is precisely the time when we don't want it.

Why the no-sex clause in high-risk pregnancies? There are several reasons why we can't engage in sexual intercourse. One is that semen contains prostaglandins, the same prostaglandins that are released during labor, which leads to contractions and shortening/softening of the cervix. Having said that, I've heard of women whose doctors have given them the green light after a period of rest after cerclage placement, and of others who've been told that it's okay later in their pregnancy (past 24 or so weeks) to have sex. Have a discussion with your doc to see if and when he feels sex is okay in your particular situation.

Another point of concern is the possibility of infection. If you have a short and open cervix, broken waters, there's a greater potential for infection. "Normal" women (sorry to keep using that word) have long, closed cervixes with an intact mucous plug to protect them from infection; however, in those of us who are high risk, this may not be the case.

A third snag is the orgasm. Orgasm leads to spasms of the uterus and can potentially trigger "true" contractions. It's common for women who have an orgasm to experience contractions afterwards. Fortunately for them, these relatively weak contractions won't have any effect on their cervix, as it is strong and long, but we don't have that "luxury."

A final reason for many couples and doctors is the "why bother taking any risk" thing. There are still the unknown components in many of these conditions that lead to an early delivery, so for many it's better to be safe than sorry. For many couples and their doctors, the decision to suck it up and avoid sex is the best choice to help maintain peace of mind. Know that you are doing everything to ensure an on-time arrival of that baby. Remember, it may seem like forever, but it's not.

So, even though there can be no hot dog in the bun, you can still engage in other activities, depending on your situation. You can always make like you're back in high school and have a heavy make-out session. Maybe you can give/receive oral or external stimulation (probably minus an orgasm; see disclaimer). Hey, there's nothing wrong with settling for massages and foot rubs during this period. There are ways to get by. It may not always be easy, but it can be done. Trust me, I was a born-again virgin twice. At one point, we didn't have sex for like eight months!

The "Wet" Dream

Countless teen coming-of-age flicks have played out the plot of the sleeping zit-faced boy dreaming of a hot co-ed...and you know the rest of the story. However, I can't remember a time when I've seen or heard the female version discussed. This just doesn't seem to be an acceptable thing for women.

I can remember occasional times when I would wake from a dream in the midst of an orgasm and then drift happily back to sleep. Later, I would have only a vague memory of it happening, but I was definitely in a better mood that day.

With my first, unsuccessful pregnancy, I have no memories of any orgasmic dreams. Fast forward to my pregnancy with my daughter, and while some would say I was lucky, I kid you not when I say I had at least half a dozen a week, sometimes two a night. I was so stressed out about this, but what are you supposed to do...not sleep? I only hoped that my "dream" orgasms were somehow different from the "real" ones and somehow less traumatic to my cervix. I never had the nerve to talk to my doctor about it. How embarrassing.

I don't know what it was...maybe the fact that I was unable to have sex, that I was completely and utterly crazed and stressed out, or that I was dealing with all the extra estrogen from the baby girl I was carrying, but I won't lie, it was kind of awesome. (Strangely, when I was pregnant for the third time with a boy, I can't remember having even one "wet" dream.)

The next morning, I would feel so guilty about it that I would be angry at myself. What if I lost the baby because of these orgasms? But what was I supposed to do? It's not like I was watching porn or anything. Some of you may be chuckling, while others know what I'm talking about. So, ladies, there's not much you can do, other than try to enjoy them while they last. (I haven't had one in several years now, so I guess those days are over.)

Taking One for the Team

Often, there comes a time when we women have to just suck it up and satisfy our partners. I guess this statement will infuriate some women. How dare I suggest this! We're the ones carrying the baby, our bodies are being stretched, we feel sick, our hormones are rampant, not to mention the enormous burden of stress we're dealing with every second of the day. Believe me, I know all this, but I'm standing my ground. Sometimes, a good old blow job will do the trick. Sure, it does nothing for you, unless you're one of the few women who actually enjoy giving one and gets excited by it. Hey, good for you.

This takes care of things on a few different fronts. First, it will help relieve stress in your partner and reduce that sex-deprived attitude, which, no matter how hard they try to control it, seems to gradually escalate until it eventually becomes major crankiness. Hey, if you do this for him, he may be willing to rub your feet more often (or even at all), make you a nice dinner of your favorite food, or even run out for ice cream at three in the morning.

Second, it may help you to experience/maintain a level of intimacy in your relationship. I know it sounds cheesy, but it's necessary, especially during this nerve-wracking time. I can remember when I was pregnant with my daughter, my husband asking me for a BJ. My first thought was, "F-You! Here I am lying here day after day, only getting up to use the bathroom, scared out of my wits that my baby's going to fall out at any time, and you want me to do what?" Eventually, though, I thought about it from his point of view and gave in. (I at least made sure he positioned himself so there was no bending involved and I could be comfortable.) It definitely helped to curb his crankiness, although this didn't become a regular occurrence; I'm not that nice.

The third and maybe the best point is, after "the act," you can turn around and rub it back in: "Even when I was on bed rest, I was there for you." I'm a fraud, really, because I didn't heed my own advice during my third pregnancy. I was too busy dealing with a toddler, working, and trying to stay sane and enjoy my pregnancy to look out for my partner. Sorry about that, dear.

> **Warning: I DO NOT condone my actions, or suggest in any way that you do what I did and cheat on pelvic rest. Every person and situation is different.**

Okay, I admit it; I did cheat, a little bit, when I was on pelvic rest. One time, while carrying my daughter, and I barely consider it cheating, I received oral and, gasp, had an orgasm. I had made it over my first hump and was around 26 weeks. Prior to that time, I could barely let out my breath for fear that I would lose the baby.

My husband thought it would be good for me to relax, so I agreed to it, and I'm not going to lie; it was awesome to have sexual contact again. Afterwards, I felt so guilty about getting oral, no penetration involved, and even guiltier about having an orgasm, but it was a nice break from the stress of everything going on. I remember it being something that helped bring us back together, even though it was for only 5 or 10 minutes. Note: it's important to avoid blowing air into the vagina, as this can cause major problems through what's called an air embolism. So, now you know…I'm not perfect, but you probably figured that out already.

With my second son, I had a preventative cerclage and no bed rest, and knowing what to expect made his pregnancy a lot less stressful. We'd stopped having sex weeks before we theoretically had to, out of fear and wanting to be extra cautious. Most doctors say that you can maintain normal sexual activities until the second trimester, but double-check with your doctor. Bleeding, high blood pressure (like in preeclampsia, if you develop it this early), and other conditions obviously change the playing field for this one.

During this pregnancy, I was much weaker in the face of temptation than in the previous one, and there were a couple times later in my pregnancy when we, how shall I say this, played around a little. I'm not sure if you're familiar with those vibrating rings you put on the guy to add to both your pleasure, but we used one of these at the tip to stop penetration. It was just enough for both of us to get pleasure out of it and, technically, involved minimal to no penetration. (We also used a condom.)

If you suffer from preterm labor, orgasms of any kind aren't recommended. An orgasm causes the uterus to contract and can lead to further uterine irritability and contractions. Also, you should never allow semen to enter your vagina, because of the possibility of infection or the triggering of contractions, so condoms are recommended. For obvious reasons, if you have ruptured membranes, bleeding, etc., you have now been committed to becoming a nun, temporarily.

My advice, if you're suffering from "pelvic rest syndrome," is that there may be safe ways to "cheat" or to cheat minimally. I know it's embarrassing, but you can talk to your doc; they've heard it all before, trust me. I cheated a little because I felt I had to do it. I tried to hold off until a good gestation and not go completely crazy, but a girl's gotta do what a girl's gotta do.

Straining During Pooping

If you have a short cervix, a cerclage, or even if you're struggling with preterm labor, high blood pressure, or bleeding, you may have a fear of bowel movements. I know I did. In my case I wanted to avoid disturbing that precious piece of string, my insides, and all that at all costs. If it isn't bad enough that you already suffer the normal effects of pregnancy, namely constipation, and have the joy of working very hard for just rabbit-like turds, you now have to worry about this.

We try to avoid straining during bowel movements to avoid excess pressure in that area and the rare possibility of doing damage, like to our cerclage. Bed rest can compound the number-two issue even further, because lying around all day does little to get the bowels moving, so I think it's pretty safe to say that many of us high-risk women struggle double-time with going to the bathroom. It's nothing to be embarrassed about, though…it happens.

So, what can you do to avoid this? All the normal stuff that's recommended for all pregnant women applies to you as well. Drink lots of water; eight to ten 8-ounce glasses daily is recommended. You can substitute some of that water with juice if you get sick of water. Eat plenty of fiber, including grains and cereals, along with fruits and vegetables. Prunes are always an option, too, you know. For those of you banned from any sort of exercise, you actually have to work against gravity to get things moving. If you need a little extra help, talk to your doctor about getting a prescription for a stool softener like Colace.

It also helps if you try to relax while you're on the toilet. Take your time. Read a book or magazine, or maybe listen to some music or meditate. If you're really struggling—and I know it sounds weird, but it worked for me—try to visualize something happening down there. You don't have to be too graphic. This will just help you ease up and relax. Try not to put too much pressure on yourself to "perform." You want to minimize pushing and straining. It may be uncomfortable, but you can always come back and try again later.

CHAPTER 13

17Alpha-Hydroxyprogesterone Caproate (i.e., 17P) to Prevent Preterm Birth. Say That Two Times Fast

Unlike the ginormous gray area around cerclages, who to place them in, when the right time is, and whether or not they truly work, the use of progesterone to reduce preterm birth in women with a history of spontaneous preterm delivery is well documented and researched. It is now widely used by doctors to help prevent and reduce preterm deliveries.

In a large multi-centered trial, 17P showed a reduction of preterm birth by a whopping 33% in a group of HIGH-RISK women. Note the caps...high-risk women. This is important. These are some great odds in our favor, for once. This drug provides a chance of reducing the risk of your baby coming early by more than 30%.[1] Not bad.

The downside is that there is limited pharmacologic data available, which means, reading between the lines, they aren't sure exactly how it works. Recently, they discovered that fetal liver cells have been shown to metabolize 17P.[1] Another study found that it improves fetal circulation by dilating the blood vessels.[2]

In a survey of obstetricians/gynecologists, 74% replied that they recommend or offer progesterone to prevent early birth. Most of them, 93%, use it in women who have had a prior spontaneous preterm birth. Around 30% also use it for dilated/effaced cervices, short cervices confirmed through ultrasound, or in women with cerclages.[3]

In another survey looking at whether published studies on the benefits of 17P had any impact on its use, they found that 67% of doctors reported the use of progesterone to prevent spontaneous preterm birth compared to only 38% at two years prior. They noted, however, that although usage had increased over this period, "there remain a substantial number of nonusers." Researchers also found that doctors tend to use it for reasons not yet proven in clinical trials.[4]

So, what does this say? 1) More doctors are using it than in the past. 2) A lot of doctors are using it, but **ALL** doctors should be considering it for woman at risk of an early baby. 3) Most doctors are using it in women where it has been shown to be effective—i.e., in high-risk women. 4) Some doctors are using it for reasons other than those where it has been proven to work.

Another study concluded that, "A substantial proportion of eligible women are not being offered progesterone for the prevention of preterm birth."[5] So, if your provider doesn't bring it up, you should. Make sure you understand why you are not a candidate for 17P or their reasoning against offering it, especially if you're in a high-risk category. It's all right to question, and if you aren't satisfied with the answer, a second opinion is always an option, even if only to make you feel better about your doctor's decision.

Typically, injections of 17P are started at about 16 weeks, after the formation of all the major organs in the developing baby. Studies found that initiation of 17P treatment at a later gestation (21–26.9 weeks) was just as effective as starting it at 16–20.9 weeks.[6,7]

More Studies

A random, double-blinded, placebo-controlled—i.e., a well-designed—study found that in women with a documented history of preterm birth, weekly injections of 17P until delivery or 36 weeks gestation showed a reduction in births before 37 weeks of 19%, a 10% reduction in delivery before 35 weeks, and an 8% reduction in delivery at less than 32 weeks. Interestingly, the babies of the treated women had substantially lower incidences of necrotizing enterocolitis, intraventricular hemorrhage, and the need for additional oxygen.[8]

Another study that looked at the efficacy of vaginal progesterone suppositories in high-risk women confirmed the previous one. Overall, preterm birth rates were 13.8% in the progesterone group and 28.5% in the placebo group. More women in the placebo group (18.5%) delivered before 34 weeks than in the progesterone group (2.7%). They also monitored uterine contractions weekly in all women and found that 23.6% of the progesterone group had "uterine activity," while in the placebo group it was more than double, at 54.3%.[9]

In a study I found quite interesting, they randomized women with short cervices (less than or equal to 2.5 cm) on ultrasound to receive either a McDonald cerclage or weekly injections of 17P. Spontaneous preterm birth before 35 weeks occurred in 38.1% of the women with cerclages and 43.2% of the 17P ladies. Analysis of these numbers showed that, statistically speaking, there was no significant difference in preterm birth between the two groups. (The 17P appeared just as effective as the string.)

When they looked at the women with 1.5 cm or less of cervix, however, they found a reduction in preterm birth in women with cerclages compared to those who received 17P shots.[10] The takeaway here is that if you have a short cervix and are a candidate for a cerclage, you and your doctor should still consider a cerclage.

Another study supporting the benefit of the use of progesterone looked at vaginal suppositories given between 24 and 34 weeks that were either progesterone or a placebo. Progesterone greatly reduced the preterm labor rate, 25% vs. 46.7%. Also, more women in the placebo group delivered early.[11]

It should be noted that, "Women receiving 17P prophylaxis [treatment] remain at increased risk for PTL [preterm labor] and preterm birth." This study sought to determine which high-risk women receiving 17P treatment would still develop preterm labor at less than 34 weeks. They found that this occurred in 22.9% of women receiving it.

Of the women with preterm labor, another early baby happened in 73.3%. Those with more than one previous early delivery were more likely to again deliver early.[12]

So, here it is again; if you have a history of preterm delivery, you're at an increased risk of delivering early again. It makes sense, even though it sucks. The key is to work with your doctor, know your history, and have the best plan in place to help you carry to as close to term as possible.

In a study that looked at the economics, they found that universal cervical length screening via ultrasound—i.e., screening EVERYONE for cervical length—and then treatment with vaginal progesterone, was the most cost-effective approach and provided the highest reduction in preterm births before 34 weeks compared to cervical-length screening in high-risk women along with vaginal progesterone, treatment with P17 in high-risk women with no screening, and no screening or treatment. They estimated that this preferred approach could lead to a reduction of 95,920 preterm births annually in the U.S. alone.[13] I'm not sure how they figured this out, but it sounds good to me, and so I think everyone should be screened. Even if just one family can be spared the pain of losing their baby or having their baby too soon, it's worth it.

It should be noted that progesterone is not suggested for use in women who are already experiencing preterm labor.[14]

Can 17P Stop My Cervix From Shrinking?

The "goodish" news on this is…well, yes…kind of. There's a study that looked at this, too, of course. In 547 women with a history of preterm birth, the women receiving progesterone had much less cervical shortening, showing an average of 1.6 mm more cervical length. In those women who had early shortening upon entry into the study (104 women), those who took 17P retained an average of 3.3 mm more cervical length than those in the non-treatment group. They concluded that vaginal progesterone (i.e., suppositories) helps to keep and maintain cervical length in high-risk women.[15]

A large, well-designed study of 24,620 women who were being seen for routine prenatal care came to a similar conclusion—i.e., that progesterone reduces spontaneous preterm birth in women with a short cervix. Although they were not specifically looking at length, as they were focused on preterm birth rates, the physics of birth state that if your length is maintained, you won't—really you can't, deliver early. The importance of this type of study is that we know that women who have a short cervix mid-pregnancy have a much greater chance of delivering their babies early. Keeping that length = good.

The preterm birth rate in the progesterone group was 19% versus 34% in the no-progesterone (i.e., placebo) group. They also found that there were no serious side effects from using this drug. Realistically, a cervix of 1.5 cm or less was only seen in 1.7% of all women,[16] so again, this type of thing is rare in the big picture.

Do I Still Need to Take It If I Have a Cerclage?

When comparing women with cerclages who had weekly 17P injections to those who had a cerclage and daily outpatient nursing surveillance only (i.e., no 17P injections), they found no difference in preterm delivery rates at either less than 37 weeks or less than 35 weeks. The number of women who suffered premature rupture of membranes was also the same in each group, around 8%.

They did, however, find that the women who were monitored daily were more likely to be diagnosed with preterm labor—about 25% more likely. Based on this, the authors concluded that any benefit to giving 17P to women who have cerclages still needs to be determined.[17]

The use of progesterone in women with a short cervix is not well supported or recommended, and it's unclear whether a cerclage combined with progesterone works better than a cerclage alone.[16] Hey, I'm not against a little extra protection, so if I had a cerclage and my doctor wants to give me P17, would I object? Probably not.

How Do I Take This Stuff?

There are two ways of receiving P17: vaginal suppositories (daily or weekly) or injections into the muscle (typically weekly and in the butt). The preferred method is actually injection, since this route is better supported by the research.

I had weekly injections of this stuff during my second pregnancy when my cervix starting shortening at about 17 or so weeks. I ended up with an ultrasound-indicated cerclage at 21 weeks and continued to take it until around 34 weeks. I didn't take it during my pregnancy with my second son, when I received a preventative cerclage.

I can tell you, this stuff is thick and is typically given in castor oil. My mom had to give me my shots in the ass, switching cheeks every other week, and it was so thick she had to use all her strength to force it out of the syringe. It really wasn't much fun; it stung like hell and left me with huge welts on my hiney, like I'd been sitting on a fat wallet located under my skin.

My advice to you is to use lots of warm compresses and to massage the injection site to help it spread and help the material to be absorbed into your system. Also, many spouses may not feel comfortable sticking a needle in your behind, so hopefully your doctor is close by (mine wasn't), or a friend or relative you trust is available to help out. I wouldn't suggest forcing someone who's a bit queasy with needles, and you really need someone with a strong, steady arm.

I had permanent marks and bruises on my butt cheeks for a couple years after I had my daughter, but for me it was well worth it. I would have tried anything and everything to keep my baby baking as long as possible. A little shot once a week is the least of your problems. Seriously, it only stung for a minute or two after the injection.

Given all the stuff we have to go through to have our babies, we all deserve medals!

Cochrane Reviews

1. They identified some "beneficial effects, including prolongation of pregnancy" but concluded that more research is needed, specifically on the benefits and harms.[19]

2. Progesterone seems to help reduce miscarriage in women with recurrent miscarriages.[20]

3. There is not enough evidence for the use of progesterone for treating women who have a threatened miscarriage (bleeding with a closed cervix).[21]

"My Braxton Hicks feel like my uterus is balling up. Even from around 13–14 weeks, I could feel the outline of a perfect tight ball in my lower pelvic area during them. With my successful cerclage pregnancy, I took 17P injections that helped so much with the contractions. I could tell when I was due for my shot because the contractions would get more frequent and stronger the day before!" ~ Janna, Ohio

References

1. Sharma S, Ellis EC, Dorko K, et al. Metabolism of 17 {alpha}-hydroxyprogesterone caproate, an agent for preventing pre-term birth, by fetal hepatocytes. *Drug Metab Dispos* 2010;38(5):723–727.
2. Barda G, Ben-Haroush A, Barkat J, et al. Effect of vaginal progesterone, administered to prevent preterm birth, on impedance to blood flow in fetal and uterine circulation. *Ultrasound Obstet Gynecol* 2010;36(6):743–748.
3. Henderson ZT, Power ML, Berghella V, et al. Attitudes and practices regarding use of progesterone to prevent preterm births. *Am J Perinatol* 2009;26(7):529–536.
4. Ness A, Dias T, Damus K, et al. Impact of the recent randomized trials on the use of progesterone to prevent preterm birth: a 2005 follow-up survey. *Am J Obstet Gynecol* 2006;195(4):1174–1179.
5. Bailit JL, Berkowitz R, Thorp JM, et al. Use of progesterone to prevent preterm birth at a tertiary care center. *J Reprod Med* 2007;52(4):280–284.
6. How HY, Barton JR, Istwan NB, et al. Prophylaxis with 17 alpha-hydroxyprogesterone caproate for prevention of recurrent preterm delivery: does gestational age at initiation of treatment matter? *Am J Obstet Gynecol* 2007;197(3):260 e1–4.
7. González-Quintero VH, Istwan NB, Rhea DJ, et al. Gestational age at initiation of 17alpha-hydroxyprogesterone caproate (17P) and recurrent preterm delivery. *J Matern Fetal Neonatal Med* 2007;20(3):249–252.
8. Meis PJ, Klebanoff M, Thom E, et al. Prevention of recurrent preterm delivery by 17 alpha-hydroxyprogesterone caproate. *N Engl J Med* 2003;348:2379–2385.
9. Fonseca EB, Bittar RE, Carvalho MH, Zugaib M. Prophylactic administration of progesterone by vaginal suppository to reduce the incidence of spontaneous preterm birth in women at increased risk: a randomized placebo-controlled double-blind study. *Am J Obstet Gynecol* 2003;188:419–424.
10. Keeler SM, Kiefer D, Rochon M, et al. A randomized trial of cerclage vs. 17 alpha-hydroxyprogesterone caproate for treatment of short cervix. *J Perinat Med* 2009;37(5):473–479.
11. Cetingoz E, Cam C, Sakalli M, et al. Progesterone effects on preterm birth in high-risk pregnancies: a randomized placebo-controlled trial. *Arch Gynecol Obstet* 2011;283(3):423–429.
12. Joy S, Rhea DJ, Istwan NB, et al. The risk for preterm labor in women receiving 17 alpha-hydroxyprogesterone caproate prophylaxis for preterm birth prevention. *Am J Perinatol.* 2010;27(4):343–348.

13. Cahill AG, Odibo AO, Caughey AB, et al. Universal cervical length screening and treatment with vaginal progesterone to prevent preterm birth: a decision and economic analysis. *Am J Obstet Gynecol* 2010;202(6):548 e1–8.
14. Berghella V. *Preterm Birth: Prevention & Management.* West Sussex, UK. Wiley-Blackwell, 2010.
15. O'Brien JM, Defranco EA, Adair CD, et al. Effect of progesterone on cervical shortening in women at risk for preterm birth: secondary analysis from a multinational, randomized, double-blind, placebo-controlled trial. *Ultrasound Obstet Gynecol* 2009;34(6):653–659.
16. Fonseca EB, Celik E, Parra M, et al. Progesterone and the risk of preterm birth among women with a short cervix. *N Engl J Med* 2007;357(5):462–469.
17. Rebarber A, Cleary-Goldman J, Istwan NB, et al. The use of 17 alpha-hydroxyprogesterone caproate (17P) in women with cervical cerclage. *Am J Perinatol* 2008;25(5):271–275.
18. National Public Radio, http://www.npr.org/templates/story/story.php?storyId=134400300.
19. Dodd JM, Flenady V, Cincotta R, Crowther CA. Prenatal administration of progesterone for preventing preterm birth in women considered to be at risk of preterm birth. *Cochrane Database of Systematic Reviews* 2006, Issue 1. Art. No.: CD004947. (Last assessed as up-to-date: April 15, 2010.)
20. Haas DM, Ramsey PS. Progesterone for preventing miscarriage. *Cochrane Database of Systematic Reviews* 2008, Issue 2. Art. No.: CD003511. (Last assessed as up-to-date: April 15, 2010.)
21. Wahabi HA, Abed Althagafi NF, Elawad M, Al Zeidan RA. Progesterone for treating threatened miscarriage. *Cochrane Database of Systematic Reviews* 2007, Issue 3. Art. No.: CD005943. (Last assessed as up-to-date: April 15, 2010.)

CHAPTER 14

Fetal Fibro...Huh?
Figuring Out Risk

Fibronectin is a protein released by the baby's membranes. It can only be found, in very low levels, less than 50 ng/mL, in cervico-vaginal secretions between 22 and 34 weeks. It IS normal to find this protein between 20 and 22 weeks, and then again after 37 weeks of pregnancy. This is why testing is done between 22 and 34 weeks of gestation, when it wouldn't be expected to be present.[1] When swabbing of the cervix confirms the presence of fetal fibronectin (FFN) after 22 weeks, a link to preterm birth has been shown to exist.[2]

FFN testing is another "tool" that is often used by doctors to help predict and manage preterm birth. Its use in predicting an early delivery is a relatively recent development, having been discovered in 1991 and approved for use by the Food and Drug Administration (FDA) in 1995. Testing costs around $200 per swab in the U.S.[1]

A high level—i.e., ≥50 ng/mL—of FFN in the cervicovaginal secretions between the target weeks increases the possibility of a preterm birth. Notice the word "possibility." The ability to detect FFN in order to accurately determine the chance of a preemie is currently only about 56%. This number even varies according to how far along you are at the time of swabbing, whether you are high versus low risk (for preterm delivery), and the number of swabs performed.[3] It is best used to predict labor within 7–10 days of the test.[1]

While this test is used to help predict the likelihood of delivering early, it is not the be-all and end-all of testing. It's more like a scientifically based crystal ball. They have found that the positive (having your baby early) and negative (not having your baby early) predictive ability varies greatly. Theoretically, a positive result, indicating the presence of FFN, means that you're more likely to deliver within the next two weeks, while a negative result means that you're not likely to deliver. A negative swab is more accurate than a positive result, as false positives are often observed.

Here is the interesting, and most important, thing to remember about FFN swabbing. A negative result has more weight and should give you more confidence/peace of mind than a positive result. "Huh?" you say.

Here's what the researchers have found. The ability of a positive swab to predict preterm delivery ranges from roughly 9% to 46%.[3] Wow, that's a big range—a 9% or even a 46% degree of confidence that a positive result will lead to preterm delivery is not that strong. I think I like those odds. It's not like they're saying, "Sorry you've had a positive FFN test, and research has shown that 80% of women with a positive result will deliver prematurely."

Remember this when you're anxiously waiting for the phone call with your results. Based on what I said before, try not to lose too much sleep over a positive test result. A large number of you who have had a positive swab will still have a baby on board in two weeks' time.

On the flip side, the ability of a negative swab to predict that you will NOT deliver within the next two weeks is greater than 90% in most cases.[3] As my doctor put it to me bluntly while I was getting my coochie swabbed, "A positive swab is not necessarily a bad thing. Most women who have a positive FFN are still pregnant in two weeks. You can *really* feel confident if it comes back negative."

This doesn't mean that just because your FFN test is negative you can start vacuuming, doing jumping jacks, and cease bed rest. Use this knowledge to help push you over the next hump. Maybe this little bit of comfort will help your morale and even help you retain a little more of your sanity in order to survive this pregnancy.

A leading expert in preterm birth, Dr. Vincenzo Berghella, states that further research to validate FFN use to accurately predict early babies is necessary before it is routinely used in everyday OB/GYN practice. He believes there is lack of sufficient proof in the current research to support the use of FFN testing in *asymptomatic* women who have had a prior preterm birth. He even goes on to say that in trials, common treatments to prevent preterm birth, such as bed rest and tocolysis (drugs to stop contractions), have not benefited women, even before the era of FFN testing, and so these should not be assumed to work when a positive FFN is found until they are proven effective through proper clinical trials.[4] Again, in preterm birth, there are too many unknowns to count.

A benefit of FFN testing is when it is used in women who are having symptoms of preterm birth before 34 weeks—i.e., those who are *symptomatic*. In one study, they found a reduction in preterm births from 36% to 13% in women who had transvaginal ultrasound (TVU) cervical-length measurements and FFN testing. Those who had lengths of less than 2.0 cm, or between 2.0 and 2.9 cm and a positive FFN swab, were admitted to the hospital, and given steroids to help with the baby's lung development and tocolysis to stop contractions.[5] As Dr. Berghella points out, there is no way of knowing which treatment or combination of treatments was effective after a positive FFN was observed in this study.[4]

How Is FFN Testing Performed?

Basically, FFN testing is like a pap smear, but with less scraping. The doctor will perform a quick swabbing and sample from the back area of the vagina. The manufacturer and the Food and Drug Administration (FDA) advise that a speculum—yes, the wonderful speculum—should be used so as to actually be able to see the exact location when sampling. Most of the research on FFN testing has been done when using a speculum.[4] (They call this "direct visualization.")

"Blind" swabbing, done without using a speculum, is not yet approved by the FDA, but research has found higher than a 95% agreement in the results when swabbing is done with or without one.[6]

Blind sampling also has a "high negative predictive value" (94.1%).[7] Having said that, of the many FFN swabs I have had during two of my pregnancies, they never once used a speculum. It was interesting to find out during my research that this practice went against the approved method of sampling. Swab results generally take as little as one hour.

The MOST important thing to remember is that FFN swabbing must come first, prior to an internal check or TVU. Sometimes, they forget that you're due for an FFN swab until it's too late, in which case you'll have to come back the next day for swabbing. It's in your best interest, unless you like going to the doctors, to mention this to the doc prior to any other internal exams. I had to remind a doc once in order to save me another 100-mile trip the next day. Hey, they're only human.

A positive test has been shown to be linked to vaginal bleeding, sexual activity, or vaginal/cervical examination within 24 hours of the test. These could all give you a false positive. Also, cervical dilation and contractions have been linked to positives.[8]

A small study found that vaginal ultrasounds did not cause the body to produce fetal fibronectin and did not lead to false positive results. Based on this, they argue that this goes against the conventional knowledge of FFN testing. According to them, ultrasound testing may be performed first, and if a short cervix is detected, then FFN testing can be performed.[9]

The following can lead to false positive results:[1]

1. Gel (like that used on the probe of the ultrasound)
2. Sex (sperm can throw off the results)
3. Manual (use of fingers) cervical exams
4. Presence of blood
5. Amniotic fluid

Remember, current practice is that FFN must come first!

Who Are the Best Candidates?[1]

According to Dr. Berghella, women who are in the intermediate cervical measurement range of 2.0–2.9 cm are the best candidates, and testing is most meaningful to them.[4] A positive FFN test in this situation can help determine appropriate treatments to prepare for the possibility of a premature baby—e.g., steroids to help speed up lung development. From previous chapters, we know that the likelihood of a preterm birth and cervical length are inversely related (the shorter the length, the higher the chance of an early baby). A woman with a long cervix would not realistically need FFN testing, as her chance of delivering within a week or so is very low.

To many, it is not realistic or cost-effective to screen asymptomatic women whether they are low or high risk, as there is no clearly defined treatment presently available. If such a wonderful, miraculous treatment did get discovered, then screening could be easily justified.

In low-risk women with no symptoms of an impending early birth, the combination of length and FFN results is the best way to determine if she is likely to have her baby early. In women carrying twins, studies have shown the FFN test to be generally useless, with doctors preferring to use cervical length to help determine the risk in multiples.

You must also have intact membranes (remember, the presence of amniotic fluid can lead to a false positive), dilation of less than 3 cm (anything over this and there really isn't a point, as delivery in the near future is very possible), and finally, a gestational age between 22 and 34 weeks, as I stated before.

Can Antibiotics Help Women with a Positive FFN?[10]

Researchers looked at whether antibiotics could reduce preterm delivery in women in the second trimester who were free of symptoms but had positive fetal fibronectin tests. (This was a randomized and controlled study, the gold standard of study design.) They screened over 16,000 women, found that 6.6% had a positive swab, and concluded that the women in the antibiotic group had the same level of preterm birth rates as other women—i.e., the antibiotics appeared to offer no benefit.

What About Those with a Cerclage?

Does having a cerclage alter or disrupt FFN testing, or, if you have a positive FFN, will your cerclage prevent preterm delivery?

One study examined how accurate FFN testing was in women who had cerclages and who had no symptoms of preterm labor between 23 and 28 weeks, compared to those who didn't have a cerclage. They found that high-risk women who had cerclages were more likely to have a false positive test. Both groups of women had a very high—i.e., greater than 98%—negative predictive value,[11] meaning that women with a negative result didn't deliver within the following two weeks 98% of the time.

In another study where FFN swabbing was done following shortening and/or funneling of the cervix which randomized the women to get an ultrasound-indicated cerclage or not, the preterm birth rate (prior to 35 weeks) was 44% in FFN-positive women with a cerclage versus 55% in the FFN-positive women with no cerclage. The rate was only about 17% in both of those who had a negative test, regardless of a cerclage or not. The authors felt that "FFN testing before an ultrasound-indicated cerclage aids in counseling patients, anticipating the outcome of pregnancies complicated by cervical shortening"[12]

FFN Testing Combined with Cervical-Length Checks: The Way to Go[1]

A combination of both a fetal fibronectin swab test and a transvaginal ultrasound cervical-length check can do wonders to help your doctors determine not only your risk, but the best course of treatment. For us, above all else, it can also provide great peace of mind.

They have found that in high-risk women with a prior early birth, a length of more than 3.5 cm and a negative FFN test at 22 to 24 weeks means less than a 10% risk of delivering early again in this pregnancy. Yippee! If you fall into this category, you know you are pretty good to go this time.

On the other hand, if you have a length of less than 2.5 cm and a positive FFN test at the same gestation time, your chances of delivering early jump to more than 60%. That stinks.

They have determined that if you're experiencing symptoms (contractions), have a short cervix (less than 2.5 cm), *and* have a positive FFN, there's a 75% chance that your baby will come within the week. Look at the flip side, though; you still have a 25% chance of not having your baby so soon, even with all that going on.

Let's consider that you're asymptomatic but have a short cervix and a positive FFN test. You still have around a 40% chance of having your baby full term. This 60% or so risk of delivering early doesn't mean that all those babies are born at 24 or 25 weeks. That number includes babies born at good gestations that have great survival rates and a low likelihood of disabilities when born in hospitals with the proper facilities.

It's good to know your chances of an early arrival so you can be prepared, just in case. They can give you steroids or move you to a better hospital if need be. It's better for your doctors to know about this possibility and be able to prepare for it, rather than simply taking a stab in the dark, right?

The Good and the Not-So-Good

+ Length of greater than 3.0 cm = no worries! Your baby isn't coming now, or even soon.

+ Length of between 2.0 and 3.0 cm = use FFN results to help determine treatment options (negative swab, good to go; positive swab, see below).

+ Length of less than 2.0 cm, or 2.0–3.0 cm and a positive swab = you need to be monitored closely. Your doc should decide whether it's time for corticosteroids, transfer to a better hospital, and/or meds to stop contractions.

Key Things to Know[1]

1. FFN is the best test available today to predict preterm birth.

2. An even better (and more accurate) way to predict an early birth is an FFN test AND a cervical-length check via a transvaginal ultrasound. (You have a 35-fold greater chance of an early birth at less than 32 weeks if you have a positive FFN test and a cervical length of less than 2.5 cm.)

3. A negative swab is a better predictor than a positive swab in women experiencing symptoms of preterm labor.

   • With a negative swab, they're pretty damn sure that the baby isn't coming soon. With a positive swab, they're only slightly (about 20%) confident that your little one will be making an entrance within the next week or so.

4. A major problem is, even with a positive FFN test and/or a short cervix, they're still not sure which treatments are best to stop an early birth.

In Summary

The main point here is…DO NOT GO CRAZY STRESSING OVER A POSITIVE TEST. You are most likely not going to deliver. The odds are on your side, even if you have a positive test, as false positives are common. Remember, only 10% of women who are showing signs of delivering early actually give birth within the following seven days, and almost 75% will actually carry to full term. These are very good odds.

The best part of FFN testing is that a negative can give both you and your doctor peace of mind. Let this test help reduce your fear and stress levels, at least for a week or so until the next round of swabbing. A negative swab means that you almost certainly won't deliver in the immediate future, so any treatments can be withheld, even if you have symptoms of preterm labor. This prevents any unnecessary treatments—at least, it should.

If you do have a positive FFN test, most likely you will receive steroids (if you haven't already) to help speed up your baby's lung maturation just in case you deliver soon. Also, if you aren't already on bed rest or pelvic rest, you can bet these will be discussed with you. Complete bed rest may not even be a sure thing, but you can probably assume that if you're one of the few who has been living with no restrictions, you will now have restrictions. Of course, all this depends on how far along you are. There is a big difference, and rightly so, in attitudes when you are 25 weeks versus 33 weeks.

FFN testing is mostly a tool to help determine your care, and for assurance. I can tell you, getting that call to tell you that your test was negative produces a huge sigh of relief. It's one less thing to worry about. You should always sleep better after a negative test, but like I said before, a positive test doesn't mean the end is surely here.

References

1. Berghella V. *Preterm Birth: Prevention & Management*. West Sussex, UK. *Wiley-Blackwell* 2010.
2. Peaceman AM, Andrews WW, Thorp JM, et al. Fetal fibronectin as a predictor of preterm birth in patients with symptoms: a multicenter trial. *Am J Obstet Gynecol* 1997;177:13–18.
3. Honest H, Bachmann LM, Gupta JK, et al. Accuracy of cervicovaginal fetal fibronectin test in predicting risk of spontaneous preterm birth: systematic review. *BMJ* 2002;325:301–308.
4. Berghella, V. MFM Consult: Fetal fibronectin: When should you screen patients? *Contemporary OB/GYN* 2009.
5. Ness A, Visintine J, Ricci E, et al. Does knowledge of cervical length and fetal fibronectin affect management of women with preterm labor? A randomized trial. *Am J Obstet Gynecol* 2007;197(426):e1–e7.
6. Stafford IP, Garite TJ, Dildy GA, et al: A comparison of speculum and nonspeculum collection of cervicovaginal specimens for fetal fibronectin testing. *Am J Obstet Gynecol* 2008;199(131):e1–e4.
7. Roman AS, Koklanaris N, Paidas MJ, et al. "Blind" vaginal fetal fibronectin as a predictor of spontaneous preterm delivery. *Obstet Gynecol* 2005;105(2):285–289.
8. Lukes AS, Thorp JM Jr, Eucker B, Pahel-Short L. Predictors of positivity for fetal fibronectin in patients with symptoms of preterm labor. *Am J Obstet Gynecol* 1997;176:639–641.
9. Ben-Haroush A, Poran E, Yogev Y, Glezerman M. Vaginal fetal fibronectin evaluation before and immediately after ultrasonographic vaginal cervical length measurements in symptomatic women at risk of preterm birth: a pilot study. *J Matern Fetal Neonatal Med* 2010;23(8):854–856.

10. Andrews WW, Sibai BM, Thom EA, et al. Randomized clinical trial of metronidazol plus erythromycin to prevent spontaneous preterm delivery in fetal fibronectin-positive women. *Obstet Gynecol* 2003;101(5 pt 1):847–855.

11. Duhig KE, Chandiramani M, Seed PT, et al. Fetal fibronectin as a predictor of spontaneous preterm labour in asymptomatic women with a cervical cerclage. *BJOG* 2009;116(6):799–803.

12. Keeler SM, Roman AS, Coletta JM, et al. Fetal fibronectin testing in patients with short cervix in the midtrimester: can it identify optimal candidates for ultrasound-indicated cerclage? *Am J Obstet Gynecol* 2009;200(2):158 e1–6.

CHAPTER 15

Choosing the Right Doc

"This is quite interesting. Can't say I've ever seen this before. I hope you'll choose to come back when you're pregnant. Nurse, come look at this!" This is what I heard as I lay spread-eagle, courtesy of a speculum examination. What the doctor was talking about were the marks left behind from my last cerclage—not the words I wanted to hear while choosing a doctor for my next pregnancy.

This was actually one of the milder run-ins I've had during my pregnancies. Actually, I wouldn't even classify this incident as anything more than a minor annoyance. There were moments during the extremely stressful and miserable days when I was losing my son when just the sight of my doctor would leave me in tears, completely distraught and so nervous that I was unable to form words. I was in a delicate state and couldn't understand how or why I could be treated this way.

Some—I can't say all—had a way of making me feel inadequate, like I was a body that was there for their experimentation only. The life of my baby wasn't even considered to be important, they were annoyed by our questions...the list goes on and on. Apparently, sadly, I'm not alone. I've heard tales from many, many women who were treated terribly, especially during what I would consider to be the worst times of their lives. It's unacceptable.

Sure, we could make excuses: "Well, it's hard to deal with these situations, the death of babies," or, "This is how they handle it." It's still

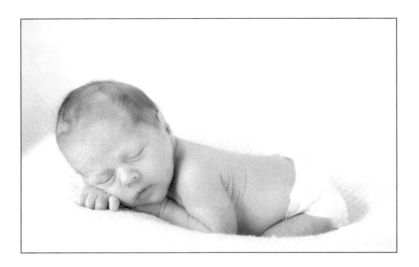

not right. Sorry to all you doctors who think you have a good bedside manner. Please take some time to sit back and think about it. Think about if this was your wife and your baby. Think about how rough and terrible an experience this is and would be for you. Maybe you're at the low end of the spectrum, because you only rush through visits because your schedule doesn't allow for more time with your patients or the ability to truly explain things. Or maybe you're at the other end. Maybe you're downright disrespectful, verbally abusive (yes, it happens), insensitive, condescending....

You may not even care about all that, because you're a damn good doctor, but I believe that eventually word will get out, and women will seek other options. To really be a good doctor, you need both the science/treatment side and the human/emotional side. To those of you who fit this bill, we thank you for your dedication and the help you give us in trying to bring our babies to term. You make such a wonderful and positive difference in our lives.

It amazes me just how arrogant some doctors can be. For example, I had set up a time to meet with a doctor to present on the benefits of having a doula (a labor companion) during labor and delivery. This was to be a 15-minute PowerPoint presentation, during his lunch hour. I showed up early, in my best suit, but wouldn't you know it, he not only ate, which I expected, but then went on to open a newspaper as I started my presentation. When I looked at him, he said something like,

"It's OK. I'm always like this. I'm good at multitasking." Not once did he even bother to look up from that damn paper. What a jerk and a complete waste of my time. He was so disrespectful; my time is just as valuable as his. He should've just declined my offer to present.

The point of that story is that your doctor should 1) be respectful of you and your partner, 2) treat your time as equally as important as his or her own, 3) give you the time of day to ask questions, 4) be capable of having an open exchange and answering your questions fully (if possible), and 5) treat you like another human being. God-like egos must be checked at the door!

A Good, Knowledgeable, and Kind Doc Is Key

> *"I felt tightness in my lower abdomen. Other than that, it was a complete surprise. I'm thankful I was in good hands at the hospital, or I would have lost both of my babies."* ~ Susan, Massachusetts (Had a rescue cerclage at around 18 weeks and delivered twins at term. Incredible!)

My #1 Piece of Advice…Interview Prospective Doctors
(If possible; this isn't always an option.)

Notice I use the word "interview," like interviewing for a job. We must remember that we are consumers, and we hire, and we can fire. Technically, our docs, midwives, nurses, techs, etc., work for us. More often than not, this message gets lost, both in the healthcare personnel we see and in us. We tend to believe we owe them, we don't feel like we have the right to question them, and we place them on a very high pedestal. Many doctors carry a "God complex" and make us feel as if we have no right to question or understand what's happening. We cease to exist as a person, becoming merely a condition that is being cared for. It's up to us to—*politely*—ensure that doesn't happen.

The ideal time to find a doctor is either before you get pregnant or very early on, to avoid being rushed into a decision or, worst case, having no time to choose and being "thrown" somewhere. This will give you time to meet with multiple providers to find the right fit for you. You may be saying, "Right fit? Who cares; I just need a doctor." Let me tell you from experience, the right fit can make your pregnancy that much less stressful, "easier," and just better all round. A good relationship is essential for high-risk women. We see our doctors and their staff (a friendly and understanding staff is a must) more than most women and end up spending more time with them than with our own family and friends. Based on our histories of loss, early birth, and previous difficult pregnancies, we can be even more needy, moody, depressed, stressed out, confused, scared, and bitchy than the normal prego lady. Let's face it; most women are not at their best when they're pregnant, so throw in a tough past or a rare condition with many unknowns, and you have the recipe for one cranky lady. Don't you want a person you can feel comfortable with?

Things to Consider when Choosing a Doctor

1. EXPERIENCE with your condition. Seems simple, right? Not so fast. Some doctors, especially in rural settings, may never see these things in their careers. They are inexperienced with premature labor, IUGR, preeclampsia, cervical length measurements, FFN, P17, cerclage placement, etc. You'll also need to consider staying within your plan, if you're lucky enough to have insurance, so you don't have to pay all those extra out-of-network costs. This may not be an option. It can't hurt to ask a doc who isn't on your plan to make special payment arrangements, especially if you really like him/her. Always ask…they can only say no.

Sample questions you can ask to gauge experience include:

- ✦ Since I have IC, I would ask: When would you place my cerclage? What type of stitch do you use? How often will you check my cervical length after my stitch? How many cerclages have you done? (If the hospital is a teaching hospital, confirm that they will be doing the cerclage themselves, not a medical student.)

- ✦ Would you prescribe P17 to reduce my risk of an early birth?

- ✦ If contractions start early, what tocolytic do you typically prescribe? What other restrictions would you consider?

- ✦ How often do you "prescribe" bed rest? What are your common bed-rest requirements (complete, partial, modified)?

✦ Will you prescribe preventative antibiotics? (If you have a history of vaginal infections like BV, this is a good one to ask.)

This list can go on and on. Depending on your risk factors and history, you should modify these questions and target appropriately. Go back through the sections/chapters that pertain to you.

"What can I do if there are no experienced perinatologists near me?" Unfortunately, those of you who live in the sticks will probably have to travel to get experienced care. Even though I live in New Jersey, one of the most populated states in the U.S., I reside in the northwest area, where there are no high-risk doctors. The hospital near me won't even touch babies less than 34 weeks. Because of this, I traveled about 50 miles each way to see my doctor during each of my pregnancies. I'm lucky that I have some of the top hospitals to choose from within an hour's drive.

Some of you will have to travel a couple hours to find a group and a hospital capable of handling your case, and some women even have to go to extremes and consider temporary housing with friends or relatives in order to be near good care. I've even heard about women getting apartments. (Note: check with the hospital, as there may be some sort of assistance available by way of putting you up during this time.) Since prematurity is always an issue with our conditions, we must also consider the hospital affiliated with the doctor or group. It's important to make sure they have a good NICU (Neonatal Intensive Care Unit) should you deliver early.

This is definitely not fun to have to deal with while you're pregnant, but it's an unfortunate reality. Further, all of this may become more complicated because of bed rest. Nothing is easy when you're high risk, right? The plus side is to remember that it's only temporary. It's possible to see a specialist during the high-risk period and then to switch to another doctor closer to home as you reach a better gestation and approach delivery.

2. Their personality, beliefs, bedside manner. Is it in tune with you/your partner?
When you interview, consider whether they appear open to answering your questions and working alongside you to determine the best course

of action during your pregnancy. Do they treat you like a person, with respect? Will they listen to your history and respond to your needs accordingly, both physically—i.e., treatment options—and emotionally, especially if you've experienced a loss or had a previous bad experience such as an emergency cerclage, premature birth, etc.? This seems simple enough, right? Unfortunately, this isn't always the case.

I experienced this firsthand during my second pregnancy, and it was why, for my third pregnancy, I interviewed several doctors long before we became pregnant. I decided I didn't need additional conflict and burden in what was an already taxing situation. At about 16 weeks into my second pregnancy, I started panicking. I just knew something was wrong and that I was going to lose this baby too, so I scheduled an office visit for a check. (I always feared my baby would fall out, since this is basically what happened the first time.) I was in tears and a bundle of nerves. The doctor, a female who had kids herself, was very short and nasty to me. My husband and I questioned the literature and the course of action they had chosen (expectant management, or the "wait and see" approach). We needed reassurance that we were making the right decision.

She seemed annoyed and said things like, "How dare you question me? I'm the doctor, not you." I typically spent all day working on my feet and was worried about the effect this would have on my cervix due to the weight of my growing baby. She said, and I quote, "Unless you're digging ditches for a living, you'll be fine," and then left the room. Bitch. My husband then stepped out into the hallway to get a drink, whereupon he heard this "professional" making fun of me with her colleagues for being upset and nervous. It was a terrible experience and did nothing to help me handle the pressures of my pregnancy. I should note that this was a very respectable group of doctors for a great hospital.

Needless to say, we avoided scheduling appointments with her throughout the rest of my pregnancy, choosing to see other doctors who were a better fit for us, and hoped to not get her on the day of my birth (which, thankfully, we didn't). (Oh, and I was right—a couple weeks later my cervix started shortening, and I was put on complete bed rest. Thank God we took preventative action, or I would've certainly lost my baby, just like the previous time. Another win for "gut feel.")

Are they harsh, short with you, condescending? If you answer yes, then move on. Do it for you and your partner's sanity. Do they take interest in discussing your history? Are they sympathetic to your past experiences? I broke down and cried during several of my interviews when I got to the part where I had to explain my history. This was embarrassing for me, as I'm a very private crier. A sympathetic doctor will hand you a tissue and respect how difficult this is for you. He or she will not rush you along or wave it away with something like, "Well, at least you can have another baby."

Another thing to consider is your birth plan. Seems crazy, right—considering your birth plan before you're even pregnant? With high-risk pregnancies, we often neglect the part where we actually give birth. We're so hung up on making it to term that we push aside the desires we once held for our birth experiences. It has been shown that a woman's birth experience and her satisfaction with her birth has a lifelong impact.[1] Finding a doctor who will support your desires will become important as you near B-day. Just because you're high risk doesn't mean you'll necessarily be high risk at birth. If you have a strong desire for a natural birth or alternative pain-relief options, you should question their openness to this. If you would like to avoid a C-section, ask about their C-section rates. It's possible to have your cake and eat it too! You just have to ask the right questions and take the time to find the right match.

During my third pregnancy, I was looking for a doctor who was not only experienced with IC, but was also open to my birth plan, which included a desire for a natural birth, since I was not satisfied with the birth experience of my daughter. I was lucky enough to find him through a doula referral. My husband and I interviewed him and then chose him to provide care for me during my next pregnancy, and ultimately I got the birth experience I desired. Thanks, Dr. Garfinkel of Morristown, New Jersey (just a quick plug).

It's equally important that your partner feels it's a good fit, especially if you have a partner who is "hands on" during your pregnancy. This is based on my experience with my husband and the doctors we saw during our loss, which has made me so adamant about why we should empower ourselves and view the doctor-patient relationship as more of an employment contract. This bit of advice comes from him, so I can't take credit for it.

We were at a critical point, with no knowledge of what was going on, and really wanted to try to hold onto our baby. (Talk of terminating was rampant.) My husband starting asking questions and demanded answers, since it seemed like no one around us was really telling us what was going on.

Multiple doctors, residents, nurses, and medical students were coming in and out of my room, checking my vagina, shaking their heads, and walking out again, with no acknowledgement of us, let alone communication. Needless to say, in his state of extreme stress, my husband got quite heated and told one doctor, "I can fire you and get someone else." The point to remember is that you have the power to choose. It's possible to do this up front in order to avoid anguish later on if you know you're likely to have a high-risk pregnancy. Heck, even if it's during a crisis, if you try to keep yourself level-headed, you can still demand a second or even a third opinion. In my extremely critical situation, we wanted answers, and we got them. Sure, at times it was NOT pretty, but in the end, after several very emotionally charged exchanges, the doctor sat down with my husband and took the time to answer our questions. By speaking up, my husband got results. It was an awfully uncomfortable situation for me, watching a yelling match between my man and my doctor during the worst time of my life, but we got what we needed in the end. Often, we have to turn to our partners to be our voice, since it's hard for us, as the mom who is carrying the baby, to deal with it all ourselves.

3. *Have they spent time looking at your records?*
Ideally, you want to have your records sent in plenty of time before your appointment to allow time for review. Let's face it; they can't possibly memorize everything for every patient, but I would expect them to have at least a rough idea of your past history/circumstances. Judge them on whether they've taken the time to look over your records or, at the very least, are interested in discussing your history.

4. *How long were you made to wait?*
I always, always judge a doctor's office by how long I have to wait. Nothing has pissed me off more than having to wait for hours on end. My time is just as important as theirs. I've switched doctors simply

because they always made me wait. Now, I do realize that emergencies happen, and in OB practices babies happen, and I can understand this, but if there's always an excuse, or, worse, no acknowledgement for your extended waiting time, I find this to be totally unacceptable. (Hey, at least apologize for the wait.)

When I interview a doctor, I always consider how long I was left to wait. Think of it this way; you'll be spending a lot of time at the doc's during a high-risk pregnancy, and if you're on bed rest or having any sorts of issues, the last thing you want is to be left in the waiting room. I was lucky in that I rarely had to wait during either of my high-risk pregnancies. I can remember being on bed rest and pulling up chairs so I didn't have to sit up, being quite the spectacle, and them taking me back right away. During my third pregnancy, I only had to wait any length of time a couple times due to a mom who was delivering—a very good reason I would say. Repeated long wait times can often be a sign of an unorganized, understaffed, or overbooked practice, not a good mix when there are periods when you may have to be there several times a week.

5. Is the front staff nice? Accommodating?

Consider how nice the front-desk people are, as you'll have to deal with them quite a bit throughout your pregnancy. Are they willing to help you with the paperwork side, insurance, disability papers, figuring out proper copays, and such? If not, you have some decisions to make. Is it easy to schedule convenient appointments? Sometimes you'll find that your schedule is unimportant, and they want to just put you in any old open time slot. If you work, can they accommodate you? The worst thing is to have to take time off for every office visit. We never know when we'll be yanked out of work, so it helps to not have to take time right off the bat.

How Do I Find a Perinatologist (a High-Risk Specialist) or an OB? A Midwife? (With Certain Conditions, a Midwife May Be an Option.)

+ Start with your insurance company. See who they have listed.
+ Get referrals from your regular OB/GYN or the local hospital.

+ Get referrals from other women (through local hospital support
  groups, lactation groups, etc.).
+ Check out the Society for Maternal Fetal Medicine site:
  www.smfm.org/index.cfm?zone=search&nav=doctor
+ Check out: www.perinatology.com/perinatologists.htm (This
  site has global listings of perinatologists.)
+ The Revolution Health site has listings. Check out:
  www.revolutionhealth.com/browse-doctors/neonatologist-and-
  perinatologist-47 (U.S. docs only.)
+ Check out the Incompetent Cervix Support Forum:
  www.ic.hobh.org/forums

"I had a doctor give me a sonogram, press on my stomach to show me the funneling of my cervix. He said, "This is what happens every time you stand up." Then he made me stand in the hallway because he needed the room for another patient. Of course, other doctors are awesome. I called my fertility specialist a few days after finding out that I had gotten pregnant naturally. He insisted I come in to make sure everything was okay and discovered dangerously low progesterone. He had a pharmacy deliver the medication to my house at 10PM that night. If he hadn't been so concerned and conscientious, I would have lost my pregnancy." ~ Catherine, location unknown

"Trust yourself. You know when things just don't feel right with your body and your pregnancy, even if it's your first pregnancy. Don't let a doctor tell you, 'Everything's fine,' just because he has MD behind his name. He might not really be listening."
~ Claudia, Louisiana

References

1. Simkin P. Just another day in a woman's life? Women's long-term perceptions of their first birth experience, part 1. *Birth: Issues in Perinatal Care.* 1991;18(4):203–210.

CHAPTER 16

The High-Risk Pregnancy Woman's Jail, Bed Rest: Beating Bed Rest Boredom and Neuroticness...or Not!

"*B*ed rest is a temporary means to a wonderful and permanent end." ~ Jenna, California

"Bed rest can be one of the longest, loneliest parts of your life—but it is temporary, and you will move past it, guaranteed." ~ Lana, New Mexico

"To women on bed rest: Hang in there, it will get better...I promise. I was a hospital bed-rest patient for seven weeks!" ~ Robin, Virginia

And from my survey, in answer to the question "How long were you on bed rest?" a feeling anyone on bed rest can understand:

"Thirteen weeks. The longest 13 weeks of my entire life, but well worth it." ~ Erin, Florida

"Four very long weeks!" ~ Ashley, Indiana (Many women do much, much more time, but any time on bed rest feels like the longest time in your life. The clock seems to stop.)

My survey found that of the high-risk women who responded (177), nearly 100% of them experienced some form of bed rest, from modified to Trendelenburg (where your head is lower than your feet). A large majority, around 70%, did strict bed rest.

Even though research doesn't support the use of bed rest, let's be real: it's one of the most commonly prescribed "treatments" in pregnancy. After reading Dr. Berghella's book, I questioned him on this. He told me that in over five years he has not confined a single woman to *strict* bed rest. So, this doctor, who specializes in high-risk women, doesn't even use strict bed rest! (He does suggest reduced/modified activity for some of his patients.) Despite that, the reality is, many of us will spend some time unable to move about normally.

When restricted to bed rest, you need to tell yourself that you are being the ultimate mother, that you are making this sacrifice in the course of trying EVERYTHING to carry your baby to term. Even though the research doesn't generally support it, you never know; there may be situations where bed rest really does help, and they just haven't discovered it yet. We know activity can bring on contractions, and we know that the weight of the baby can have a negative impact on your cervix if it's weak, so you can see how rest (maybe not strict bed rest) could help in certain situations. (Obviously for those of you with high blood pressure, the need for bed rest is quite clear.) Listen to your doc, discuss it, and tell them that you understand that the research doesn't support bed rest. You may find a good reason for having to do bed rest,

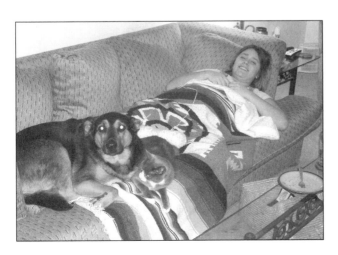

Me on bed rest. Many weeks in and many more to go. Giving my best fake smile for the camera (and definitely NOT looking my best). See, I'm not lying when I say I learned to crochet. Thank goodness for my dog and cat. They were my only company for thousands of hours.

or you guys may come to an understanding whereby maybe you aren't on *strict* bed rest, and you just have to reduce your daily activity.

There are numerous books dedicated to dealing with the issue of bed rest: how to cope, tips to pass the time, ways to set up the house, and overall survival techniques. I would recommend these to those of you looking down the barrel at long periods of bed rest, or even to those of you looking at a stint of a couple weeks. If nothing else, you'll pick up a few tips to help pass the time.

Some of the tips I remember hearing about from my bed-rest time, a few of which actually came in handy, were 1) learn to knit or crochet, 2) watch those movies/shows you've been meaning to catch up on, 3) file/organize your recipes, 4) break up the day by moving from bed to couch, 5) set up a living area in bed or by the couch (refrigerator, work station, etc.), and 6) write to your friends.

Now, I'm a slacker who did very few of these things. I had very good intentions starting out, but they never materialized. About the only thing I did during my "jail time," all four and a half months of it, was learn to crochet. The sad part was, I didn't even finish that blanket until my daughter was a year old. I must admit, though, it did help pass the time.

Starting out on bed rest, I had all these plans for things I could accomplish and organize...my recipes, pictures, tax documents. Needless to say, those same items are still on my to-do list six years later.

As it turned out, I spent most of my time depressed and unmotivated, and ended up wanting to just sleep the time away. I wished I could've just woke up at 24 weeks, then 28 weeks, then 32 weeks. I found out quickly just how un-tired you become when you do nothing all day. I spent the wee hours of the mornings usually watching infomercials because I couldn't sleep.

Not only is bed rest entirely boring, isolating, demotivating, and depressing, but it is also extremely scary, stressful, anxious, self-depreciating, and difficult, to say the least. I hated it when I left work to go on bed rest and my co-workers said, "Lucky you; I wish I could go relax for a while," or "Enjoy this free time to relax." If only they knew.

Every day, I cried in fear for the baby in my womb, sadness for my dead son, and scared at the possibility of losing another baby. I cried because of loneliness, self-pity for the situation I found myself in, the isolation I felt from all my friends, who had so quickly forgotten about me and moved on, and the distance I felt from my husband. The world had moved on without me, and it was hard to accept that everyone had seemingly also forgotten about me being locked up in my own home.

In short, I can't sugarcoat it for you…IT SUCKED! Aside from the death of my son, it was the worst experience of my life; but it led to the best experience of my life, the birth of my daughter, and therefore it was sooooo worth it. Seriously, I wouldn't bullshit you on this.

Depression Happens. You Just Need to Recognize and Deal With It

As I said just before, I was majorly depressed while I was on bed rest. I don't really think anyone else really understood why I was so upset about lying around in bed all day—after all, how hard can that be? They had no idea.

Unless you've been through this experience, I don't think you can understand what it's like, day in, day out. It's really, really hard. That said, if you find yourself way down in the dumps for days on end and find that you need a little extra support beyond your usual circle, there are places you can go to get it, places like Sidelines High-Risk Pregnancy Support Group (a non-profit), who will match you up with someone who has been in a similar situation, or chat forums, like the IC forum, where you can interact with others who are or were on bed rest. There are even local support groups, so contact your doctor or hospital.

Do It for Your Baby: Every Day Inside Helps

From those who have been there to you:

> *"One of the best things my doctor had me do was tour the NICU. I saw babies at 26, 29, 30, and 34 weeks old. It was amazing to see the difference in their size. While it was difficult, and I can remember crying all the way through in my wheelchair, it was the best thing for me to remember during the LONG days on bed rest. It gave me motivation and kept me focused. My heart goes out to all moms on bed rest."* ~ Klea, California

> *"Remember, you are not alone. Remember that what you are doing is so important to your baby."* ~ Joan, Nebraska

"I spent five weeks on strict bed rest with my twins. It was often hard to accept that I was not having a 'normal' pregnancy, but reminding myself that I was the ONLY person in the world who could keep those babies growing inside of me kept me going." ~ Christine, Pennsylvania

"Some days are minute-by-minute, moment-by-moment, so rest on the days that you are lucky enough to have go by hour-by-hour." ~ Lynn, Pennsylvania

"Every day you get through is another victory. A few weeks or months of your life on bed rest will be nothing in comparison to the years you will have to love and enjoy your child. If you overdo it and something happens to your baby, you will never forgive yourself, and you will have to live with that guilt; it's never worth it." ~ Jennifer (location unknown)

"When you're on bed rest, ask for help and visitors. You don't have to be alone. So many people have asked me how I can cope with four to five months of bed rest. It's pretty easy, actually; I'm willing to do whatever it takes to get my baby here safely. I'm not saying it wasn't difficult at times, especially once I had to go on bed rest with a toddler. But like every parent, you do whatever you have to do to keep your children safe and healthy." ~ Lindsey, Virginia

"If you are pregnant and on bed rest, hang in there. Follow your doctor's instructions. You are doing the best thing for your baby by being on bed rest. The longer your baby stays inside your belly, the better. Arm yourself with books (NOT about babies), movies, games, TV shows, small craft projects, friends, family, good food, and a phone. If you have to go into the hospital, ask someone to bring you some SOFT toilet paper. People want to help...let them." ~ Betty, Georgia (did 16 weeks of bed rest to have her baby after the loss of her son at 24 weeks)

"While on bed rest, during the dark hours when worry took over of me, I focused solely on the doctors handing me my son for the first time, healthy and full term. I visualized this over

and over; I refused to let my mind think the worst." ~ Joan, Canada (It brought tears to my eyes when I read this quote; such a lovely bit of advice. She did 24 weeks of bed rest.)

What the Research Says: There Is No Point to Bed Rest

Bed rest has not been shown to work to prevent or treat preterm labor, even though it is advised in about one in five of all pregnancies in order to prevent early labor or to treat a bunch of conditions. There are risks associated with bed rest, not to mention the extra financial burden on the family and the ENORMOUS emotional strain. It's important to note that there are NO randomized controlled studies, the "gold standard" studies the professionals turn to for answers, which look at bed rest compared to regular activity in women with a short cervix. A good study is needed in order to accurately assess the potential benefits of bed rest.[1]

In one study, they looked at women who had preterm labor and a negative fetal fibronectin (FFN) swab and compared those on bed rest who were allowed to use the bathroom/shower with those who were allowed to live their lives normally, including working, and found no difference in the number of preterm births before 37 weeks.[1]

"I spent five weeks on modified bed rest. I had to lie down on my left side for two hours in the morning, two in the afternoon, and two in the evening. The rest of the time had to be spent with my feet elevated. After that, I spent one week in the hospital on full bed rest, with bathroom/shower privileges, on mag sulfate. Then, I spent an additional three weeks at home on full bed rest with bathroom/shower privileges and was on a terbutaline pump. My baby was born one day after they removed my pump and took me off bed rest—at 36 weeks 2 days. The doctors called me a classic preterm labor case." ~ Kristen, Minnesota

"I was on a combination of modified and complete bed rest with shower privileges for 21 weeks. It was a very difficult time, but so worth it when our little miracle man arrived at 38 weeks. The first 10 weeks of bed rest were the worst—we didn't know if what I was doing was making a difference, but when I hit viability we knew it was." ~ Janna, Ohio

One of the tips you will see in all bed-rest books is to have a routine. I also did a bit of the routine thing, and I believe it helped to break up the day. I would stay in bed until 1 or 2 pm, then I would shower, lying down of course (I took long showers), and finally I would make my way to the couch. By the time I made it to the couch, it was already well into the afternoon. I guess part of me felt that I was tricking my brain into believing the day was shorter by staying in bed so long. Hey, we do what we have to in order to survive, right? That ended up being my routine, and you will just have to see what works for you.

> *"With my first pregnancy I was on complete bed rest, in Trendelenburg with no bathroom privileges, for nine days. (Peeing in a bed pan while upside down is quite tricky.) With my second pregnancy I was on complete bed rest at home for 4.5 months. I was allowed to shower, go to the bathroom, and maybe go to the kitchen for a quick snack or drink, but no cooking, cleaning, or leaving the house, other than for doctor's appointments. I am currently on bed rest with my third, with similar bed rest to with my second. It is definitely trickier this time because we moved to a new house with a lot of stairs. I am allowed to use the stairs once a day. I've kind of adopted an every-other-day routine of staying in bed versus coming downstairs and laying on the couch. On days I stay in bed, my husband will bring me breakfast before he goes to work and will pack my lunch in a cooler and bring it upstairs for me. I had hopes of keeping my 17-month-old at home with me, but that did not work out, so we had to put him in daycare full-time. If I do have to watch him on my own while my husband is out running errands, we will usually get in my bed and put on a movie or read books. That way he is much more confined to a smaller area (our bedroom) and is much easier to keep track of."* ~ Lindsey, Virginia

One Day at a Time

> *"Four and a half months. My doctor did not come right out and tell me this would be the case—he took me along one week at a time. If I'd known it would be four and a half months, I probably would have gotten a lot more depressed. Being on bed rest*

was such a foreign concept, and having to take leave from work was embarrassing, as people didn't understand the seriousness of it. Through amazing support, I made it one week at a time, resulting in the birth of my beautiful full-term twins." ~ Susan, Massachusetts (At her second-trimester growth scan she was found to be dilated and one of the twins had dropped, and yet she made it...and so can you.)

It's All Right to Vent

"I found the months of bed rest more endurable if I actually allowed myself scheduled time to have a pity party. I got a drink, sad book, or sad movie and let myself cry and whine for one full day. Then I felt refreshed and ready to handle the next weeks again. Acknowledging that what you are going through is difficult and stressful is not a sign of weakness, but a sign of strength in that you know what you need and you allow your-self to experience all of those feelings." ~ Shaylene, Nebraska (Amazing advice here, ladies.)

"Let your feelings out or else they'll explode and won't do any-one any good. Keep yourself busy on bed rest, trying to learn, taking up a new hobby, etc." ~ Deb (location unknown)

You Can Do It

"You become a mother the moment that you find out you are pregnant. Worrying is part of the job. But so are hope, faith, and unimaginable love. Those three things are what we all need to hold on to, especially during the difficult times." ~ Jenni, New Jersey

"Try to relax. Many women have been in your shoes and have had very successful outcomes." ~ Tracy (location unknown)

"Going on bed rest when a doctor recommends it is a very hard thing to do. It means going the extra mile for your child, mak-ing sure you do all in your power to make sure your child has a good beginning, no matter what." ~ Sarah, Maryland

The Effects of Bed Rest Don't End at Birth

Adjusting back to normal life is no walk in the park. Life is no longer the same as you once knew it. You have a new baby now. Your body is sore from being inactive for so long, your muscles have wasted away, you have the "normal" postnatal issues to deal with on top of all that other high-risk/bed-rest stuff, and now you have to take care of a baby who demands so much attention. Don't think that as soon as the bed-rest curse is lifted, everything will instantly be back to normal again.

Understand that this will take some time to adjust to, not only mentally, but physically as well. Don't beat yourself up for not being able to do everything you'd hoped you could do. This is completely normal, and eventually you will be good to go!

"I'd just completed the survey, and as I hit send, I thought of something I wish someone had told me that no book really touched on: depression. I was frustrated beyond belief while I was on bed rest (and the books talk about that), but I thought that when I could get up and get control of my life again, I'd feel better. And in some ways it was better. But there was also the whammy when I got up that I was not in the great shape I was when I was 'put down.' I used to work out daily, but bed rest stopped that. Although I knew I had gained weight, I didn't really understand all the other ways bed rest and pregnancy impacted my body. Once I was released from bed rest at 38 weeks, I had no energy to do any of the things I'd dreamed of doing during all those weeks on bed rest. I thought that with all that 'rest' I'd be ready to go. Wrong! Most women have nine months to slowly gain weight and to feel their body change, but on bed rest your body changes and you feel many of those changes all at once, at 9 months.

The joy of the new baby helped keep me up, but the post-baby weight, months of no exercise, the lack of sleep, and the C-section all made me quite depressed. It took a long time to feel good again. I know a lot of women go through something similar after having a baby, but I think it's magnified with bed rest.

Also, a kinda funny story: while I was on bed rest, Martha Stewart was released from jail and put under house arrest. Sit-

ting on the couch one day, I heard her interviewed, saying some-thing about how house arrest is harder than jail because you see people in jail. When you're in jail, people know it's hard for you, and they come and visit you. During house arrest, people think your life is back to normal—but it isn't. You may be in your home, but you can't do what you want to do and you can't go see the friends you want to see. It's more isolating than jail, because you're so alone. Now, Martha isn't the most reason-able/relatable person in the world, but I remember feeling like she said it so well—and I still had it worse." ~ Tara, Virginia

Cochrane Reviews

1. There is not enough evidence to know for sure if bed rest helps pre-vent miscarriage. The authors point out that most of the time the cause of the miscarriage is not over-activity, so bed rest may not be the best strategy for prevention. It should be noted that they only found two studies with a total of 84 women as participants and "this is a main factor to make this analysis inconclusive."[2]

2. There is not enough evidence to prove or to **disprove** bed rest in helping to prevent preterm birth. Even though it is common practice to "prescribe" bed rest, there is no evidence showing its benefits. (Only one questionable study was found and included.) The reviewer's conclusions actually advise against routine use of bed rest "due to the potential adverse effects that bed rest could have on women and their families, and the increased costs for the healthcare system." They state that research is "mandatory."[3]

References

1. Berghella V. *Preterm Birth: Prevention & Management*. West Sussex, UK. Wiley-Blackwell, 2010.
2. Aleman A, Althabe F, Belizán JM, Bergel E. Bed rest during pregnancy for preventing miscarriage. *Cochrane Database of Systematic Reviews* 2005, Issue 2. Art. No.: CD003576. (Last assessed as up-to-date: April 15, 2010.)
3. Sosa C, Althabe F, Belizán JM, Bergel E. Bed rest in singleton pregnancies for pre-venting preterm birth. *Cochrane Database of Systematic Reviews* 2004, Issue 1. Art. No.: CD003581. (Last assessed as up-to-date: April 15, 2010.)

CHAPTER 17

Medical Pregnancy, Natural Birth ... Can This Be Possible? *ABSOLUTELY!*

O MG ... you've done it ... you've made it! After all the time spent worrying, wondering, praying, bordering sanity-ville, and isolated from the world, you're FINALLY at a point where now *all* you have to worry about is labor. Or maybe the thought of a C-section, as required by certain conditions, is giving you the jitters. This should be the least of your worries after all you've been through. Seriously, I mean that. Labor/birth is such a short time period in relation to the rest of your journey. You've made it through that, and you can make it through this, too. So relax and try to savor this moment. This wasn't an easy ride, and it probably wasn't a particularly fun ride for either you or your family, but you did it. Give yourself a pat on the back. Soon, you will become just another "ordinary" pregnant lady.

For some conditions, there's no end to the high-risk period. You're struggling right up until the moment your baby arrives. This includes all you preeclamptic/hypertensive girls, babies showing signs of stress/trouble, and those of you having placenta separation/bleeding issues. Sorry girls, you guys won't get a break to be "normal."

Some of you who are carrying multiples may be able to deliver vaginally. (Twins positioned favorably can be birthed safely under the care of a trained doctor.)

Those of you who suffered from PPROM may only get a brief moment to catch your breath. As soon as your baby's lungs are ready, you'll probably be delivered. There's no point risking infection now that you made it to a good gestation, is there? (Hopefully, labor will now be allowed to progress naturally, instead of a C-section. There's no need for an unnecessary C-section if you can avoid it, so speak with your doctor.)

If you're interested in having a more "natural" birth—even remotely interested—though you've had a pregnancy that was far from normal and natural, this chapter is for you. It will discuss some issues and things to consider, and provide some pointers. If you're really into a natural birth, I would highly recommend further reading on this subject to give you inspiration and more complete guidance. (Check out the resource section on my website, www.hrpwhyme.com.)

Stopping Tocolytics

You've made it to the "safe" zone, and depending on your situation, assuming you're at or near term, the drugs that have been preventing labor will be stopped. Yeah! As long as your baby is stable, labor will be allowed to happen . . . hopefully. (Tell your doctor you prefer this.) You can smile now. No more nasty side effects from those tocolytics.

The End of Bed Rest

By this point, those of you who've been banished to the bed/couch are now permitted to re-enter the real world. Even though you probably won't feel too energetic after so many months of bed rest and the resulting muscle atrophy, you should try to get out and do a few things for yourself before the baby arrives. Go get a massage and/or facial, have some lunch with friends, go shopping, even if you can't buy clothes for yourself, and shoot for some pre-baby time alone with hubby.

With my daughter, by the 34-week mark, my doctors had lifted many of my restrictions. I was now able to make small trips out for lunch or shopping. I didn't quite have the energy to do my normal activities, but it was a huge emotional weight lifted off my shoulders just to be able to interact with the world again.

From this point on was when I really believed and felt like, I was actually pregnant. Maybe that doesn't make sense, but prior to this time, I'd been so focused on her not dying or being born too small that I'd never enjoyed the "pregnant" aspects of it all. The only fond memories of being pregnant with her was at this end period, but no matter what, I can say without a shadow of a doubt that it was worth all of it. I would have dealt with a hundred times more stress and anxiety to have my children here with me today.

Fulfilling Your Dream of a Natural Birth (If You Don't Have This Dream, I Politely Urge You to Consider It If You Can.)

I'm going to switch gears 100% from the rest of the book. Up until now, it has been all about this study says this, and that study says that, this medical intervention has shown promise in prolonging pregnancy, and that drug is able to stall labor for 48 hours. The reality is, there are a lot of us who, against all odds, make it to term. To the low-risk highway we come. But now what?

You've probably never even considered this as a reality or taken time to fantasize about making it to this point, among all the worry and fear, not to mention tests and doctor visits. Well, do yourself a favor and reconnect with your inner thoughts, the ones you had before all of this high-risk stuff—to your birth visions before any of the bad what ifs became a reality, back to when you were naïve about the fact that babies can be born early, or that babies can become sick and even die.

You've had a hundred doctors visits, enough ultrasounds for a dozen pregnancies, and more swabs of your coochy than you ever thought possible. Maybe you've even had machines to monitor contractions, shots in your ass, a spinal, a hospital stay(s), intravenous medications, a fishing line tied into your insides and then cut out, or many months spent on bed rest with your muscles wasting away. Finally, the time has come for the big event, the one you've been waiting for forever. Is it really possible, and does it even matter at this point if you have a "natural" birth? There's one simple answer to both those questions...YES! Yes, it is possible, and yes, it does matter if it's important to you.

Our doctors have been there for us, helping us to carry our babies as long as possible, but now is the time we want them to back off. (Hopefully, you found a doctor who meshed well with you and your needs/desires.) How can that be? If you're lucky enough that your situation allows for it, minimizing medical intervention is now the key to obtaining a more natural birth. This does seem like an odd suggestion after a pregnancy that has focused on medical treatments and management, but believe me, once you've made it this far, it's time for that mentality to disappear. (Even if your baby is coming early, you don't necessarily need to have an elective C-section. See the preemie chapter.)

When I say natural birth, I don't mean you'll be giving birth in the middle of a field of sunflowers on a warm spring day, wearing a flowing white dress, a crown of flowers, and Birkenstock sandals. Okay, I admit that was my own preconceived notion of a natural birth back in the days before I bore children of my own. I thought it was a hippie thing, this concept of a natural birth, and many other women may, on the surface, also believe this stereotype.

Reach deep down inside and think instinctively. Go back to your animal nature. You may find that, after putting aside all the fear drummed into our heads by the media, friends, and society as a whole, natural birth isn't all that bad. The fear of childbirth is perpetuated in many societies, especially in the U.S., but this is not so in other cultures. These cultures embrace childbirth, and you can too. Really! I'm not some crazy hippie. I live in New Jersey, so that would be an oxymoron.

There are many ideas floating around out there about what a natural birth is. For some, it's birthing in the comfort of their own home, surrounded by loved ones. For others who are lucky enough to enjoy this privilege, it's giving birth in a birth center that adopts a woman/family-centered approach and believes in freedom of choice. But for the vast majority of us who are interested in a natural birth, especially those of us who are high risk, it means having a hospital-based birth, without an epidural or other pain-management medicines. It can also mean just holding off on an epidural or other pain meds for as long as you can, going into it with the aim of seeing how long you can last. It may mean allowing labor to happen naturally without the aid of Pitocin (a synthetic drug used to induce labor). All these are perfectly acceptable options. It's your body and your baby, so the choice is yours. (Well, it should be, anyway.) Being high risk, a home or birth-center birth is not an option, so we have to make the best of getting what we want in a hospital birth, which can be quite tricky.

To me, a natural birth means being educated about your choices and having the freedom to decide what you want. It's about not being bound to an uncomfortable hospital bed, thrashing around, unable to handle the pain of your contractions. (Lying flat on your back, unable to move, is the worst way to handle contractions.) It's about not being pushed into the use of pain meds in order to pacify you and keep you quiet purely for the ease and convenience of everyone else. It's also about not having unnecessary medical interventions simply for the sake of "managing" your labor/birth.

It is being able to walk around and, use a toilet, a birth ball, a tub, or other measures to manage your pain, without prejudice or bias from those around you, like nurses or doctors. It's being allowed to have whoever you want to be present during the birth of your precious miracle. It's about having total and complete support during your entire experience with the right person (or people). If you threw this idea of your birth experience right out the window as soon as you realized you were high risk, it may not have to be that way. Believe it or not, all this can happen, but it's up to you. Having a doctor/midwife who will support your wishes is also essential.

Now, if you say, "I don't want to feel any pain; as soon as I walk into that hospital, hook me up to that epidural IV," that's okay, too, although I do hope you will still read this and maybe reconsider, even if it's just for a little while. You never know, you might find that it's not as bad as you thought after all.

As I said earlier, some of you will have no option other than a C-section, but others will still be able to have a vaginal or even a "natural" birth. During my first pregnancy, I wanted a natural (drug-free) birth. As soon as I saw the line on my pregnancy test, I knew that I wanted to go to a midwife and have a water birth in a hospital. The thought of laboring in the water just sounded so comforting to me. I really don't know where this idea came from. Maybe I watched too many episodes of *A Baby Story*.

I don't think of myself as a trendy yuppie; none of my friends were doing it, and I'm not against the use of pain relief or drugs, but for some reason, somewhere along the way it became very important to me to have this "natural" birth I envisioned. Sure, I was scared I wouldn't be able to do it—shit yeah, I was freaked out about the pain—but I always left my mind open to an out, just in case I needed it. Having said that, I just knew I had to try it. In the hope of having an experience like this, I went with a midwife, but as you know by now, that dream didn't become a reality...at that time.

Fast forward to pregnancy number two, which was now considered to be high risk. I was now so wrapped up in having a healthy baby that I put aside all thoughts of a natural birth, and even any thoughts about birth altogether. I now went to a maternal fetal practice that had six doctors who specialized in high-risk obstetrics, and my dream of a natural birth was soon a foggy, distant memory. When it came time to have the baby, I was induced immediately after my water broke. I was uninformed about my options, very placid, and had a support team that didn't really know how to support a woman in labor. During that pregnancy, I'd never thought about the actual birth or considered the options like I had in my first pregnancy. I just went along with what the doctors suggested, far from an active participant, not knowing anything or caring about the birth I'd once obsessed over.

I never questioned the doctors or pushed for what I wanted. (This is not the fault of my doctors; many women are actually happy with this type of approach to birth.) I didn't know enough to ask that they hold off on putting me on Pitocin, to let my own contractions have a chance to kick in; I didn't know enough about how to deal with the immediate intensity of the contractions brought on by the Pitocin; and I didn't know anything about the benefits of movement and changes in position as opposed to trying to deal with the pain while lying flat on my back in bed. Within hours, I was screaming for an epidural. I was very disappointed in how it went, because it was nothing like I'd imagined. (Being on strict bed rest, I was unable to take any sort of birth classes.)

With my third pregnancy, there was less stress about the health of the baby or my ability to have a full-term baby, as I had done it before. Having done my research between babies and chosen a doctor who could take care of both my medical needs (i.e., cerclage and such) and my birth needs when it came time, I was ready to re-explore my dreams. (My doctor was open to natural birthing options.)

Even though I had to be induced with Pitocin because of gestational diabetes and a history of shoulder dystocia, my awesome doc respected my wishes and worked with me to administer it gradually. I got to labor, with the help of my doula, my husband, and my best friend, using a birth ball, on the toilet, in the tub, even on the cool, dirty hospital floor, but anywhere to avoid being flat on my back, struggling through the contractions. I delivered an 8 lb 8 oz baby, drug free except for the Pitocin, feeling every bit of the pain and, crazy as it sounds, being ecstatic about it. There was no struggling through pushing with an epidural and no forceps and head damage like with my daughter. Three to four pushes and pop, he was out. It was life-changing, and all within the confines of the hospital walls. Who'd have thought.

I'm no superwoman, by any means. I don't run marathons; in fact, I can barely run a mile without feeling like I'm going to throw up. I don't eat organic foods or focus on healthy foods, and I love all sweets, pizza, burgers, and pasta. What I do know is that I can look back and be happy with my decisions, and know that I did it.

I feel that the birth of my daughter could have been different if I'd approached it differently ... and better. Based on her position, being sunny-side up, it wouldn't have been easy to have a drug-free birth, but

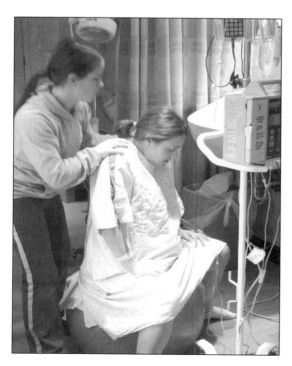

Dealing with contractions with the help of my doula, Jessica.

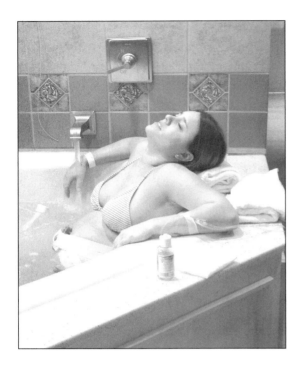

Laboring in the tub in the midst of transition. Just 15 seconds earlier I was thrashing around and yelling my head off. Water is a wonderful thing. (My doula, though not seen in this pic, was right next to me.)

I'll never know. I'm just lucky that 1) we decided to have another baby, 2) I had another healthy baby, and 3) I got to have the birth experience I'd always wanted by doing all I could to ensure this reality (interviewing docs, doing research, having a doula). Had I not had another child, I may have always regretted the lack of enthusiasm I had toward the birth of my daughter. So, the takeaway message is, no regrets... push for what you want. Try to get what you want, and understand that if things change along the way, forcing you to switch directions, that's okay, too. At least you'll know that you tried.

It's NOT as Bad as You Think: What to Expect

Many of you are probably shaking your head and thinking, "What, is she nuts?" Now hear me out. Yes, some labors are rip-your-head-off painful, and long, drawn-out affairs. But, many women have labors that they find to be bearable without pain meds, experiences on which they later look back fondly. Can you believe that?

In the famous midwife's book *Ina May's Guide to Childbirth*[1], many women tell the stories of their natural birth experiences. True, many of these women were real hippie women living in a commune, but nonetheless, these are very inspiring, empowering, and moving stories of birth. (I read this book shortly before my own "naturalish" birth to motivate me.) I'm not saying you won't have any pain, although some women do report that they experienced little to no pain, if you can believe that. There will be pain at some point, but with the right tools in your tool bag, you can do it! [Seriously, for many the crazy intense pain of the transition phase of labor (as it's called) is actually very short, lasting only about 15–30 minutes.]

Going into the birth of my son, I knew that if I was going to make it, I needed the support of someone who believed in natural birth, someone who knew what to expect during the course of labor, and someone who was knowledgeable about positions and relief measures. I thought of my husband staring at the TV during the labor with my daughter and knew that the only way I was going to do this was by hiring a doula. (A doula is a trained labor support companion who provides emotional and physical support. Check out www.dona.org if you'd like to find one near you. Hey, if you live in the Northern New Jersey area, email me. I'm now a doula.) I interviewed several until I found the right person to match my personality. (It's very important to have the right mesh and chemistry with your doula.) Note: Some insurance companies will now pay for all or parts of doula services, so call. The research for doulas is very positive.

During labor, she was my rock. Just looking at her, knowing she was close by, made me more at ease. She kept me positive, always giving me words of support, offered me position changes and massage, and took charge when the going got tough. Without her, I would've caved in within a heartbeat, and my birth experience wouldn't have been anywhere as close to as wonderful as it was.

Even being on Pitocin—at a very controlled rate, thanks to my doc—the contractions were manageable, and I felt pretty good. I could smile and joke between contractions and even pose for photos. I sat on the toilet and bounced on a birth ball to open up my pelvis and help the baby drop down into position. It wasn't until I hit transition that I was ready to bail. Looking back, I now know what transition is all about, and this reaction is extremely normal during this phase of labor. This is the toughest phase of labor, because the contractions are now longer and stronger, with no rest periods, in order to dilate the cervix the final couple of centimeters before pushing can start. Remember, transition is the hardest phase but also the shortest.

Going through it, I felt like my insides were being ripped out. I feared each contraction and yelled for an epidural, until I heard the magic words, "Wow, you're just about fully dilated. That explains why you're acting like this." Before I knew it (it seemed like hours, but in reality it was only about 20 minutes), I was ready to push. Pushing was a breath of fresh air after the brief torture of transition. Sure it hurt, but I can't even begin to explain it. The relief of pushing was awesome. Since this wasn't my first baby, and my body knew instinctively what to do, especially since I still had feeling from my waist down, it wasn't another agonizing three-hour pushing session like my daughter's birth. A couple of pushes, and out he flew, literally.

Shit, if I can do it, anyone can. I can't stress it enough; do your birth research, nail down a good coach or two, and be open with your doctor early on about your desires so you can feel him/her out. As the majority of births, at least in the U.S., are now being "managed" medically, it's pretty much up to you to 1) know your options, 2) make sure your hospital and doctor will be supportive of your desires and not a hindrance (this is actually the hardest to cover), 3) be in the right frame of mind so as not to undermine yourself on the big day (get rid of those repressed fears, talk about them, don't set your standards so high as to beat yourself up, and try to go in excited and relaxed), 4) be an advocate for yourself on B-day, and make sure your support team will do this when you can't, and 5) know that it may be tough, hopefully for just a bit, but that YOU CAN DO IT! (Note: in labor sometimes the shit hits the fan and things happen that change your birth plan. Don't be too disappointed; you tried.)

I only wish more of us, after all the turmoil of a rough pregnancy, could enjoy the wonders of a great birth. We deserve that at least, after all we were robbed of during a difficult pregnancy. What's the point, you ask? Drug-free-birth babies, assuming your baby is at or near term, are more alert, are able to nurse immediately after birth, and have been found to be generally more relaxed, calm, and peaceful than babies who were exposed to various drugs (narcotics, epidurals, etc.). You avoid the side effects of any drugs, which can affect both mom and baby, such as those from epidurals, narcotics, and Pitocin. If you're interested in reading more about the long list of benefits for both mom and baby, please check out some additional resources dedicated to this topic. I could go on and on, not only about considering a natural birth or abstaining from drugs, but also about how to have a great birth experience, but then this book would be over 500 pages long!

Achieving a More Natural Birth

According to Jennifer Block, author of the incredibly scary but true book *Pushed: The Painful Truth About Childbirth and Modern Maternity Care*[2], there are several items necessary to achieve a less medical and a more natural birth, which are derived from the familiar Cochrane Collaboration. These include:

+ Labor starts on its own. (It's not medically induced with meds.)

+ During labor, women are allowed (and encouraged) to move however they want.

+ Avoidance of routine medical interventions, which are only to be used when there's a real medical need. (This includes augmentation with Pitocin, breaking the waters manually, etc.)

+ Women must have continuous support, both emotional and physical.

+ Pushing shouldn't be done while you're flat on your back. (Think about it; this routine procedure doesn't make sense. It goes against the laws of physics; you know, that thing called gravity.)

+ Momma and baby need to be kept together after birth. (No routine separation immediately after birth for this and that. This helps to establish not only breastfeeding, but a strong emotional bond.)

If you would like to educate yourself about the issues in maternity care, I highly recommend this book. Sometimes, ignorance is bliss, which is what I came to realize after reading this intriguing and thoroughly researched book. If more women would take an interest in these issues and take a stand, then some big changes could happen within our medical system.

Stuff to Impress Your Doc With

According to Cochrane Reviews:

✦ Artificial breaking of waters to shorten labor, or reduce the need for a C-section, is not supported.[3]

✦ "Since the evidence shows no benefits or harms, there is no justification for the restriction of fluids and food in labor for women at low risk of complications."[4]

✦ "Women should be encouraged to give birth in comfortable positions, which are usually upright." They found the pushing stage to be shorter, a reduction in assisted deliveries (forceps/vacuums), and a reduction in episiotomies in upright positions.[5]

✦ Walking upright in the first stage of labor, the dilation stage, has been shown to reduce the length of labor. "Women should be encouraged to take up whatever position they find most comfortable in the first stage of labor." Lying on your back causes the weight of the uterus to reduce the strength of contractions and doesn't optimize them for dilation/descent of the baby down the birth canal.[6] Translation: lying on your back strapped to a monitor is no good. (Ask for a portable unit.)

References

1. Gaskin IM. *Ina May's Guide to Childbirth*. New York, New York. Bantam Books, 2003.
2. Block J. Pushed: *The Painful Truth About Childbirth And Modern Maternity Care*. Cambridge, MA. Da Capo Press, 2007.
3. Smyth RMD, Alldred SK, Markham C. Amniotomy for shortening spontaneous labor. *Cochrane Database of Systematic Reviews* 2007, Issue 4. Art. No.: CD006167. (Last assessed as up-to-date: April 15, 2010.)
4. Singata M, Tranmer J, Gyte GML. Restricting oral fluid and food intake during labour. *Cochrane Database of Systematic Reviews* 2010, Issue 1. Art. No.: CD003930. (Last assessed as up-to-date: October 1. 2009.)
5. Gupta JK, Hofmeyr GJ, Smyth RMD. Position in the second stage of labour for women without epidural anaesthesia. *Cochrane Database of Systematic Reviews* 2000, Issue 1. Art. No.: CD002006. (Last assessed as up-to-date: April 15, 2010.)
6. Lawrence A, Lewis L, Hofmeyr GJ, et al. Maternal positions and mobility during first stage labour. *Cochrane Database of Systematic Reviews* 2009, Issue 2. Art. No.: CD003934. (Last assessed as up-to-date: April 15, 2010.)

CHAPTER 18

The Amazing and
Miraculous Preemie Baby

"*H*aving a preemie can be very lonely, so make sure you reach out to other preemie moms who understand. Only those of us who have had a preemie or lost a child can understand the pain, grief, and guilt.*" ~ Rachel, California

"*If you ever feel something's not right, even if you're not very far along, NEVER brush off symptoms or wait too long before getting checked out. Should you have a preemie, learn everything you can and keep a journal. Keep a disposable camera at the hospital to take lots of pictures, and never assume the doctors are doing everything in the best interests of your kiddo. Docs will always give you the worst-case scenario, so take it with a grain of salt. Ask the nurses if you can have things like the tiny diaper they use, the small blood pressure cuff, pieces of hair if it is shaved, etc. Later, you can make a scrapbook, which is very therapeutic. There are many things from the NICU you'll forget; it's called the NICU fog.*" ~ Cindy, U.S.A.

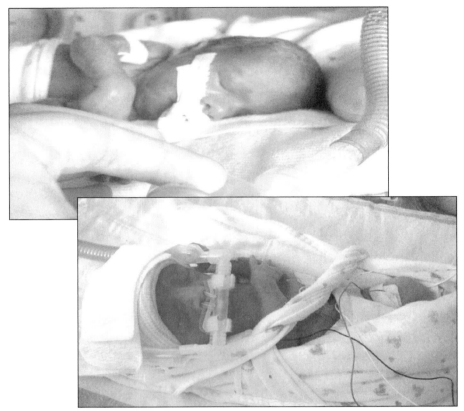

Baby Lyra, born at 26 weeks and 6 days weighing just under 1000 g. Both she and her twin are doing great today. Photos courtesy of Chris Sternal-Johnson (daddy).

Looking at the reality of a preemie baby, especially a micropreemie born at 28 weeks or less, is extremely scary. It will unquestionably be the roller-coaster ride from hell. When I was in the hospital with my first son at nearly 23 weeks, the likelihood of a very sick baby with severe developmental problems became a reality. The meetings with the neonatologist left me in a state of frenzy and tears. All those numbers . . . less than 1%, no chance, blah blah . . . Unfortunately, I never made it to viability, which in New Jersey, where I live, is 24 weeks.

This, as I've since seen/heard firsthand, is not always the case. Miracles can and do happen every day. Babies as young as 23 weeks, weighing in at around a pound or even less, can now be saved in the best NICUs. If you have a premature baby, I would highly recommend other resources to help you cope with life in the NICU, what to expect, as well as the specifics on the problems and treatments encountered when having a premature baby, because this chapter can only begin to skim the surface of these issues. (Resource suggestions can be found on my website, www.hrpwhyme.com.)

The families that have traveled the path of a premature baby, balancing life and death at every moment, know just how difficult it truly is. Even though the survival rate of late preterm infants, those born at 34–36 weeks, is in the high 90s percentage-wise, they still have a death rate that is four times higher than babies born at term.[1] So even if your baby comes just a little early, there still may be hurdles to clear.

I didn't put that last bit in to scare you—okay, maybe I did, just a little. I need to drive home the point that you want to avoid having a preemie at all costs, even if it means having to stay in the hospital for several months. Try to do whatever you can to "hold" that baby inside, because every additional day counts. Often, this isn't possible, and there's nothing more you can do, but at least you'll know you did all you could for your baby, and that's worth a lot.

Many women just don't understand how delicate a situation this is. They may think they don't have to follow their doctor's orders. They might think, "Oh, I'm sure I can go shopping and do some housework, even though my doc advised me to stay off my feet." They just don't understand how important it is to keep the baby inside their womb for as long as possible. They might believe that an early baby is just smaller and will grow once it has been born, failing to comprehend the possible developmental implications when they're born too soon.

One study looked at the rate of complications in preemies born at 30–34 weeks in 1997, and then went back to re-evaluate them at five years of age. When the gestation increased from 30 to 34 weeks, the death rate decreased from 8.1% to 0.4%, while complications of concern, such as respiratory distress syndrome, fell from 43.8% to 2.6%, infection from 7.2% to 2.6%, and severe brain injury from 5.5% to 1.3%. Those four extra weeks *in utero* made a huge difference. Infants born at 33 or 34 weeks rarely suffered from necrotizing enterocolitis (death of intestinal tissue), bronchopulmonary dysplasia (a chronic lung condition that affects either premature babies or babies who were on a breathing machine after birth), or hospital-acquired (a.k.a. nosocomial) infections, although they did still require ventilation to help breathing/oxygenation, antibiotics, and possibly nutrition supplementation.

When they were re-examined at five years of age, the kids who were born at higher gestational ages had less cerebral palsy (6.3% at 30 weeks compared to 0.7% at 34 weeks) or mild to severe cognitive disabilities (35.3% at 30 weeks compared to 23.9% at 34 weeks).[2] It's important to remember that this study was based on babies born in 1997. Technology, as well as our understanding of how to care for premature babies, has come a long way since then.

A Swedish study looking at the survival of extremely premature infants—i.e., born before 27 weeks—found that an overall incidence of 3.3 babies per 1000 were born at this gestation. The survival estimates were 9.8% at 22 weeks, 53% at 23 weeks, 67% at 24 weeks, 82% at 25 weeks, and 85% at 26 weeks. They found a lower risk of death of the baby in women who'd had tocolytic treatment or antenatal corticosteroids, or in babies who had surfactant treatment within two hours of birth, and those born at a level III hospital.[3]

If you're in this unfortunate situation, whereby the early birth of your baby seems imminent, you'll be bombarded with lots of figures, and the less far along you are, the more you'll be having this type of conversation with the neonatal specialists, causing your head to spin. Expect to feel shock that this is happening and confusion over the decisions that will have to be made and the treatments that will have to be undertaken for your tiny baby. This will all be very overwhelming to digest at once. It can be very hard to stay positive, but please try, even if it's all you can do to hold it together. Many, many families have pulled through this to have healthy, wonderful preemie babies... so maybe you can, too.

What Are the Various NICU Levels?[4]

Let's face it; the better and more experienced your hospital is in caring for preemies, the better your baby's chances are. In a couple of large studies, they found that level III care was shown to increase the overall survival rates of premature babies. Those hospitals that routinely cared for these tiny babies, and hence had a higher volume, also had lower death rates.

NICU Level Descriptions:

Level I: Provides basic newborn care.

Level IIA: Has limited specialty care.

Level IIB: Has the additional ability to provide positive airway pressure or mechanical ventilation for up to 24 hours only.

Level IIIA: Can care for babies born after 28 weeks and who weigh more than 1000 g, or 2 lb 3 oz; is capable of longer-term mechanical ventilation; and is able to perform minor surgeries.

Level IIIB: Able to care for babies who come before 28 weeks and who weigh less than 1000 g; can provide more difficult breathing support and good imaging, and have specialists on-site and specialists able to perform complex surgeries.

Level IIIC: Does all the above, but can also provide the highest level of life support and has specialists who are able to perform open-heart surgeries.

Babies do better when they're transferred while still in their mom's uterus, rather than after they're born. All women who are believed likely to deliver soon and who are carrying very low-birth-weight babies should be moved to a level III care center, according to the American Academy of Pediatrics and the American College of Obstetricians and Gynecologists. It's important for providers to avoid moving women who'll likely deliver during the actual transfer (not good), but sometimes this isn't possible. In reality, less than 25% of these babies are actually born in level III facilities, since there just aren't enough of them.

Amazing Babies[5]

(Note: read the stories quoted throughout this book. There are some really amazing babies here too.)

The earliest baby on record was born in Ottawa, Canada, in 1987. James Elgin Gill was born at only 21 weeks and 5 days, and weighed 1 lb 6 oz, a good size for that gestation, which probably helped him to survive and go on to be quite healthy.

Amillia Taylor was born in October, 2006, in Miami, Florida, at 21 weeks and 6 days. At birth, she was only 9 inches long (23 cm) and

weighed a measly 10 oz (283 g). Oh my ... can you even visualize how
tiny she was? She had digestive and respiratory issues, suffered from a
brain hemorrhage, and spent about four months in the hospital before
she was released.

On record for some time as the smallest baby was Madeline Mann,
a 26-weeker who weighed just 9.9 oz (280 g) and was 9.5 inches long
(24 cm), until Rumaisa Rahman, who was born at the same hospital at
25 weeks, came along in September 2004. She weighed just 8.6 oz (244
g), was only 8 inches long (20 cm), and has a twin sister. Their mom
suffered preeclampsia, which forced doctors to deliver the babies early.
Rumaisa stayed in the hospital for more than four months until she
was released weighing 2 lb 10 oz (1.18 kg). Both twins did well but
later had to undergo laser surgery to correct eye problems.

The Wonderful Steroid

Time and time again I've told you how great antenatal steroids are for
our tiny babies. The use of steroids has saved many, many babies by
helping to speed up the development of their fetal lungs so that when
the baby is born, they can help the baby breathe on its own sooner,
reduce dependence on breathing machines, or even allow them to skip
breathing help altogether.

Respiratory distress syndrome is a very common problem faced by
preemies, and steroids have been shown to dramatically reduce its
occurrence. There's no disputing how wonderful this treatment is for
premature babies. It's been said that steroid use is "a rare example of
a treatment that yields both a cost savings and an improved health outcome." Though the benefits have been known for over 50 years, the
use of steroids was slow to catch on.[4]

Doctors have suggested that, "All women being treated for preterm
labor between 24 and 34 weeks should be given antenatal steroids."
It's best given as two doses of the steroid betamethasone in your muscle, 24 hours apart, although four smaller doses can be given 12 hours
apart. They found that, when sampled 40 hours after treatment, the
steroid was undetectable in the baby's cord blood, and these drugs
haven't been found to be harmful to either mother or baby when a single round of treatments is used. The only short-term side effect in mom

is an increase in sugar intolerance. The preferred steroids are dexamethasone and betamethasone, although some research has suggested a preference for betamethasone due to a reduction in intra-ventricular hemorrhage with its use.[4]

The 2008 expanded health data found that steroids for fetal lung development were received by 1% of all moms. Surfactant replacement therapy, another treatment used to help early babies' lung function, was given to newborns at a rate of 3.7 per 1,000.[6]

A study that looked at the effect of the use of steroids during pregnancy on the survival of babies born at 23 weeks gestation found an 82% reduction in the likelihood of death. That's incredible! Sadly, though, they found that this wasn't the case for multiples. (The overall support for treatment in women carrying multiples is just not there yet.) There was no effect on the incidence of other common problems related to premature delivery, such as necrotizing enterocolitis (15.4% vs. 28.6%) or severe intraventricular (brain) hemorrhage (23.1% vs. 57.1%).[7] (Statistically, these differences were found to be non-significant, even though they may appear to be quite a difference.)

A consensus of the National Institutes of Child Health and Infant Development concluded that a single round of steroids leads to a significant reduction in death, respiratory distress syndrome, and intraventricular hemorrhage regardless of gender or race in premature babies.[4]

What about routine use of repeat (i.e., rescue) treatments? No. In the past, it was common practice to give multiple doses/courses of steroids. This is when another dose is given seven or more days after the first treatment. However, guidelines from the National Institute of Health have recommended only a single course for women who will most likely deliver within seven days and who are between 24 and 34 weeks, due to concerns about side effects from multiple doses.[8] Repeat doses are not suggested until more trials have been done.[4]

Ethics Surrounding These Tiny Babies

"Have your own faith and follow your heart. Don't let doctors force you to make quick decisions." ~ Evette, New Jersey

The ethics of how early is too early to save babies have been debated around the world. When I delivered my son in 2004 in the state of New Jersey, the cut-off point where they would intervene to save him was 24 weeks. Any earlier than that, and they wouldn't attempt any intervention after birth. Unfortunately, I didn't make it to 24 weeks.

Due to increased survival and better knowledge and technology, many countries and states are now considering lower limits of survival, like 23 or even 22 weeks, although some countries still consider gestations of 25 and 26 weeks necessary to be considered "viable." In an article that looked at this issue, they found the following guidelines:[9]

Sweden (2004)

+ They will consider, case by case, babies between 23 and 25 weeks gestation for treatment.
+ Parental consent must be obtained for treatment.

USA (2002)

+ For babies less than 23 weeks or less than 400 g (14 oz), do not resuscitate. (According to *Preterm Birth: Prevention and Management*, 23 weeks is the "limit of viability."[4])
+ There are no regulations for higher gestational ages.

Australia (2006)

+ Increasing obligation to treat between 23 + 0/7 weeks gestation and 25 + 6/7 weeks.
+ Exception to be made if parental consent is refused after appropriate advice/counseling.

In Japan, the viability limit as defined in the Japanese Motherhood Protection Act was changed from 24 to 22 completed weeks of gestation in 1991. This change was based on survival rates. The survival rates of Japanese babies born at 22 and 23 weeks between 2002 and 2004 were 31% at 22 weeks and 56% at 23 weeks.[10]

According to the medical textbook *Preterm Birth: Prevention and Management*, the World Health Organization (WHO) still recommends using 28 COMPLETED weeks, or almost 29 weeks, as their limit of viability, although they do recognize that this varies by country and region according to many factors.[4]

So, think of this: a 28-weeker born in the U.S., in a pretty good hospital, has about a 90% survival rate. Now think of this baby, born in a tribal community in Africa, that lacks running water, never mind medical care or an NICU. What's the chance of survival there? So sad.

For babies in that 23–25-week range, the toughest question faced by both parents and doctors is: Do we try to save them, or do we let them die to minimize their pain and avoid the possibility that they may be extremely sick and/or disabled? Questions on the future quality of life for these children are central in these discussions. In many circles, it's felt that letting these babies die and not attempting resuscitation or extreme care is the most humane decision.

As a parent, I can't imagine having to make this decision. In my case, the decision was made for me, because of how far along I was and the presence of infection. Was I angry at the time that they would not attempt to save my boy's life? Damn straight. I was downright pissed off and extremely bitter. When I think back now, however, do I think this was the right thing to do? Yes. But how can I say that, you may wonder? I now know that at almost 23 weeks, the chance of my baby's survival was low. Can babies be saved at this gestation in this day and age? Yes! And some of these very early babies end up having only minor disabilities or none at all. I know that I had a very bad infection, which had spread up through my placenta, so my baby probably would've struggled to live for even a few hours. Even if he had survived, how would his quality of life have been? Not very good. We had many things working against us, and I know he would have suffered terribly and had major disabilities, even if he had been able to survive. I don't think I could've lived with that.

I'd always thought that he'd died peacefully during birth, and it wasn't until several years later, when I requested my records so that I could switch doctors when I became pregnant with my other son, that I learned this wasn't the case. I was so out of it that I don't remember what happened after he was born. I closed my eyes and didn't want to look because I was so scared. Now, I read that he'd been born alive, with a heartbeat. This was devastating to me, and I wished I'd held him until he passed. How long did he live? It briefly made me question my decision. Should I have demanded that they try to save him, or try to make it another week instead of jumping to induce? It took many years of guilt before I could accept this. Some of you will find yourselves having to make similar tough decisions. All I can say is, do what's right for your baby, you and the situation. Don't rush into making any decisions.

In one French article, they talk about a "gray zone," those babies born at the margin of viability, which is 24–25 weeks in France. There, as in many other areas of the world, if a baby is born before 24 weeks gestation, the only option is to provide care to prevent pain and suffering until the baby passes on.

They acknowledge the tough decisions about whether to provide intensive care or let these babies die—i.e., withhold resuscitation and intensive care at birth. As they say, this involves complex ethical issues, because they recognize that some of those babies receiving resuscitation will survive and grow to be normal, healthy children, while others will be severely disabled. They cite the following factors (at a given gestational age) as providing a better chance of survival: higher weight at birth, being a singleton baby (i.e., not one of twins or higher multiples), being female, having gotten prenatal corticosteroid treatment *in utero*, and birth at a place equipped to handle these little ones.[11] Each of these factors should be considered by you and your doctor when discussing your options.

Sadly, I know that a few of you reading this will be forced to make difficult decisions for your babies, who'll be born at this cusp. This will be the hardest decision of your lives. It will be agonizing and will cause enormous turmoil within you, at so many levels. No one, not your doctor, not your family, can tell you what the best decision is. You'll need to dig deep inside to figure out what's best. Use your head and your heart.

What the right decision is will differ between families. Some families don't care about the odds of life, death, or extreme disabilities. They're simply willing to do everything for their child, no matter how it turns out. Others may not be able to have a child, knowing that the risk of debilitating disabilities is so great, and may choose to withhold aggressive treatments. No matter what, it's up to you and your spouse/partner to decide, as you're the ones who'll have to live with your decision. (Unless your baby is below viability, in which case, most times, even if you demand treatment, it's not possible.)

These tiny babies are truly special. Weighing in at around a pound or less, it's surreal to see one with your own eyes, but at the same time it's an amazing wonder. It's hard to really understand the impact of these tiny beings unless you've actually seen them. (I have, and it's amazing and incredibly frightening. To see a perfect baby, just so tiny, is scary.) My only hope is that there will be fewer and fewer babies born too early in the years to come because of an increasing understanding of prematurity and how to stop babies from coming too soon. They can make it and grow to be normal, healthy children.

The best predictor of survival is the age of your baby, or how many weeks gestation your baby is. Weight is also an important consideration—the bigger your baby is, the better—as is your baby's gender; girls tend to do better. Knowing all three of these is best when considering your baby's survival chances.[4] Like everything, this isn't an exact science. One baby at 24 weeks may do much better than another baby at that same gestation. Every day, every week that goes by is better for your baby, so take it day by day. If your baby does come early, you then need to take it hour by hour...and keep your hopes up.

According to the 2010 Premature Birth Report Card[12]

U.S.A. scores a D. "One in eight babies born in our country is premature. The rate of premature birth in America is higher than that of most other developed nations." (See the reference for the March of Dimes Web site so you can look at individual state report cards.)

A "Tool" Used to Calculate Survival of "Borderline" Babies (22–25 Weeks)

See the website www.nichd.nih.gov/about/org/cdbpm/pp/prog_epbo/epbo_case.cfm.

The following is taken directly from the website.

NICHD Neonatal Research Network (NRN): Extremely Preterm Birth Outcome Data

Can I use the data to determine individual outcomes?

If you choose to use these data to determine possible outcomes, please remember that the information provided is not intended to be the sole basis for care decisions, nor is it intended to be a definitive prediction of outcomes if intensive care is provided. Users should keep in mind that every infant is an individual, and that factors beyond those used to formulate these standardized assessments may influence an infant's outcomes.

EXAMPLE:

Gestational Age (Best Obstetric Estimate in Completed Weeks):	24 weeks
Birth Weight:	1000 grams
Sex:	Male
Singleton Birth:	Yes
Antenatal Corticosteroids:	Yes

Estimated outcomes for infants in the NRN sample are as follows:

Outcomes	Outcomes for All Infants	Outcomes for Mechanically Ventilated Infants
Survival	90%	89%
Survival Without Profound Neurodevelopmental Impairment	80%	79%
Survival Without Moderate to Severe Neurodevelopmental Impairment	64%	64%
Death	10%	11%
Death or Profound Neurodevelopmental Impairment	20%	21%
Death or Moderate to Severe Neurodevelopmental Impairment	36%	36%

Comments: The calculation is based on a large research study. Note that this takes into account the age of the baby, the baby's weight, whether the baby is a boy or a girl, a single baby or one of multiples, and whether mom received steroids. Also important is that they stress that these values are based on a baby who receives care at a level III NICU, and may not be the same at a lower-level hospital.

Hint: remember all the advice on risk and statistics. You never really know.

The Pre-Viable Brush Off

Unfortunately, if you're in the advanced stages of preterm labor, dilated with membranes bulging, waters broken, bleeding heavily, or you're suffering from severe preclampsia/eclampsia prior to viability, as it's so coldly termed in the medical world, some doctors will be quick to write you off. I will never accept the use of the term "viability" and baby in the same sentence. They've seen these sickest of babies come into the world, struggling and with severe disabilities. You may be advised to 'terminate' or be induced to deliver the baby now. Remember, this is your decision, and it's up to you to weigh the consequences, good and bad, of any decision you make. Don't be rushed, or pushed, into something you won't be able to live with for the rest of your life. It's okay to take some time to think about it, gather your thoughts, and even to decide against your doctor's wishes, not that I'm saying you should do that. You have the right to another opinion or two. (See Ruth's amazing and tough journey later in this chapter to have a healthy son she adores.)

As you've seen throughout this book, there are quotes from women who've been in these situations, walked in your shoes, and went on to carry their babies past this critical gestation, some of them well beyond this zone. So, again...there's hope. After this magical point in your pregnancy, doors will suddenly open up, and options will now be considered and discussed. You'll now get closer care and attention. Your baby is suddenly thought of as a full-fledged patient.

From a mom's viewpoint, this can be quite difficult and frustrating. To feel like your baby is not yet a person in need of care is wrong. After all, to us, this is not just a statistic, but our precious little baby who we've been dreaming about for months, maybe even years. Not that I think the approach many doctors take is right, or that I'm defending anything, because I have been in this situation, but I can understand why it's like this. They see the reality of babies born too soon at these very early gestations. Doctors, by nature, also don't typically go around giving hope or focusing on the good that can happen. That's what I'm here to do, to remind you to hope (and even pray if you need to). Keep your chin up, girls.

My advice, if you're in this situation, is to try to clear your mind so you can think rationally about your decision. Don't rush to terminate or induce labor because you feel pressured. Take time to weigh your options, do some research, get second opinions, and ask around if you have to. Know that you may be one of the lucky ones who'll be bringing her baby home, healthy and plump. Should you choose the unimaginable, know that you did everything you could to protect your baby and that sometimes terrible things like this happen. It's not your fault.

What Can I Expect During Delivery of My Tiny Baby?[4]

There's one thing you can be sure of, and that is an exponentially increased level of stress beyond that experienced by "normal" women. You'll be running the full gamut of emotions. If your baby is coming really early, there will be the worry about the health of your baby, and the vibe in the room will feel very strange. There'll be a team of people moving about around you, and you'll feel like a side thought, because all their efforts will probably be focused on preparing for the baby. There's no question that this will be a very trying experience for you. You're being robbed of the birth day you've dreamed of…but you can do it.

We know that if your baby is very premature, you can expect to be transferred to a level III Neonatal Intensive Care Unit (NICU) before the baby is born, if that's at all possible. Studies have shown that if an abnormal heart rate is observed, it's best to perform a C-section quickly, because a heart rate beyond the normal 160 beats per minute at 22 weeks can be a sign of infection. Constant monitoring of the baby's heart rate during delivery has been shown to improve outcomes in babies that are less than 3 lb 5 oz. Doctors generally use troubling patterns as a signal to deliver quickly.

In terms of anesthesia and pain relief, the safest type for your preemie is regional anesthesia, like an epidural. The use of narcotics should be avoided in preemies, since delivery often occurs quickly, so there's typically not enough time for them to wear off. These drugs can have negative effects on the baby, like sedation, breathing, or heart rate troubles. It's recommended that general anesthesia (being knocked out) only be used in emergency deliveries, where there's no time for other options, or if the woman can't handle regional anesthesia for other reasons. They've also found that the use of an episiotomy, forceps, or elective C-section delivery to get your premature baby out quicker in order to limit the trauma from the birth itself doesn't provide any benefit to the baby or improve outcomes. "Vacuum should never be used before 34 weeks."[4] This is linked to several problems, even bleeding in the brain.

Some of you may have heard about asking your doctor to hold off clipping the cord for a bit after the baby comes out, to allow all the stem cells to flow back into the baby. Well, now they've also found that holding off on cutting the cord by up to two minutes is better for preemies. This practice has been linked to fewer transfusions and fewer brain hemorrhages. So ask to please hold off cutting the cord if they can.

Now, just because you're having your baby early doesn't mean you're guaranteed a C-section. Studies that have looked at elective C-sections, meaning those performed other than in an emergency situation, as opposed to a vaginal delivery, have concluded that "vaginal delivery is preferred" in babies that are head down.[4] If a C-section is performed for a preterm baby, it's recommended that in order to reduce the chance of injury to the baby, a low vertical or classical uterine incision is best. (This is not the horizontal, along the bikini line, incision typical of C-sections.)

Remember, if your baby shows signs of distress, an emergency C-section is best. To deliver any baby early, meaning before 39 weeks, there must be a damn good reason. Even babies born near term, at 34 to 36 weeks, have a higher chance of cerebral palsy and mental retardation.

How to Help Care for Your NICU Baby

✦ Pump milk to give your baby all the benefits of your antibody protection. Pumping milk will make you feel like you're connected and doing something for your baby, even though the baby can't be home with you. Pumping is hard work; don't get me wrong. It gets easier with time as you establish your milk supply (after around 6–8 weeks). The only way to survive pumping is to get (or rent) a good electrical pump (hospital grade). Early on it's best to stick to pumping around every three hours to really establish your milk. During this time your supply can easily wane if you stretch too long between pumpings. You don't need to crank it up so high as to hurt your nips; just relax and even think about baby or look at a picture to naturally allow let-down occur. This takes practice, so don't beat yourself up. Even a half ounce is liquid gold to your baby.

✦ Talk to your little one. Your baby knows your voice from the time spent in the womb, so talk to him or her. (A study has shown benefits in 27–28-weekers who were played recordings of their mom's voice.[13])

✦ If you're able to, give your baby skin-to-skin contact, known as Kangaroo Care. Research has shown the benefits of this skin-to-skin contact.

✦ Take care of yourself. It's just as important for you to be well rested and healthy. It's a long road, and you need to care for yourself so you can be there for your baby. Don't feel guilty about doing "you" things while baby is in the NICU. It's okay to take a break from the hospital. A little relief can help to recharge you mentally.

✦ Develop a NICU routine. Educate yourself about the NICU environment, common treatments, machines, and common preemie problems. (This will help you to relax while you're there; otherwise, trust me, your baby will sense your stress.)

✦ Get involved in your baby's care at your comfort level. This could simply be diaper and gown changes, or even more advanced feeding tube changes. Being a mom at some level will help your confidence and help you to bond with your baby.

What Can I Expect?

Early problems for premature infants[4,14]

✦ Inability to breathe, or breathe regularly, on their own because of underdeveloped lungs. (Respiratory distress syndrome is the most frequent severe result of being born prematurely at any gestation.)

✦ Necrotizing enterocolitis* (Death of intestinal tissue. This only happens in 7% of very early babies.)

+ Sepsis*, which is caused by bacterial or fungal infections that can begin anywhere in the body. (This is more common in babies born after PPROM than from preterm labor or for other reasons.)

+ Body temperature regulation, where baby can't maintain his or her own body heat.

+ Feeding and growth problems because of an immature digestive system.

+ Jaundice, which is yellowing of skin and possible brain damage due to buildup of bilirubin, a blood breakdown product.

+ Anemia, where not enough red blood cells carry oxygen to tissues.

+ Intracranial hemorrhage (bleeding into the brain).* (Severe brain bleeding only occurs in 11% of very early babies.)

+ Retinopathy of prematurity (an eye disease, which can cause blindness).

+ Severe neurologic disability. (Only 25% of babies who come at 25 weeks or less will suffer from this. Think of this as meaning 75% of babies won't have this problem.)

Problems premature infants might face as they grow older[14]

+ Apnea (episodes of stopped breathing), which may require special monitoring, even at home.

+ Bronchopulmonary dysplasia, a chronic lung disease that may or may not improve as the child grows.

+ Hearing or vision problems related to immature nerves or side effects of treatment.

+ Developmental delays and learning disabilities from brain damage related to immaturity.

+ Very preterm babies (those born at less than 28 weeks) are still at high risk for long-term neurological disorders as they grow up. (A study found this when following up kids at 6–10 years of age.)[15]

---

*Common in very early babies; not so common in those babies born close to term.

Cochrane Reviews

1. Summary: steroids…they work. They help to speed up baby's lung development, hence reducing death, breathing problems and other problems at birth including respiratory distress syndrome (RDS), cerebroventricular hemorrhage, necrotising enterocolitis, breathing support, intensive care admissions, and infection in the first 48 hours of life. They're also effective in women who have premature rupture of membranes and pregnancy-related hypertension.

   Further study is needed to determine "optimal dose to delivery interval," which drug is best, what the results are in multiple pregnancies, and the long-term effects.[16]

2. "Repeat dose(s) of prenatal corticosteroids reduce the occurrence and severity of neonatal lung disease and the risk of serious health problems in the first few weeks of life." They also acknowledge that the long-term effects, risks, and benefits are unknown.[17]

   How can this be? This review contradicts a statement made by the other reviewers, which goes to show that even within a set of reviews, there's still conflicting and unclear information. How's a doctor ever supposed to make sense of this? Should they or shouldn't they repeat doses?

3. Giving thryrotropin-releasing hormone (TRH) with corticosteroids to women at risk of very early birth in an attempt to reduce breathing problems in the baby doesn't improve the outcome and can cause side effects in mom.[18]

4. "Vitamin K given to women before a very early preterm birth does not decrease the risk of bleeding in the brain and associated neurological injury in babies born very preterm."[19] (The belief was that vitamin K would help with coagulation.)

   • "Vitamin K is the most common 'drug' administered to babies born in the western world." It is routine practice to treat preterm babies with it. There is much variability in how much is used, where to administer it (route), and the formulation/type used.[20]

5. "Evidence does not support phenobarbital treatment to women giving birth before 34 weeks to decrease the risk of bleeding into the baby's brain."[21]

Statistics

Sorry, more numbers, but in this situation you'll be told lots of this stuff, so here it is. Note the range of numbers—i.e., it's not exact, and they don't know for certain where your baby will fall.

Table 1: Odds of a Premature Baby's Survival by Length of Pregnancy[5]

Length of Pregnancy	Likelihood of Survival
23 weeks	17%
24 weeks	39%
25 weeks	50%
26 weeks	80%
27 weeks	90%
28–31 weeks	90–95%
32–33 weeks	95%
34+ weeks	Almost as likely as a full-term baby

Source: March of Dimes, Quint Boenker Preemie Survival Foundation.

Table 2: Outcomes for All Infants[22]

Gestational Age (in Completed Weeks)	Death Before NICU Discharge	Outcomes at 18 to 22 Months Corrected Age		
		Death	Death/Profound Neuro-developmental Impairment	Death/Moderate to Severe Neuro-developmental Impairment
22 weeks	95%	95%	98%	99%
23 weeks	74%	74%	84%	91%
24 weeks	44%	44%	57%	72%
25 weeks	24%	25%	38%	54%

Table 3: Outcomes for Mechanically Ventilated Infants[22]

Gestational Age (in Completed Weeks)	Death Before NICU Discharge	Outcomes at 18 to 22 Months Corrected Age		
		Death	Death/Profound Neuro-developmental Impairment	Death/Moderate to Severe Neuro-developmental Impairment
22 weeks	79%	80%	90%	95%
23 weeks	63%	63%	76%	87%
24 weeks	40%	41%	55%	70%
25 weeks	23%	24%	37%	54%

The Dos and Don'ts of the NICU: For Medical Professionals

(Don't be afraid to speak up to get what you want or need. The NICU can be a very scary place.) Reprinted with permission from www.premature-infant.com. For more information and resources on preemie babies, visit this site.

Do: Ask me what I like to be called. I may or may not want to be called "mom."

Do: Send me a Polaroid of my baby when I can't get out of bed because I have had a C-section.

Do: When referring to my baby, please don't call him "your baby" (as if he is your baby) or "the baby." He is your patient, but he is my baby. The best possible way to refer to my baby is by calling him by his first name.

Do: Give me a tour of the nursery soon after I arrive, so I know where the pumping room is, where to store breast milk, the lounge, bathroom, etc. (Remember, if I am groggy or having a difficult time coping, I might need a second tour later.)

Do: If you are the nurse caring for my baby, acknowledge me when I come in the room, so I know who you are.

Do: Tell us when I can speak with the doctor.

Do: Promote attachment between parents and their babies. Show me that you are confident I will not cause my child any harm.

Do: Tell me how to read stress cues so I know the best time to touch my baby and when to stop.

Do: Show me how to do things that I can do to help care for my baby.

Do: Realize that once I am able to do some kind of activity for my baby, it is really stressful to have a staff member decline my doing it because they are unable to help.

Do: Acknowledge when we do things correctly, praise us, thank us!

Do: Tell me how to touch my baby in a developmental and soothing way.

Do: Allow me to hold my baby as early as possible—it is the best part of being a parent.

Do: Help me to do Kangaroo Care as early as possible. Please check on me during this time to make sure I am okay.

Do: Encourage us to make a tape to leave in the isolette; singing, talking, or telling stories for my baby. Tell me what I can do to decorate my baby's bed.

Do: Create an environment for my baby that seems healing and supportive (i.e., no harsh lights or minimal noise, but cluster care when possible).

Do: Take pictures (with a Polaroid or with a disposable camera I have left for you) of our babies when we're not there or when we're cuddling or spending time with our babies. We may not think to get our cameras out at those special moments, and we may be missing some big ones when we can't be there.

Do: Talk to my child and explain that you are about to touch them.

Do: If you find it necessary to shave my baby's head for an IV, please save a lock of hair from the "haircut."

Do: Provide support without judging.

Do: Realize that every parent is different and responds differently. Find out how we want to deal with things.

Do: Understand that parents, like our children, will have "crisis days," and they may not coincide with the status of my baby.

Do: Work to build genuine connections with parents. Even when there is nothing concrete or specific that you can do, your presence, attention, and compassion bring strength and comfort.

Do: Help parents of preemies build a community by removing obstacles preventing families from finding comfort in the experiences of others. Do what you can to create an environment in which parents can talk and support one another.

Do: Provide honest information and clear explanations. Please allow us to ask questions.

Do: Let us know when tests are being done on our babies (even if it means a quick call to home) and explain what they're for—in parents' terms.

Do: Let us know that we are allowed to read our baby's chart.

Do: Give us access to as much information as possible. Have a parent library with current books, videos, and a list of websites available. We would love to be able to buy books right there in the hospital—please encourage your gift shop to stock a supply of books and resources that we may purchase to help us through this process.

Do: Give us complete information that is significant to future possible outcomes (concerning all drugs, procedures, and alternatives that we can choose from).

Do: Realize that the truth is always easier for us to deal with in the long run. If a bleak prognosis can be expected, that prognosis won't be any easier if it comes as a complete and total shock later on.

Do: Respect parents enough to allow them to feel all their jumbled emotions without running away or minimizing what they feel.

Do: Talk with us about other things than our baby to help us pass the time and get our minds off things (maybe even ask us about the birth or things unrelated to our baby). It's nice to be treated as a friend.

Do: Support us if we are unable to breast-feed/express milk and must use formula for whatever reason.

Do: Refer me to a lactation specialist if I am having trouble lactating or feeling uncomfortable with pumping milk or breast-feeding.

Do: Please respect my efforts in pumping my breast milk and breast-feeding my baby. Thaw only what breast milk is necessary for each feeding—it is a precious commodity.

Do: Do ask me if I would like to have a screen put up when I am trying to nurse my baby, as it is a very exposing experience with these tiny babies. Please check in with me often when I'm behind the screen, especially when the alarms are going off.

Do: Make sure to let me know when my supply of breast milk is running low so I can make sure to bring some in.

Do: Dress my baby in her own clothes whenever possible.

Do: Find out our schedules so we can be there for feedings, baths, and maybe even a quick holding during weights and isolette changes.

Do: Give credence to a parent's intuition about their child. If I tell you, "Something is wrong," act on that information as if it were true.

Do: Congratulate us on our baby's milestones. (Diapers finally taped on, larger diapers, changing to a new type of bed, going to a lower oxygen setting, getting off the vent/CPAP, wearing clothes, learning to suck/swallow, being held, etc.)

Do: If you have not cared for my baby before, please read the chart carefully and note what times I usually come by.

Do: Put graduate pictures of former patients in the waiting room.

Do: Laugh with us.

Do: Cry with us.

Do: Treat us like real parents.

Please Don't . . .

Don't: Move the baby without telling me ahead of time, or at least meeting me at the door.

Don't: Tell me how I should be feeling or that I "need to be patient."

Don't: Dismiss or diminish my concerns. I am not used to seeing my baby have bradycardias *[a drop in heart rate]* or color changes.

Don't: Assume that I don't care for or love my baby if I don't touch him. I may be very scared or overwhelmed.

Don't: Tell me my baby had a bradycardia because I was touching him, feeding him, or doing something wrong.

Don't: Please never treat me as if I am stupid. All of the medical terms and information are very difficult to understand and comprehend at times, especially since I am probably feeling a tremendous amount of stress.

Don't: Write harsh judgments about me in the nurse's notes, unless the information you are recording is known to you without question from both observation and communication.

Don't: Assume anything about me or my family if we are unable to visit regularly. My family may be very loving and supportive, but cannot come to the NICU for other reasons.

Don't: Sound annoyed or make insensitive comments when I call to check on my baby. The phone is sometimes my only connection to my precious baby.

Don't: Do the tasks that I have already been doing (bath, diapers, feedings, etc.) if you know I am on the way to the nursery. It takes away what little parenting I can do.

Don't: Act as if breast-feeding is not crucial for my baby. There is enough scientific evidence of its importance to preemies that I should be encouraged to breast feed. However, if I am unable to produce milk, please do not make me feel inadequate by comparing me to all the other mothers who have no problem with lactating.

Don't: Please be careful to not share information about a baby with the wrong person. Please check and double check that you have the correct information with the correct parent.

Don't: Talk about a baby in a negative way when the parents are gone. It is morally wrong, very unprofessional, and may also hurt other parents' feelings (wondering what they say about their baby when they are not here).

Don't: Try to instill your personal views (philosophies, religion, or ethics) on us. Allow us the same freedom to choose and have our views as you were allowed to choose and have yours. (This includes miracles happening in the NICU.)

Don't: Be afraid of my emotions or of your own.

Don't: Let me travel this difficult journey alone.

Edited by: Dianne Maroney (author of *Your Premature Baby & Child)*, Andrea O'Brien, and Sheri DeBari.

Ruth's Journey to a True Miracle – Jacob

"It seemed like an eternity when we were going through it. The entire high-risk pregnancy, severe hemorrhaging, bed rest, PPROM, and placental abruption was not only terrifying, but felt like years in our lives. Once we'd delivered, we spent the next four months in the NICU, and that felt so long too, but the day we brought our baby boy home, life started again. Then, it seemed like our journey until his homecoming had been a matter of minutes. These times ARE trying, they ARE difficult, and they ARE scary. No question. But they don't last forever— it just feels that way at the time.

My whole pregnancy had been full of scares. I needed to take progesterone injections the whole way through, just as I'd had to do during my first pregnancy, and at 7 weeks 2 days I started hemorrhaging severely. I was bleeding constantly and losing huge clots. This was due to subchorionic hematomas and continued until 18 weeks, when my waters broke, and the hemorrhaging started again, lasting until delivery.

When we went for a scan at 11 weeks, we found out that I was pregnant with twins, and that one of them had already died. The doctor then spoke with us in detail about the scan results and explained that our twin had stopped growing. He was so kind and gentle in how he spoke. He told us that there was nothing we could have done to prevent this, and then told us about the potential risks to our other baby.

I was 18 weeks and 5 days when I began to leak amniotic fluid early in the morning. It was green, the consistency of oil, and smelled strongly (not the sweet smell of the fluid in my first birth). I told my husband and then I phoned my mum, as I was worried. I decided it was time to go into the hospital, as the leaking was continuing and I was getting uterine tightening.

I was admitted with PPROM (preterm premature rupture of membranes). They were concerned about infection, and we were told by one of the nurses that I had chorioamnionitis. She told us that it was very serious, and I needed to be in the hospital for treatment, as women still died from this condition. This was such a shock to us. The doctor who did my observations conducted a speculum exam, wherein she witnessed the amniotic fluid pooling and leaking, and confirmed that it was my waters with a test strip. She also performed an ultra-sound, which showed low fluid levels. She was hesitant to say whether or not I would be able to maintain the pregnancy, but after some firm pressure for answers, she told us that our chances were not good. She said that most women went on to deliver their baby very quickly, and at this gestation our baby would pass away shortly after birth.

It was a very strange thing to suddenly hear myself telling Mum, in a very serious tone, that I would have this baby early. I told her that what I meant was I would have this baby very early, that it would spend a long time in hospital, and would then come home healthy. I'd had no intention of saying those words, and I surprised myself by say-ing them. The doctors didn't believe that I would be leaving the hospi-tal pregnant, let alone birthing and taking home a healthy baby.

The nurses who looked after me through the night were lovely, and were also quite honest about the usual outcome of situations such as mine. I continued leaking fluid and contracting throughout the night, our baby was moving so much and kicking so strongly, and in the morning I was visited by a team of doctors. Needless to say, it was completely devastating to hear the distressing news they brought. The doctors insisted that my pregnancy would not continue. "You will be delivered today," was the phrase we heard. They assured me that I would not be leaving the hospital pregnant.

My thoughts then turned to staying pregnant and to giving our baby the best chance I could. I asked if I could remain pregnant with the help of antibiotics, and I was informed that the treatment for this infection was delivery. They were pushing strongly for my consent to have our baby medically removed. I was terrified. They also informed me that the longer I waited, the lower the chance I had of retaining my womb, and therefore the potential for a successful pregnancy in the future.

The doctors insisted that our baby would not survive, even if they were able to keep me pregnant. They were lovely, speaking with my mum and me in great detail about the complications a very premature baby would encounter, and told us that in my condition, it was impos-sible for our baby to be born at a gestation that would facilitate sur-vival (24 weeks plus is considered viable here).

They continued to push for my consent, but I told them that I was sorry, but I could not accept the help they were offering. They had no hope for our pregnancy. One of the doctors told me kindly, but without optimism, that sometimes miracles happened. When the doctors came back to speak with us, they explained in basic terms that if we did not consent, my husband would lose us both, so he could choose to lose either his baby or his baby and his wife. I felt so sad for the doctors, as this was the best advice they had for us. Given the complications I was experiencing, it was the right course of action for them to have initiated.

I had asked the doctors for more time, because I knew our baby was still alive, and I could not bring myself to consent to having our child terminated. They told us that they would send me for another ultrasound, since I was being so hopeful for my pregnancy.

I was having trouble accepting what they had told us, and I think my husband was, too. Before Mum and Dad left, I asked Dad to pray for me. He asked me what I wanted him to pray for, so I asked that God give us our child, which is what we so desperately desired. I also asked that should God decide to take our child to be with Him, that He would allow my labor to progress quickly without medical intervention, that He would take that decision and that distress out of our hands. It would have been such a mercy to lose our baby without consenting to a termination.

As soon as Dad had prayed, my amniotic fluid, which had been leaking constantly, stopped leaking altogether. I also had no further contractions, although I did not know this right away, as they had been coming at random. Since I was nearly 19 weeks pregnant, the doctors decided to give me the full anatomy scan. When we arrived, the doctor asked us why we were coming for the ultrasound, and I told her that my waters had broken. She spent some time searching for the tear in the amniotic sac but could find no evidence of it. She asked if we were sure it was my waters (as other fluid loss can mimic amniotic fluid). When I told her about the testing that had confirmed that it was, she looked very surprised and told us that I had a "perfect" level of amniotic fluid, the optimum 10 cm surrounding our baby.

The doctors deliberated for a while, then came back in to speak with us. They told us the results of the ultrasound and said that everything looked good. We spoke at length with them about our situation, and they explained that they wanted me to stay overnight so they could *monitor me, but that if I didn't leak any fluid overnight, I could go home in the morning. I knew that I wouldn't leak anymore, as God had answered our prayers. Since we had our nine-month-old daughter at home, I wanted to be released from the hospital, but the doctors were not comfortable with this; however, after some discussion, they signed off on my release from the hospital, as they had no medical reason to keep me there.*

We were all overjoyed that I was able to leave, and I was in tears. There were so many emotions I was experiencing; shock, relief, happiness, amazement. Words cannot fully describe the feelings I had. How grateful we were.

The next few weeks went smoothly, in spite of the continuing blood loss, which had started again soon after my waters broke. Then my waters broke for the second time at 23 weeks 6 days. According to the doctors, my waters could not have broken again; however, my membranes certainly had ruptured again. I have since asked several of the doctors about this and received varying replies. Some have suggested that the rupture was high in the sac and that I had a constant amniotic fluid leak until I delivered. These doctors can't explain why I stopped leaking fluid after my dad prayed, only to have a second gush five weeks later, nor can they explain the lack of evidence of a tear from the ultrasound scan. Not one of them can explain why I tested positive with the test strip and had a speculum exam and an ultrasound confirming that my membranes had ruptured.

I spent the next nine days on restricted bed rest and was seen daily by a team of doctors and medical students, too. Thankfully, I was given the two steroid shots that accelerate lung maturation. Several times during my stay, I was taken to the Labor and Delivery suite after threatening to go into preterm labor. The labor room had been set up with pediatric bed warmers and all the necessary equipment for a preterm birth, which was very unnerving.

The pediatrician was lovely and spoke to me for a long while. He explained all the common complications and likely outcomes of preterm babies, the statistics that change so dramatically with every day a woman stays pregnant, our options for deciding whether or not to attempt to revive our baby, and when it becomes a legal requirement to intervene. We had the right to decline any interventions for our baby. He left me with a handful of booklets detailing all that we had discussed and a very heavy heart. I did not want to process all that he had told me. It was made very clear that our chance of having a healthy baby at my gestation was somewhere in the 1–2% range (becoming a 2–3% range at 25 weeks). I had been told it does happen but not to expect it, hope for it, or make a decision to intervene without carefully considering our baby's long-term quality of life. It was one of the hardest discussions I ever had to make. Everything inside me wanted to believe that our baby would be in that small range of healthy outcomes. I did not know how we could live with ourselves if we did cause our baby long-term suffering by choosing to have the baby kept alive. On the other hand, I did not know how we could live with ourselves if we allowed our baby to pass away at birth because we did not choose to ask for the necessary medical interventions.

The doctors all encouraged us to make our own choice and explained that they would support us where needed. They told us very clearly what their choices would be and also let us know that it was a co-decision between parents and doctors. They could not make choices for us, nor could we for them, so at least a part of our decision would be based on how our baby reacted to the help that the doctors would offer, if we wanted it. They told us that we could change our minds at any time until the point of delivery, and then we could change our minds based on how our child responded to the treatment already given. I made the initial choice to have "every and all" intervention available to keep our baby alive. It was a hard decision to make. I spoke to my husband regarding what the doctors had said, and he agreed that we should ask them to do everything possible for our baby. It was quite a daunting decision, as we knew it was very likely that we would have a baby with severe problems should I birth early. Knowing that it would be our choice was difficult, as we never wanted our baby to suffer, nor did we want to lose him.

The consultant discussed the option of a Caesarean, as our baby was breech and unable to turn due to low fluid levels. With a baby of this gestation, women cannot have a LUSCS (lower uterine segment Caesarean section). This is the most common type and is a small cut along the bikini line. It is a less serious surgery that heals faster, with fewer complications, and also enables a mother to opt for a vaginal birth with any subsequent pregnancies. If we chose the Caesarean method of birth, I would need a classical Caesarean. This is a vertical cut through the muscles and uterus, with a horizontal cut across the skin. It looks the same on the outside, but makes a future vaginal birth impossible. It is also a more serious procedure to recover from, and there are more risks to this type of Caesarean.

I had been in the hospital for over a week when I decided that I wanted to go home. I had not gone into preterm labor already, as the doctors had thought I might. I was not enjoying the bed rest, but I was thankful that the doctors believed it would help my pregnancy.

The following day, 25 weeks into my pregnancy, I was sent for another ultrasound scan. My fluid level was down to 3 cm. Later that day, I ended up going into spontaneous labor as a result of hemorrhaging.

I was taken to Labor and Delivery, and less than 10 minutes into the surgery, I heard a cry. It was our son! We had a baby boy. What a joyful sound it was to hear his voice. It wasn't the way we had expected to welcome him into the world, but here was our son, Jacob Kenneth, alive and in the best care possible. We were well aware that we had a very small chance of having a perfectly normal baby, and yet we were so happy at the moment of delivery that we had chosen this path. The pediatrician quickly wrapped Jacob and began breathing for him with specialized equipment. He was very thoughtful and brought Jacob to me briefly before leaving with his team to start his critical care.

What a shock it was to see him. I had seen a girlfriend's baby delivered at 31 weeks and had thought that Jacob would be just a little smaller, but he was a lot smaller, weighing in at just 720 g (1.6 lb). I had never seen such a small baby. It really came as a surprise, and it took me a few seconds to realize that I was looking at the tiny face of my beautiful son. Seconds later, I was left with the medical staff as my husband and newborn son were taken to the NICU.

The Lord continued to bless us throughout our NICU journey as Jacob experienced many of the typical micro-preemie problems. He began in an isolette on high-frequency oscillatory ventilation (HFOV), a machine that vibrates air into the lungs 300 times per minute. A regular ventilator used for preemies would have burst his lungs. He received treatment with nitric oxide and surfactant for his lungs. Morphine and high doses of caffeine were administered to keep him sedated and pain free and to help his respiratory system.

He had constant saturation/desaturation levels (sats/desats), which is when the blood oxygen levels are too high or too low, and he had As and Bs, a term for apnea of prematurity and bradycardia (bradys). These are periods of no breathing and a slowed heart rate. Jacob also had cyanosis episodes, where he would turn blue from lack of oxygen. There were times when he had tachycardia, which is an increased heart rate; he suffered from pulmonary hypertension (high blood pressure in the arteries supplying the lungs) and pulmonary hemorrhage (bleeding from the lungs); and he also had a minor brain hemorrhage. Jacob had nine blood transfusions during his stay, one of which was needed after he bled out from an IV line that he had dislodged. This led the doctors to test him and find that he had a factor IX deficiency, which caused melena (blood in the stools) and hematuria (blood in the urine).

He was on the mechanical ventilators (which breathed entirely for him) for several weeks before graduating to CPAP (continuous positive airway pressure), which he remained on for several months. The CPAP machine has a tube that provides oxygenated air through prongs that fit into the baby's nose. The pressure is constant and helps the baby to breathe by keeping the airways inflated, but does not control the breathing itself, as the ventilators do. Jacob had several episodes of sepsis, requiring him to be re-intubated on the mechanical ventilators, and went through many courses of antibiotics.

He also had a symptomatic PDA (patent ductus arteriosis). The PDA is a blood vessel, called the ductus arteriosis, which connects the pulmonary artery with the aorta when a baby is within the womb. It is essential for circulation in the baby, which receives oxygen from the mother. After birth, the vessel usually closes, but in some preemies it remains open (patent) and mixes oxygen-rich blood from the aorta with oxygen-poor blood from the pulmonary artery. This strains the heart and increases blood pressure in the lung arteries. Jacob did not respond to medical treatment as most PDA babies do, and needed his fluids to be restricted to reduce the pressure.

Jacob experienced NEC (necrotising enterocolitis) symptoms several times while attempts were made to prime him with breast milk.

NEC is infection and necrosis of the intestines, so he was placed on "nil by mouth" for weeks to avoid developing this problem. He was fed via TPN (total parenatal nutrition), which is given by an IV line, before he was finally able to digest my expressed breast milk through a nasogastric tube. He also had retinopathy of prematurity (ROP), thankfully only progressing to stage 1 and needing no treatment. Jacob also had chronic lung disease of prematurity (CLD), also known as bronchopulmonary dysplasia (BPD), which results in long-term respiratory problems.

In his first few days of life, I could fit my wedding ring over his leg, and his ID bands were strapped to him, as they were too large to fit his arm or leg, even on the smallest setting. There were IV lines in most limbs, as well as an umbilical line. He appeared very red, as though burned, and I could see his veins and his eyes under his skin. I was very blessed to be able to hold my son only weeks after he was admitted into the NICU. It was a wonderful experience.

At King Edward Memorial Hospital, we are able to practice Kangaroo Care, which involves placing a mostly naked baby against a bare chest (covered with a hospital gown). This practice markedly reduces the incidence of desats and bradys, as the baby is much more relaxed. It also helps the baby to maintain temperature and mothers to produce more breast milk with a change in her hormones. The process involved in having him removed from his isolette and handed to me was rather involved. It took two nurses to do this safely, one to hold Jacob and the other to bring all the wires and cables. Both of them had to be present in case of emergency with such a small baby.

It was a shock to hold him for the first time, as there was no weight to him at all. It didn't feel as though I was holding a baby. He was soft and covered in lanugo, very boney, with no fat on him at all, and yet so strong in his movements. I was taught how to do his daily care, which initially involved mouth care to moisten his mouth and treat him with thrush medication, taking his temperature, changing his electrodes, saturation monitors, and his nappy. As he grew and became stronger, I was also able to bathe him and do his hat release (massaging the scalp and ears to help prevent deformities from the CPAP hat). When they are very small, as he was, these are done every six hours to avoid over-handling. Cuddles are also limited, and I had to ask to hold *my son. I could touch him very carefully without over-stimulating him, and was restricted to this most days.*

The four months he spent in NICU were like living in a different world. As an NICU mum, I learned to speak medical slang with the doctors and nurses and learned far more terms than I had ever wanted to. I knew when I could safely turn off the constant screams of the alarms and when I needed to call for help. Being a mum is an experience that is hard to define, but being an NICU mum is impossible to explain.

I struggled through many days watching my son suffering through the procedures of the NICU. The three-hourly blood tests have left scars on his heels and on the backs of his hands, and he has a burn mark from an IV line. Jacob went through many painful procedures, such as lumbar punctures, hormone function tests, X-rays, and ultrasounds. There are many good days and many bad days for our NICU babies, and the term "roller-coaster ride" is a very fitting one. I had heard the phrase "two steps forward, one step backward" many times in relation to preemie babies, but I think the best way to sum up the constant exhaustion, fear, stress, good news and bad news, milestones achieved, and extreme changes in our son's health would be to quote one of his first NICU nurses. She told me that, "in NICU, we do not take things day by day. We take them instead hour by hour." There is really no better way to say this; each and every passing hour could bring wonderful news or dismal news. It could range from heartbreak to joy. Fortunately, the Lord had certainly blessed me with the strength, the patience, and the resolve to be a NICU mum.

I could spend even more time writing about all of Jacob's prematurity issues, and of his time in the NICU, but what I will write about is our son now. The Lord has helped him to become a perfectly healthy eight-month-old boy (4½ months corrected), despite the doctors' insistence that he would have major problems. Jacob has come such a long way since his delivery. We are fortunate to have our boy looking very normal and not deformed from the intensive care he needed. Many of his preemie peers have significant physical reminders of their stay in NICU. I had prayed through my hospital stay for a baby unaffected by prematurity, and here we have our son at home, healthy and beautiful, just like a baby birthed at term." ~ Ruth, Australia

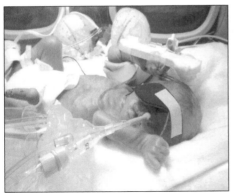
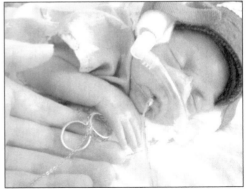
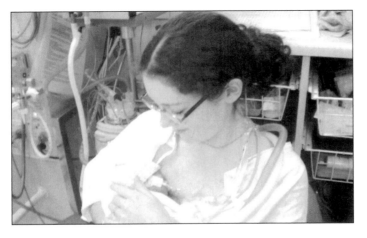
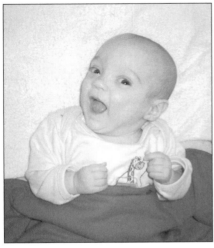

Top: (left) Jacob the day of delivery at 25 weeks + 2 days, weighing just 720 grams. (right) Graduated to CPAP. Middle: Mama holding her tiny boy (Kangaroo Care). Bottom: A happy, healthy, baby!

References

1. Tomashek KM, Shapiro-Mendoza CK, Davidoff MJ, Petrini JR. Differences in mortality between late-preterm and term singleton infants in the United States 1995–2002. *J Pediatr* 2007;151(5):450–456.

2. Marret S, Ancel PY, Marpeau L, et al. Neonatal and 5-year outcomes after birth at 30–34 weeks of gestation. *Obstet Gynecol* 2007;110(1):72–80.

3. Blennow M, Ewald U, Fritz T, et al. One-year survival of extremely preterm infants after active perinatal care in Sweden. *JAMA* 2009;301(21):2225–2233.

4. Berghella V. *Preterm Birth: Prevention & Management.* West Sussex, UK. Wiley-Blackwell, 2010.

5. Quint V Boenker Preemie Survival Foundation, http://preemiesurvival.org/info/index.html.

6. Menacker F, Martin JA. Expanded health data from the new birth certificate. 2005. *Natl Vital Stat Rep* 2008;56(13):1–24.

7. Hayes EJ, Paul DA, Stahl GE, et al. Effect of antenatal corticosteroids on survival for neonates born at 23 weeks gestation. *Obstet Gynecol* 2008;111(4):921–926.

8. Bernstein PS. Conference Report, Autumn in New York – confronting preterm delivery in the 21st century: from molecular intervention to community action. *Medscape Ob/Gyn & Women's Health* 2000;5(2).

9. Hentschel R, Reiter-Theil S. Treatment of preterm infants at the lower margin of viability – a comparison of guidelines in German speaking countries. *Dtsch Arztebl Int.* 2008;105(3):47–52.

10. Nishida H, Sakuma I. Limit of viability in Japan: ethical consideration. *J Perinat Med* 2009;37(5):457–460.

11. Moriette G, Rameix S, Azria E, et al. Very premature births: dilemmas and management. Part 1. Outcome of infants born before 28 weeks of postmenstrual age, and definition of a gray zone. *Arch Pediatr* 2010;17(5):518–526.

12. March of Dimes, 2010 Premature Birth Report Cards, National Center for Health Statistics 2008 Preliminary Data, http://www.marchofdimes.com/padmap.html.

13. Krueger C, Parker L, Chiu SH, Theriaque D. Maternal voice and short-term outcomes in preterm infants. *Dev Psychobiol* 2010;52(2):205–212.

14. Torpy JM. Premature infants. *The Journal of the American Medical Association (JAMA)*, 2009 301(21), http://jama.ama-assn.org/cgi/content/full/301/21/2290.

15. Brévaut-Malaty V, Busuttil M, Einaudi MA, et al. Longitudinal follow-up of a cohort of 350 singleton infants born at less than 32 weeks of amenorrhea: neurocognitive screening, academic outcome, and perinatal factors. *Eur J Obstet Gynecol Reprod Biol* 2010;150(1):13–18.

16. Roberts D, Dalziel SR. Antenatal corticosteroids for accelerating fetal lung maturation for women at risk of preterm birth. *Cochrane Database of Systematic Reviews* 2006, Issue 3. Art. No.: CD004454. (Last assessed as up-to-date: April 15, 2010.)

17. Crowther CA, Harding JE. Repeat doses of prenatal corticosteroids for women at risk of preterm birth for preventing neonatal respiratory disease. *Cochrane Database of Systematic Reviews* 2007, Issue 3. Art. No.: CD003935. (Last assessed as up-to-date: April 15, 2010.)

18. Crowther CA, Alfirevic Z, Han S, Haslam RR. Thyrotropin-releasing hormone added to corticosteroids for women at risk of preterm birth for preventing neonatal respiratory disease. *Cochrane Database of Systematic Reviews* 2004, Issue 2. Art. No.: CD000019. (Last assessed as up-to-date: April 15, 2010.)

19. Crowther CA, Crosby DD, Henderson-Smart DJ. Vitamin K prior to preterm birth for preventing neonatal periventricular haemorrhage. *Cochrane Database of Systematic Reviews* 2010, Issue 1. Art. No.: CD000229. (Last assessed as up-to-date: April 15, 2010.)

20. Clarke P. Vitamin K prophylaxis for preterm infants. *Early Hum Dev* 2010;86 (Suppl. 1):17–20.

21. Crowther CA, Crosby DD, Henderson-Smart DJ. Phenobarbital prior to preterm birth for preventing neonatal periventricular haemorrhage. *Cochrane Database of Systematic Reviews* 2010, Issue 1. Art. No.: CD000164. (Last assessed as up-to-date: April 15, 2010.)

22. National Institutes of Health, Eunice Kennedy Shriver, National Institute of Child Health & Human Development, NICHD Neonatal Research Network (NRN): Extremely Preterm Birth Outcome Data http://www.nichd.nih.gov/about/org/cdbpm/pp/prog_epbo/dataShow.cfm.

CHAPTER 19

Your Baby Died…
Not You

It's been almost seven years since my angel, Ashton, grew wings, yet the wound is still there, and at times it still feels like a gaping hole. Just saying it makes me cry, even after all this time, so if anyone were to ask me about the experience, I would say that yes, it still hurts; yes, I still cry; and no, I will NEVER be completely over the loss of my beloved son. Those of you who have lost babies will, to some extent, understand how I feel.

I can remember watching the Sunday morning news once, and the guest was an elderly woman. She was talking about the loss of her baby some 50-plus years ago, and how she still thought about her baby often. At the time, I had only lost my son about a year prior, but it struck me that what she was saying was true. For those of us who have lost a baby, or even babies, we will carry that burden with us for the rest of our lives.

What I want to say to you is that it's only a burden if you let it be. It's how you come to terms with your loss(es) that's important. This can make or break you as a person. Here was a lady expressing her grief to let others know that it's okay to still feel the pain of your baby or child's death some 50 years later, but she was also saying that your life *does* go on.

I can honestly say that the urge to cry doesn't come very often any-more, not like in the months or years immediately following his death, when I couldn't stop crying. This was so embarrassing for me, as I am not one of those people who likes to publicly display her emotions, especially tears.

I can now mention him or think about him and be okay with it. I no longer feel guilty about laughing or enjoying my life. I have found a sort of peace with—even acceptance of—his death, and I have found a way to pay tribute to him, and to all the other babies who never had a chance, through this book.

What to Expect During Delivery When You Know Your Baby Won't Make It

> *"Each of my three pregnancies that ended in a miscarriage was normal. I did not feel anything. I saw my doctor and my perina-tologist every two weeks because of my previous miscarriages. On one of my peri checkups, they told me that I was fully dilated. I had no pain or anything. What was more painful was that I had to deliver the baby, knowing that he would not make it."* ~ Blanche, Arizona (has an incompetent cervix)

There are no words to describe the feeling of knowing that you have to go through labor and that your baby is most likely going to die. That was the scariest moment I have ever experienced—enduring eight hours of labor knowing that I had to push out a dead or dying baby was like living my worst nightmare or something far worse.

You will experience such a range of emotions, from denial, to extreme grief, to anxiety, to downright panic. At times, the only way I made it through was to almost ignore the reality of the situation. Much of that night was a haze to me (and I wasn't on any narcotic drugs or anything, just an epidural).

That said, I survived, although it barely felt like it at the time. I made it through, and so can you. It helps if you surround yourself with trusted loved ones and nurses who are sympathetic to your situation.

While we were waiting for my body to fully open up so I could push out my tiny baby, it helped to have people around me who were supportive and even trying to make me laugh. It's amazing what laughter can do to ease the tension and pain, even in the worst of life's situations. Thanks to my father for this. He managed, or should I say tried, to make me laugh in the midst of all this. It helped to feel normal during those long hours, if only for a nanosecond.

After your baby is born, you'll probably be asked whether you want to hold him/her. Your desire to hold your child may vary depending on whether or not your child is born alive. Some people are not be able to bear the thought of holding their dead child, while others want to, because it's the only time they'll get to spend with their baby.

Initially, I didn't want to hold my son, so they took him away. I couldn't bring myself to even look at him, because I was too scared. I thought he was going to look like an alien or something. I'm so happy my nurse convinced me that he was not scary, that he was a normal, cute baby, only smaller, and that it would help me to see him. I would have really regretted for the rest of my life not holding my son if I hadn't taken her advice. I wasn't ready to hold him right away, but I eventually did a few hours later. My advice is that if you can, hold your baby. It can really help to bring a sense of closure.

If the baby is born alive, some parents choose to hold their baby until they pass on, and I can't think of a better way for your baby to take his or her final breaths than in the arms of the people who love him or her.

The Early Days

About the time the shock of reality registers, you'll be leaving the hospital, looking around at the other new mothers carrying out their new bundles of joy. You, on the other hand, are a shell of the woman you were. The world has stopped. Your body has become deflated, with nothing to show for it, and your baby is left behind in the cold mortuary.

The physical pain of having lost your baby literally rips your insides apart. I am sure the experience was slightly different for each of you. The days and weeks following your baby's death may have been a blur of activity and pain. Maybe you gave up on everything, not even daring to take a shower and get dressed to face the day. Perhaps you threw yourself into things, keeping yourself busy in order to run from the pain. You may not have let yourself grieve, thinking that you had it all under control.

Some of you may have cried quietly, others of you may have screamed like you've never screamed before, and yet others may have been so drugged up that the whole early part was a fog. You may have seriously considered death for yourself, unable to even fathom how you might go on and live life. Regardless, the turmoil that went on inside all of us is the same. We are all united in some strange way by the loss of our children.

There is no way around it: the early days suck. I would have rather taken a knife and plunged it into my heart than to have lost my son, and yet I survived, and I'm glad I did. Part of me is now ever so slightly grateful for the experience, as it has changed me in ways nothing else ever could.

During this time, you have no choice but to take it slow, day by day, and you need to let yourself grieve. However you need to grieve, do it. I spent several hours each day in the shower crying, looking down at my deflated belly and tending to my leaky breasts, which should have been feeding my baby. I hid in the shower, as this is a place of comfort for me. I felt that those around me were sick of my constant crying, so I retreated to the solitude of my shower so they wouldn't know I was crying again.

These will be some of the hardest days you will ever have to experience. It may bring you closer to your family, or it could drive you apart. You may feel that none of them understands, even your significant other. After all, how could they? You were the one who was carrying this angel.

> *"The pain of loss is so hard. Day by day it gets a little easier, but you will never forget your lost little one. Cling to your family and friends through this tough time and know that you will make it through."* ~ Cheyenne, Ohio (lost a child at 24 week.)

People Will Say the Stupidest Things

You may find that some of your friends will avoid you, while others you never thought would be there for you will pull through just at the right time. Let's face it; many people don't know how to respond and don't know the right things to say. Knowing this can help you to understand why some people seem to be abandoning you, or why things can now feel awkward.

Some people will say what seem to be the most insensitive things. "Don't worry, you can always have another baby," or, "Guess it just wasn't meant to be." You get the idea.

There are two ways to handle this. You could 1) fly off the handle and tell them what an asshole they are, or 2) calmly explain how you're feeling and that you understand that they probably didn't mean any harm, that they don't know what it's like.

Shortly after my loss, my friend and I were talking, and she said something like, "I know how you feel; after my abortion." I was flabbergasted. I didn't have an abortion. I had carried my baby, who was my future hope, for almost six months. We wanted this baby more than anything. I didn't choose this. How could she liken my experience to her abortion? I was completely insulted. All this went on inside my head because, just as quickly as I heard her words and was ready to freak out, I understood that she was just trying to help me and share a commonality.

You may not have even been full term when you went to the hospital, but some people will think you had your baby and now you're both home and fine. I was approached several times after the death of my son. When we got home from the hospital, my neighbor saw us and yelled, "Oh, you had the baby? Congratulations!" I just ran inside, leaving my husband to explain. When I returned to work a month after my loss, many people asked how the baby was doing. I felt worse for them, because I would break down, apologize, and walk away. They would stand there dumbfounded, feeling really bad, and apologizing.

"I had been enrolled in a Healthy Pregnancy program through my insurance company. Shortly after the loss of my daughter, a representative of the program called and asked, "Is your due date still the same?" and I responded, very coldly, "No. My baby died." I then had to explain what had happened. But I felt like everyone should know and be sensitive, even though that

wasn't realistic. I realized later that part of the grieving process is thinking that you should be the center of everyone's attention. That was exactly how I felt at the time." ~ Amy, Nashville (lost her daughter at 23½ weeks)

They mean no harm. Most people, even if they have kids, lose track of time. You may barely have been showing, but people still assume you've had the baby. Many people don't think that bad things like this happen. My only advice, as a way of avoiding these types of situations, is to have someone else—like your spouse or a close friend—tell others what happened.

Some people will surprise you during your grieving process. There will be those people who really comfort you during this time, people you never thought of who will provide that type of support. Two people in particular surprised me after our loss. The first was a friend—not particularly close, but one of those people I'd known forever but didn't talk to on a regular basis—who actually didn't even have any kids at the time. He sent me the loveliest card with a beautiful little poem. It said so much to me, and I remain extremely grateful for it to this day. I even told him so several years later.

The other person was a coworker in my building who also sent me a card. We weren't close at all. He said that he knew how rough things were right now, but that things would get better, and sunny days would be coming again sometime. He also opened up to tell me that he had lost a baby as well. That meant so much to me. Unfortunately, I never got to tell him how much his card meant to me.

Time Can and Will Heal

I never used to believe that old saying "Time heals all wounds." I thought it was a load of shit. After this experience, though, I have come to really believe those wise words. I have been very fortunate in that I have not experienced much loss in my life, and it never occurred to me that I could lose a baby, but I did.

After the loss of my son, I very slowly picked up the pieces and tried to move on. Shortly after the loss, my husband and I decided that we needed to leave town and get away for a break. As I am a person who loves the beach and sunshine, we decided to head south. We packed up the car and tried to just drive away from our grief. Did this work? Actually, it did, a bit. For us, it helped to be surrounded by the beauty of the ocean during this difficult time. Back home it was dark, gloomy, cold, and snowy. Did we run away? Yes. But I still grieved during much of our eight-day trip. And that was okay.

In the early days, the sound of an ambulance was enough to remind me of my ride to the hospital and my loss, and the scent of a certain soap brought me reeling back to being in the hospital. The oddest things would trigger my memories, and there was no controlling my emotions. I was angry, I was bitter, but most of all I was sad. Not only was I struggling with this, I was also struggling with the natural changes your body goes through after birth: the bleeding, my milk coming in, the body shape changes, the jelly stomach, and the hormones.

I had a hard time laughing, too. If something struck me as funny and I started to laugh, I would stop myself, because I felt guilty for laughing. If my friends asked me out, I would say no, because I felt guilty to be moving on with my life. It took a lot of internal convincing to tell myself that it was okay to laugh, that it was okay to go have fun. I had to tell myself that my baby wouldn't want my life to stop just because his did.

I can therefore say with good authority that you need to have this little talk with yourself, too, if you're struggling with living your life after your loss. If you've turned to booze or drugs, which so many do, you need to seriously look at yourself and ask, "Am I really happy with what I am doing?" I can assure you that your answer will be a resounding "No!"

This chapter is not a guide on how to handle your loss, because there are other books out there dedicated to that. What I am here to tell you is that you're not alone. What you're feeling and thinking is completely normal. You need to let out your thoughts and feelings with someone you trust. Life can and will be good again, but it can only be good again if *you* let it be good again. The ball is in your court.

"They say what doesn't kill us makes us stronger. I heard that a lot after the loss of my twin girls, and one day I came back with, 'Well then by now I should be the HULK.' But it is true."
~ Mercedes, New York (her babies became angels at 23 weeks)

"After experiencing a loss, time helps. It will take months or even years, but eventually you will be able to tell your story about your loss without breaking up and crying after just one sentence. During the first few days after a loss, it feels like you have been hit by a freight train. The best help for me was education. I immersed myself in reading about pregnancy loss. I experienced two losses and eventually gave birth to twins (high-risk pregnancy). Education is key. My advice is, be a strong, educated advocate for your unborn child(ren)." ~ Gail (location unknown)

"The loss of my sweet baby Olive haunted me for an entire year. I still cry and think about what she would look like and how it would be for my daughter to have her as a sister. The pain lessened with time, and I accepted that my baby was not meant to be here on earth. Although, my second child was born at 24 weeks, she is alive, smart, and perfectly healthy! Time was the only cure for my pain. I had to first stop blaming myself and the doctors for her death and let her go. She sent me a beautiful daughter, and who knows, it may just be my Olive in disguise."
~ Melissa, Louisiana

Closure

There are many ways in which we try to find closure in our losses. You may seek answers from your doctor to the question, "Why did this happen?" Often, however, there won't be any sure answers. Many have suggested planting a tree in memory (I did this) or making things like memory boxes and the like. These are great ways to remember your little one. Do something totally different, something that's you. Will it erase the pain? No, of course not. But it can help to complete the circle.

One of the ways to closure is how you choose to honor your child's body. I had my son cremated. Now I wish I'd had a memorial for him, so others would know that he was real. At that time, I just wanted to get it over with and then try to forget, but that backfired. How can a mother forget her child? His ashes sat in what was supposed to be his room for well over a year, and I would often take them down and hold them or look at them.

My husband and I finally decided that the closet was not a good resting spot for the love of our life, so we brought him to a beautiful spot in the woods, overlooking a valley, that we liked to visit occasionally, and threw his ashes down the side of the mountain. It was a very solemn experience, and I didn't feel like it unified my husband and me very much. We kind of just sat there in silence grieving, each lost in our own thoughts, and I don't think we even talked until the walk back, but the experience definitely helped to bring some closure into my life. It took me a long time to want to let go of those ashes, but when we were ready, it felt right. The point is, find closure however and whenever you want. This is a very personal matter of the heart, and only you and those close to you will know what and when is right.

I continue to find closure by remembering my son, and occasionally I let my daughter know about him. For me, that's very important. Both my kids will know about their brother when they're old enough. I never want to forget him. He may have only touched my life for a short period of time, but his influence on me has been huge.

If you find that you're not getting any sort of relief from the pain or the tears, or if you're suffering from depression some time after your loss, it may be best to seek out help. "Help" may not necessarily mean a counselor, but it may mean speaking with someone who has been there, having a buddy to confide in, or going to a support group. Or it could mean professional help. You deserve it for yourself and for your lost baby to not let this be your downfall. Don't let the death of your child be the death of you. You can't do that. Remember, the ball's in your court.

As I was writing this, I found two useful websites. One, www.facesofloss.com, is a place where others who've suffered a loss post their stories. While I don't suggest reading other people's stories when your wounds are still raw, I do recommend writing your story as a way of closure and posting it on a site such as this. The other site I found, www.grieveoutloud.org, will actually match you with someone who has also experienced a similar type of loss. I had never heard of this before, and I really think this could be a wonderful asset for those of us who are suffering quietly.

> *"I comfort myself at times by thinking that one day I will meet my little boy in heaven, and we will have a chance to be together then. I just have to wait until then."* ~ May, New Jersey

> *"I was not allowed to grieve my first baby, but I did name her Ava Oceane. With my twins, my husband and I bought a locket and made hearts with the letters A and B to represent our babies. It wasn't until I got the chromosomal test results back that I learned the sex of my twin daughters. I'm still grieving pretty bad, but what has helped me was to create some type of memorial (my locket) and to name them. Also, when someone asks if I have children, I say, 'Three daughters in Heaven, Ava, Faith, and Hope.'"* ~ Mary, Alabama

Here are excerpts from a mom who lost her son and "writes" to him to help deal with her loss:

> *"Can't sleep. We found out about a week ago the results of your autopsy. I hadn't really given it much thought. I've been trying to keep myself busy, trying to move on...but it's hard. Shit keeps coming back...The pathologist said you were perfectly healthy, but you died because my cervix dilated prematurely and you got infected. It fuckin sucks. When people say dumb shit, it just adds fuel to my fire. I know I shouldn't let it bother me, but some people just don't have any sense. One person in particular told your dad and I to "get over it," less than a month after you died. I don't think anyone could know how we could possibly feel, unless they've given birth to a lifeless baby and held him/her in their arms.*
>
> *After you were born I had a constant reminder that you were no longer with us. My body was all out of whack. I was engorged with milk, leaking, cramping, and bleeding. It was an unforgettable experience. They say that losing a baby can cause problems at home, that it either breaks down a relationship or*

makes it stronger. When your dad found out I was pregnant, he was so happy. It seemed like he loved me even more. I was worried that when I lost you, something would change between me and your dad. Thankfully, it brought us closer.

I want to, someday, make you a little brother or sister. I'm so scared, though. I never want to go through what I did when I had you. I don't want another baby of mine to suffer inside of me. I'm looking at your picture right now. I still find it amazing that we created you. Sometimes I just stare at your picture and try to imagine how you would have looked grown. I wish I was still pregnant with you.

It's a new year. I try to tell myself to move on and start fresh. Now that I know the reason you died, I'll hopefully avoid any future problems. If I am lucky enough to make you a little brother or sister, I hope that you watch over him or her. I will never forget you, and you could never be replaced. I miss you and love you very much, Anthony. Until we meet again, visit me in my dreams." ~ Verity, Las Vegas (She ended up giving birth to a healthy baby boy after six months of bed rest.)

A Story of Placental Abruption

"I found out I was pregnant on January 30, 2009. It was by far the happiest day of my life. I thought about all the wrong and good that I had done and promised myself to try to be the best mother to the little one growing inside of me. As the weeks went on, I desperately wanted to know what I was having. In April, I found out I was having a girl. I went home to my husband and said, 'Isabella Maria.'

He looked at me and said, 'Who's that?'

'That's going to be your daughter's name,' I told him.

He shrugged and said, 'Okay, Isabella Maria.' We were overjoyed. From that moment on, it was 'Isabella, Isabella, Isabella.' I didn't have any problems during my pregnancy. I took relatively good care of myself, I didn't overindulge, and I wasn't very active, due to my constant need to sleep and relax. My excuse was always, 'But I need to. It's for the baby.' At 33 weeks 5 days, I saw my doctor. I heard Isabella's heart beating at 140 beats per minute, and she was kicking up a storm. My doctor said, 'That baby is healthy.' My blood pressure was creeping up a bit, however, so he wanted to see me the following week, which would have been the day of my baby shower.

I went home to take a nap, and when I woke up I felt these horrible pains. I never thought it was anything serious, but I was brought to the hospital and felt sick to my stomach. They put me in a private room because they thought I had a stomach bug. I remember sitting on the bed when I felt something very wet come out. I thought, 'Oh no, my water broke!' But no, it definitely wasn't my water; it was bits of my placenta, mixed with a lot of blood.

The nurses hooked me up to IVs and got an ultrasound done, which confirmed that my daughter no longer had a heartbeat. She was gone. After hearing the news, I can't remember exactly the chaos surrounding me afterwards, but I do remember thinking, 'Please God, take me, but don't take my Isabella. She hasn't begun her life yet, so take me and save her. She will have a wonderful life,'

Sadly, what was done could not be undone. I had asked to be put out, but they advised me that they couldn't, because I would either wake up brain dead or not at all from all the blood loss. I had to have seven units of blood (our body only holds eight units). They did an emergency C-section, and told me that my placenta had detached, something that happens in 1% of all pregnancies, so I'm told. I remember being in the hospital for four days and thinking, 'Yes I'm in pain from my C-section, but I'm in more pain because my heart is broken and I feel empty inside. I would rather be with my Isabella.' My body stressed out so much that three days after I was initially released, I had to be hospitalized again due to my blood pressure. I've learned to accept the fact that I can't change what happened; however, I am now trying to use my experience to help other women."

~ Kim (location unknown)

Strain on Your Relationships

It's no secret that the loss of a child is one of the top life events that can drive a couple straight to divorce. It's also no secret that men and women grieve very, very differently. My loss definitely put a wrench in my marriage for quite some time. My husband preferred to numb the, pain by surrounding himself with friends and alcohol, while, as I mentioned earlier, I cried and holed up.

We had trouble talking about it, because I always wanted to obsess about it, the details, how I felt, my fears, while he wanted to forget all about it. We didn't bond over the experience, like you sometimes read in books—far from it, actually. It drove us a long way apart. I became angry with him over how he was reacting, and he withdrew.

It wasn't until one night when he came home late—again—and we fought that he finally broke down in tears. It only occurred to me then that he was also struggling with the loss of his son and with what he had seen me go through. Over time, things got better, although we never really talked about everything like we probably should have. I still have trouble saying the name of our dead son to him, though I'm not sure why. Maybe we're still in the "time heals all wounds" phase, and we'll eventually get to a place where we can talk together, comfortably, about our son.

If you're in a similar situation, try to honestly explain to your partner what you're feeling and going through. Be open with what you need in your relationship to help get you through this. At the same time, *you* need to listen to *his* feelings and needs, because even though you were carrying the baby and dealing with the loss as a mom, he's grieving as a dad as well. This is such an important thing to understand, and it will only help your relationship as you go through difficult times together.

It's common to experience troubles in your relationship during stressful times, and the death of your child(ren) is no exception. Try to lean on each other and share the burden of grief. If that doesn't work, each of you can find friends to lean on. Just try not to become too distant toward each other. I've heard of many couples not surviving this.

Hopefully, those of you reading this are thinking, "You must be crazy. My partner is my rock, and we are dealing with this together."

For those of you with whom this rings true, just keep doing what you're doing. Lucky you. For the rest of you, I can say from experience that it will get better. It isn't easy, but with some determination you can make things work.

A Miscarriage (Meaning an Early Loss) Is a Loss, Too

Miscarriage can almost be more difficult to grieve publically than an infant or late-pregnancy loss, as some people may not view the baby as really being a baby or person yet. People seem to expect a woman to "get over" a miscarriage pretty quickly—some may even think a week or two is too long. You may hear things like, "You're *still* dealing with that?" only a month after you miscarried, possibly even from family members. It is for this reason that miscarriage is often a lonely, private grief. Many women either don't know how to talk about it or can't bring themselves to face the cold negativity that surrounds grieving a miscarried child.

You may experience many different emotions in the aftermath of a miscarriage, and a lot of that will depend on how far along you were when you miscarried. For example, a woman who didn't even know she was pregnant until she found out she was miscarrying may be confused as to what exactly she is feeling. She should have been celebrating the discovery of her pregnancy, but now she doesn't know how to feel, since the pregnancy ended before it began.

Do not let other people make you feel invalidated in your grief. You have a right to grieve the loss of your child. Make sure that you do what you need to do in order to go through the grieving process. There are many different ways you can express your feelings. One possible way toward healing is art therapy.

Art therapy doesn't have to be limited to the graphic or fine arts, either. You could also write poetry or compose a song (if you're at all musically inclined); whatever you feel you need to do, do it.

Another thing that may be helpful in the healing process after a miscarriage is naming your child. It may sound crazy at first, since you probably didn't even know if it was a boy or a girl, but a lot of women have a certain intuition about the sex of their child, so if you had that intuition, go with it. If you didn't, you could always choose a unisex name, something that could be used for either gender. Even if you never tell anyone that you had a miscarriage, knowing your child's name for yourself can be very healing. It can give you a connection point with the child you never knew.

> *"I started having some mid-cycle spotting off and on for about 3–5 days. Then, I had some severe lower abdominal pain on the left side, accompanied by lower back pain and some nausea. I didn't want to get out of bed. I wasn't sure what was going on, since I'd just had a period about a week and a half earlier. I went to the doctor two days later, and they ran a pregnancy test, which came out positive. The decided to test my hormone levels in my blood. That was Friday. By the following Tuesday, I knew that I had lost the pregnancy. It took me a while to figure out how to feel about it, and I think that going through the miscarriage brought up a lot of feelings I hadn't dealt with after the loss of my first daughter, Genna. A friend had suggested art therapy, so I did a watercolor painting, which helped a lot. And my husband and I named our baby. I'm still figuring out my emotions."* ~ Amy, Tennessee (had a miscarriage 2½ years after losing a child at 23 weeks)

> *"The alarm bell would be the moment I did not feel the nausea. It felt like someone turned off a switch and I was not sensitive to smells anymore. I did not have to vomit. I did not feel sick to my stomach. I went to a doctor appointment, and they found the heartbeat. I experienced light spotting. Then, within two days, the heartbeat stopped. I was told during the ultrasound that there was no heartbeat. This happened with both losses."*
> ~ Gail (location unknown)

PART II

CHAPTER 20

Stories of Hope and Amazing Babies

These stories were submitted by women from around the U.S., and a few from around the globe. Their stories are written from the heart and describe in deep feeling the true reality of what it's like to go through such a difficult experience, sometimes more than once. Many of the gals came back to me and told of how hard it was for them to actually sit down and put all that they'd gone through down into words. To relive the despair, grief, sadness, and fear all over again was extremely difficult. Many found it to be a "therapy-like" experience that helped them to cope and gain closure.

I'm extremely grateful to all of them, each and every woman who took the time to do this, often at the risk of paying a heavy emotional price, for taking that step and sharing their stories in order to help other women and families cope and remain hopeful for their pregnancies and their babies. (Even those, that due to space, couldn't be included in the book. These stories and more can be found on my website at www.hrpwhyme.com.) I have to warn you that you may not want or even need to read all of these stories. Some will bring tears to your eyes; in fact, I cried reading damn near every story.

Depending on your situation, it may not be the best time for you to read these. I can't tell you for sure, but I want to put the warning out there. The point of these stories is not to scare or sadden you, but to provide hope, as each of these stories has a "happy ending." Yes, many women have lost babies, as I have, but their story doesn't end there. They go on to beat the odds.

I've placed "happy ending" in quotes because, as we all know, having a healthy child doesn't erase the pain of our lost babies. Our angels will never be forgotten. We have to remember to enjoy each and every minute with our healthy babies, treasuring them. We're often forced to sacrifice ourselves, mentally and physically, and sometimes our jobs, family relationships, freedom, sexuality, and even our sanity…the list goes on and on. In the end, however, you'll realize that it's all worth it. It's so clichéd…but it's true. To this day, I look at my sleeping children and know that everything was worth it to have them here. I love them more than I ever thought was possible. (My daughter will be 30 one day, and I'll still try to sneak in to watch her sleep. She's truly a miracle to me.)

I hope these stories will make one thing abundantly clear to you…you're not alone. Far from it, actually. Women and their families are suffering quietly around the globe all the time. If you need additional support or you lack a support system (this applies to dads/partners too), there are resources out there, such as Sidelines (www.sidelines.org), March of Dimes (www.marchofdimes.com), and other Internet-based support groups (like Incompetent Cervix Support Forum ic.hobh.org/forums/, preemie baby groups, etc.) that can offer support during this tough time. There are also church, community, and hospital-based support groups located all around the globe. Don't be afraid to reach out, and most importantly, don't be too proud or independent to ask for help, even if it's to wash your dirty underwear, clean the bathroom, or request help with meals.

Not One, but Two Babies

By Jamie and Geno Rodriguez

Keywords: hospitalized bed rest, infertility, losses, multiples, premature babies, preterm labor

It is interesting to reflect back on my pregnancy journey. When I first thought about contributing to this book, I was excited; in fact, I was elated. I had a powerful journey, one that I wanted to share with others to inspire hope. When I decided to write, however, I began to feel slightly scared about taking myself back to that place filled with so much fear, a place where the day-to-day was unknown. I had protected myself for so many months, and I wasn't sure I was ready to go back. This is my attempt at revisiting the past. As much as my story is painful and sad, it is also incredible, inspiring, and powerful.

I met my husband on the first day of my sophomore year of college. The attraction was strong, and I knew he was the one. That's where our story began. Eleven years later, he is still the most amazing man I have ever met. We dated all throughout college and shared every joy, every tear, and every beer! We triumphed together, we challenged one another, and we grew into adulthood together. Not too long after college, we got engaged and then we got married. No one was surprised. We were meant to be together.

We started entertaining the idea of having a baby right away. I was ready. He was kind of ready. We decided we wouldn't "try" right away, but we wouldn't prevent it. This was September 2006. By December, we still weren't pregnant, so we then started actually trying. We took temperatures, had sex nightly, monitored cycles, ate healthy, etc. February came around, and we'd still had no success, so we decided to go to a fertility specialist. The doctor monitored my blood and put me on a cycle of Clomid the next month. It worked, and I got pregnant. We were elated. I still remember that positive pregnancy test, seemingly the millionth one I'd taken to date, and the first positive. I called everyone I knew. We picked out names and baby furniture and talked about childcare...and that was only the first day. In subsequent weeks, we planned a trip to New York for Mother's Day, so excited to finally present the "pregnant me" to his family.

Our first night in NY, however, I started bleeding. I panicked and did what any young Jewish woman would do; I called my mother, then the doctor. They both told me not to panic, monitor my discharge, and go to the hospital if anything changed, the bleeding increased, I got a fever, etc. The bleeding continued overnight, so in the morning, I went to the hospital. On Mother's Day, instead of celebrating my new role, I mourned my first loss. The baby we had planned for was no more. I was seven weeks. We were devastated. And to make matters worse, the hospital handled it horribly. The facility was disgusting, the people were rude, and the doctor wouldn't even let my husband in the room when she delivered the news. Actually, the only positive was the orderly who came to clean the blood off the floor from the patient BEFORE me. He told me that his wife had just suffered a loss as well. I can still picture his face. No comforting nurse, a jerk of a doctor, drug addicts screaming outside, and an orderly with a halo.

Our first loss was a setback, but we weren't going to be defeated so easily. It's amazing how once you suffer a loss, all of these other people come out of the woodwork and share their experiences. This was not so comforting at the time, but it did make me realize that I was not alone, and it normalized the experience. I was also surprised at how people from outside (i.e., anyone but my husband and me) handled the loss. Close friends, family members, and coworkers trying to say all the right things, said everything wrong. I heard comments from "At least you were early," to "I'm sure this is God's will," to "Don't worry, you're young and you can try again." None of this made me feel better; it made me feel worse. Early or not, I needed to grieve. I am fairly confident God does not want me to be barren—yes I can try again, but this child is gone. Relaxing my muscles is not going to jump start my uterus. An angel who could have been ill, passed in the womb, or who passed even after she took her first breath, still left me alone, frightened, and needing to mourn.

True to my personality, we jumped right back in the saddle. I'm not so sure how ready my husband was, but I was so obsessed and focused. We started again, sex, sex, and more sex. The next month passed, and my period was late. I took a pregnancy test, and the results were positive. SCORE! However, by the time I'd made it to the hospital to confirm, the results were negative. It was a chemical pregnancy. In many ways, we'd moved on so quickly from the last loss by focusing on the next, but having a chemical pregnancy brought back all of the raw emotions we'd worked so hard to forget. So, how did we decide to process and tackle our emotions, you may ask? Naturally, we bought a dog. If I couldn't have a baby, I wanted a second bulldog. This is NOT something I recommend, however. Barkley was cute, charismatic, and looked great in a bonnet, but no matter how hard you try, no puppy or expensive purse can fill your emotional void.

So we threw ourselves into work, travel, and our marriage. Soon, however, more and more friends popped up pregnant, and it was hard to take their journey alongside them. I wanted to be them. We took a break from trying and went on a family trip to the Dominican Republic. Though I was not rotund, vomiting, and sporting the pregnancy glow, I looked great in a bikini, drank margaritas, and convinced myself that this was enough.

July passed, as did August and part of September. We had been trying for over a year, but still no luck. I started to look back at my pregnancy calendar. I had neurotically tracked every period, every act of intercourse, every temperature reading, every medicine, every doctor, etc.. . . okay, no judgment, please. As I was leafing through the pages, I realized I hadn't had my period this month, or last. This was odd. I hadn't even noticed. I pulled out the last packet in the pregnancy test box. Too bad Costco doesn't sell a jumbo box of pregnancy tests. It would have been a best seller. POSITIVE. WHAT? How did that happen? Oh wait, that night in the Dominican Republic...

We rushed to the fertility specialist and had a blood test. I knew the nurse pretty intimately by then, because this was not my first time at the rodeo. The hour wait was agonizing. HCG levels confirmed it...prego was me! We saw the doctor a few days later, got some pictures, and had a prenatal visit. I was ecstatic; my husband was neurotic. We were 14 weeks, so we told everyone. The chances of miscarrying after the first trimester were extremely low, so I was safe. Or so I thought.

The next week was horrible. Monday morning, I got a call to say that my mother's cancer had returned. Tuesday, my Dad was admitted to the hospital because he needed to get his gall bladder removed ASAP due to an infection. Wednesday, I woke up to my normal routine, but I felt different. I thought it was due to the stress, but I had this feeling that something was wrong. I tried to ignore it, because, after all, I was in my second trimester, the "safe zone," but it kept nagging me. I called the doctor, who at this point was on speed dial, but unavailable, and left a message asking her to see me again. She called back and was fairly confident that I was fine if I wasn't bleeding or cramping. I begged, cited my history, and, I'm pretty sure, made up a few other symptoms. I didn't care...I needed to be reassured. I made the trek to the hospital, which was an hour away, and my doctor checked me out. My cervix was closed, the mucus was the right color, weight gain was appropriate...I was fine. I asked for an ultrasound. She said no. I begged, but she still said no. I cried; she still said no. Then I pulled an Oscar-worthy performance, full of arms flailing, snot flying, and whimpering. At this point, my husband joined me. She said yes.

I remember sitting on the cold table and having the technician move the wand around my belly. I looked at the screen, and it looked different. Instead of seeing a baby kicking, I saw an image floating and immediately became alarmed. I asked the technician what was going on, and all she said was that she was going to switch to a vaginal ultrasound to see the image more clearly. No good. Then she quietly excused herself and said she was going to get the doctor. We cried; we knew. Our baby had died. Round 3, another failure, another loss. I went home, still technically pregnant, knowing that I had to return to the hospital to have a D&E the next day. Walking around like the living dead, housing a dead child, was almost too much to bear. I cried and cried and cried. The procedure the next day was miserable, though I must say the doctors and nurses were unbelievable. They talked with me, consoled me, and one of the nurses cried with me. When everything was over and I came to in the recovery room, I was numb—physically and emotionally. I grieved, convinced I was never going to recover. This was my bottom. It took me months to get back on my feet. I would not sleep alone, I would not shower in the light because I did not want to see my body change back, I shut out all my friends because no one understood, and I wallowed in my own misery.

Around December, we decided to call the fertility specialist again to discuss options. We also started exploring the adoption route. The fertility specialist was a complete bust, and adoption was also stressful. Extended waiting lists were discouraging, and the price tag of $50,000 for an out-of-country adoption and the process through which we could save money and time by ordering a minority child was nauseating. We also toyed with surrogacy, but again, the $100,000 price tag was a little too steep for us, with no guarantees.

Shortly before the New Year, we met another fertility specialist. We were a year and a half into this painful process, and three losses later, we were desperate. It was then that we met Dr. Gionfortoni. He was incredible. He educated us, comforted us, soothed us, and inspired us. He stuck with us, was sensitive to what we had been through, and made us laugh along the way. We were hopeful, but the months passed, and nothing. To make matters worse, my body was so out of whack from all the pregnancies that I couldn't even menstruate appropriately. My ovaries were not cooperating, and my emotions were all over the map, a pleasant side effect of the hormone treatment. My house was kept at a steady 50 degrees, but I was still hot. I was also moody, and my husband and I got into some pretty intense arguments on who was more at fault, my sluggish ovaries or his dumb sperm that just couldn't find their way. They say men are sensitive about the size of their genitals, but whoever said this obviously never crossed paths with a man trying to get his wife pregnant. In our house, my husband would go from 0 to 10 in a millisecond if he felt his sperm troops were under attack.

Nevertheless, we kept going. I took Clomid and some other oral medicines, and we did shots and exploratory procedures. I lived one hour away from the doctor, but I drove there almost daily to monitor the growth of my follicles. I would ovulate, I would be given the trigger shot, we would have sex, and nothing, month after month after month. Furthermore, our bank account was running low. By early summer, I was done. I was ready to adopt and just reconcile that this was our new plan.

A woman said to me somewhere along the way that the goal was to be a mother, not just to get pregnant, and to not lose sight of the goal. She was right. I wanted to be a mom, and adoption would grant me that privilege.

My husband begged and prayed, however . . . just one last cycle. We did this cycle like most others, except I was not as focused, as I was under a tremendous amount of pressure with my PhD program and work. I went to the doctor every day, and he told me that for some reason, he couldn't stimulate the follicles to grow. The cycle was a wash. We pleaded; we had no more money and no more emotional energy. This was it. We couldn't do it again next month; there wasn't going to be a next month. He added one last medicine to the regimen of shots being jammed into my butt cheek every night by my loving husband and told us to come back in a few days. If this didn't work, it was over.

The week flew by, as I was preparing for a work trip to Massachusetts, where my parents lived. I stopped by the doctor on my way to the airport, prepared to be told that once again it hadn't worked, but nope, there were four HUGE follicles ready to bloom. Say what? My doctor explained the risks, and encouraged us to consider jumping ship, because the chance of multiples was high, etc. We didn't hear any of that, however. All we heard was chance. I ran out of the doctor's room, jumped on a plane, and headed to Massachusetts. When I landed, I called my husband. We had to use our last trigger shot, and he had to fly from Virginia to Massachusetts to join me so we could consummate the deal. We paid the hefty last-minute ticket price, and he was on his way. I explained to my mother how to give me the shot (hubby wasn't in town yet) and then nicely, if somewhat indirectly asked Mom and Dad to give us some privacy so we could make sure Mr. Sperm met the eggs...in their house. Gross.

I'll spare you the details, because we want to keep this G-rated, but I can tell you that it was stressful and not super enjoyable. We wanted to be sure we'd done everything right and given ourselves as many chances as possible, so during the designated 12-hour period, we had intercourse again and again and again. It was mostly painful, because at this point I had developed Ovary Hyper Stimulation. I was bloated, retaining water, and moving my body killed me, but I didn't care. I wanted my baby. Time passed, and 10 days later I was still in pain. I dragged myself to the doctor and begged to be put out of my misery. He suggested taking a pregnancy test. I said it was too early; we were only 3.5 weeks into the cycle. He recommended we try anyway, so we did it, and I happened to glance over at the test about a minute in...a nice sold line. We screamed, cried, and hugged the doctor. We were pregnant! We did an HCG test for confirmation, and it was definitely high. Only 3.5 weeks in, my HCG level was almost 200. BOO-YAH!

When we went back for our six-week ultrasound, we were on pins and needles. We'd told virtually no one about the pregnancy, a trend that actually continued until I was about 22 weeks along, even though I was enormous and very noticeably pregnant. People would ask, and I would deny it. I think the losses created such a sense of fear that we were too nervous to publicly acknowledge anything. I can still remember the six-week appointment quite vividly. I sat down, got changed, got the ultrasound, saw the smile on the doctor's face, then the frown on the doctor's face, and then the questioning began. It ended with, "No worries, Mom. The babies are fine . . . all three of them." Triplets? We were having triplets. WHAAAAAAAAT?

We almost fell off our chairs. Unfortunately, our joy was somewhat short lived, as the doctor immediately brought up the issue of selective reduction. Though we could appreciate his perspective, we could not imagine terminating any of our babies, the ones we had worked so hard to get. We were lucky in that the situation was dealt with for us, because when we came in for our 11-week appointment, we discovered that I had miscarried one baby. That was loss number four for us, and it reaffirmed that we were in no way out of the woods yet. My doctor told me that I was likely a habitual aborter. What the heck did that mean? There was no time to be sad, though. I still had twins that I needed to grow.

Eventually, I graduated from the fertility specialist to a brilliant man he referred us to named Dr. Thomas Peng. We owe him everything. His bedside manner, medical knowledge, and willingness to guide us were incredible. He did not discount a single worry, processed all our neurotic questions, and did not give up on us, even when we drove him crazy. He saw me weekly throughout my entire pregnancy and gave us ultrasounds every other week. He talked us through them and explained every little detail. Now, I am super doctor-savvy, because I've spent most of my life advocating for my health, and never have I met a man who was so bright, so warm, and so empathetic. He was a guiding light.

The first five months of pregnancy with the twins were pretty challenging. I vomited and vomited and vomited. Whoever called it morning sickness totally lied, because I had morning, day, and night sickness. I was pretty good about not complaining, because I'd wanted this for so long, but it was hard. I would see glowing pregnant women loving every second and feeling great. I loved my babies, but I didn't love losing my lunch. At times, the worry was overwhelming, too. I was convinced that every day would bring more heartache and loss, and my husband was going crazy. I remember one fight we had about me not taking my prenatal vitamins. I'd stopped taking them (under doctor supervision) because they were making me sicker, and 99% of the time I would vomit them anyway, but my husband told me the twins were going to have spina bifida as a result. He also told the doctor to talk to me about my cell phone usage, because he was afraid the kids were going to come out deaf, and he was concerned about me jumping into our pool, because the babies might drown. Do I need to continue? This was my husband's way of trying to control a situation over which he was powerless. It drove me nuts, but it was just step one of him developing into the incredible father he remains to this day.

Around 21 weeks, I finally started feeling better, although I remember vomiting on the way to register for baby gifts. Who does that, by the way? By the time you're at the baby-nursery planning stage, you should be chowin' down on Big Macs and selecting wipe warmers, not taking Zofran and pulling over to yak in some stranger's yard.

In week 23, I went for my normal checkup. Dr. Peng was extra thorough that day because after 20 weeks, things with twins sometimes get crazy. Just as we were preparing to leave, I asked if he could double-check my cervix, because I'd read all about the incompetent cervix online. (FYI, a large percentage of stuff out there is totally not applicable to your situation, so if you're pregnant, fight the urge; do not diagnose via WEB MD.) He checked me via a vaginal ultrasound and saw some funneling of my cervix. He remained calm, but told me that this was enough of a concern that he wanted to admit me to the hospital overnight for observation, but not to panic. So, off we went, panicking as usual.

Fortunately, all went as planned. There was no hospital drama, and I was discharged the next day. I was put on bed rest and given some oral anti-contraction meds. Dr. Peng also had my insurance give me a home contraction monitor, which they rejected, but he said he didn't care; the office would pick up the cost for me. My best friend's wedding, which I was in and really looking forward to, was not quite how I envisioned it, but I was getting used to that by now. I was a blimp, sat in my chair the whole night (modified bed rest), and could not partake in any of the festivities. But I was safe, so were my babies, and I got to see my best friend walk down the aisle. I was content.

Instead of staying the whole weekend, I went home the next day. My doctor was fairly strict about the bed rest, and we weren't going to take any chances. I got home, hooked up to the monitor, and relaxed. Then the phone rang. It was the nurse. She asked me if I'd felt the eight contractions I'd had in the last 20 minutes. Uummm...no. We went to the hospital immediately, at which point the drama set in. Upon arrival, we had to sign paperwork for a DNR for our babies, because they weren't viable yet. Upon examination, I was in active labor, 90% effaced and 2 cm dilated. I was only 22 weeks pregnant. If they couldn't stop the labor, our babies would die. The doctors were kind, the nurses unbelievable, but we were hysterical. We'd made it so far, and now it was all about to come crashing down. I had to be medicated for my anxiety, because I was crying and shaking uncontrollably, and nothing would put me at ease. Fortunately, my miracle worker, Dr. Peng, did it again. He got the contractions under control with a weird medicine cocktail and stabilized me enough so I could be moved out of Labor and Delivery after about a week and up to anti-partum, where I spent the last three months of my pregnancy, unable to get out of bed.

This was by far the most trying time of my life. Everyone assumed it was a three-month vacation, but I can assure you it was anything but. I took numerous trips back and forth from Labor and Delivery whenever I went back into active labor, I had pretty painful Braxton Hicks contractions, developed a whole other host of medical issues that were gastrointestinal in nature, plus some heart problems, and how can I forget the gestational diabetes? In short, I was miserable...thankful, but miserable. And I was so scared, petrified for my life, the life of my babies, and the sanity of those around me. For three months, I woke up every day in crisis mode, ready to fight.

I will say, though, that there were some key things that got me through. To begin with, my husband was unbelievable. He was able to pull some strings because he worked at the hospital, and he got me moved into a double room where he occupied the other half. How many husbands would move into a hospital room to live with their wives? How many husbands would stay up and rub hemorrhoid cream on their wives late at night because they were on Ambien and couldn't even function, let alone complete a task that required fine motor skills? My husband would stay up and have UNO contests with me, take care of our virtual farm on Farmville, hug me when I was hysterical, micromanage the nurses to ensure that I got the best care, visit during every lunch break, and eat McDonald's and hospital food-court food so he wouldn't have to leave. He washed me in the shower as I sat in the chair and loved me through all the madness. He was and still is unbelievable.

My parents were also great. They flew to visit, sent gifts constantly, and motivated me every step of the way. They didn't judge and gave me the space I needed to do what I needed, which was living this journey with my husband and with the staff at the hospital. Too much connection with the outside world made me miss it, which made my stay harder. My dreams and hopes for this pregnancy had changed dramatically, and I had to mourn that loss as well, but once I did, I got to enjoy the uniqueness of my experience, which was actually pretty darn cool. My family was able to push their own egos aside, recognize that they couldn't provide me with what I needed at that time, and encourage me to focus on me. Not many others would be able to do that, and I am grateful for this.

The staff at the hospital also carried me through. Not only was Dr. Peng my guiding light, but the nurses, the other doctors, the cleaning lady, the woman who brought me my lunch, the pastor on staff, and everyone else was so committed to my care. The nurses became my best friends. They would stay up late with me and chat, spend their lunch breaks in my room showing me the newest video on YouTube, sneak me food from their holiday parties (let's not forget I missed Halloween, Thanksgiving, Hanukah, and Christmas), and tell me stories of crazy patients past. They all laughed with me, cried with me, and totally entertained me. The chaplain came daily to process all of my feelings and validate my emotions. The other doctors and medical students went above and beyond the call of duty. They would visit me before and after their shifts to checkin. Even if they weren't covering my case anymore, or weren't even assigned to the hospital anymore (residents moved around a lot), if they were around, they stopped by to let me know they were thinking of me. The cleaning lady came every day at the same time and told me stories of her own daughter, life, and pregnancy. It sounds crazy, but these little things made the loneliness manageable. And then there was Sidelines. My buddy knew every emotion, every feeling, every medication, every pain, every sorrow and every joy, because she'd lived it years before. She truly understood me, and carried me when I was convinced I couldn't do it anymore.

And just like that, three months passed, and then they were kicking me out. Yes, that's right, the hospital was divorcing me. I was 34 weeks pregnant, and now our home for the past three months was cutting me loose, because although I was still pregnant, I was out of the danger zone and ready to be released. So, naturally, we were in a panic. We lived an hour away. What if I went into labor? What would we do? I was already 100% effaced and 5 cm dilated, and I was convinced that if I stood up the babies would fall out. So, being totally insane, we booked a hotel near the hospital. I was also devastated, in a weird, unexplainable way. I wasn't ready to let go of this network of incredible people that had become my inner circle. As a way to stay sane and strong, I'd cut myself off from everyone around me and really put everything into my new life that I'd built over the last three months, but now we had no choice...we were out.

The babies, though, had a different idea. At 3:15 am on our last night in hospital, I woke up and found that I'd peed the bed. I struggled out of bed and waddled to the bathroom, still sensing a light leak. Weird. My husband stirred, and I told him I'd peed the bed. He jumped out of bed to check (he'd earned his honorary MD through this experience), and then suddenly it was like Niagara Falls as my water broke. BABY BIRTHDAY! It was time. After all these months of fear and excitement, we were finally there. Oddly, I was surprisingly calm, because I knew we'd made it. We'd gone from a point where every hour counted, hoping for just one more day, to practically normal. I was 34 weeks, which was still a bit early, but trust me, when you go in at 22 weeks, 34 weeks seems like light years away. And then, at 5:05 am and 5:06 am, Gabriella and Lucas were born, weighing 4 lb 5 oz and 4 lb 7 oz, respectively. They were perfect, unbelievable, and everything I could have hoped for. That moment when they held them up above the curtain, that first cry, was the single best moment of my life.

Our twins are now two years old and are the best things that could have ever happened to my husband and me. They say the funniest things, and are perfect spitting images of us, both in looks and personality, and they complete us in a way that I never knew possible. They are so great that, two years on, they inspire me to maybe…and I say maybe…consider doing this again.

I share my story because I know I am one of the lucky ones. My doctor told me afterwards that never in all of his years of practice had he been able to keep someone pregnant as long as me with symptoms as serious as mine. I can't tell you how many times we wanted to give up because the pain was just too much to bear, but we made it. We got through. We have our miracles now, and they were worth every heartache, every tear, and every hemorrhoid. It is not easy, and it certainly was not fun, but I did it. I emerged victorious, and I gave my children the gift of life. Most of all, I gave myself them, which completed my life.

The most important lesson learned along the way is to not be afraid to advocate for yourself. Follow your gut and do not accept sub-par care. Doctors need to treat both the physical and the emotional you. Don't settle for one that can't do both. Don't judge outsiders, either, because their sometimes ignorant comments really are kind-hearted. They just don't know any better, so just smile and remind them that they're lucky they don't know what it is like to be in the throes of infertility and loss. For those of you who were/are in my shoes, welcome to the exclusive club that no one wants to be a part of.

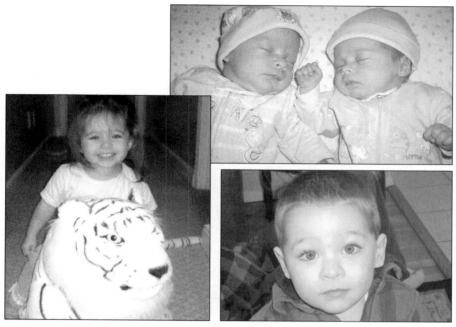

Update: They got quite a nice surprise (i.e., no IVF!). At the time of writing, Jamie is nearing her due date with NO bed rest and NO preterm labor. (She is taking progesterone.)

Mommy's Intuition Is Best

By Jamie Dickey

Keywords: bed rest, cerclage, incompetent cervix, placenta previa

It was our first pregnancy. I had found a great husband and we decided we were ready to start a family. We went about the normal routine of taking my temperatures daily, charting when I thought I was ovulating. Lo and behold, in only two short months, I saw the word PREGNANT appear in that little window.

I was SO excited. I set the test out on my husband's towel while he was in the shower, bubbling over with excitement, waiting to hear his reaction. The first thing he said was, "Why is there a Winnie the Poo washcloth with a thermometer that reads pregnant in here?" As soon as he said it out loud he knew, and he rushed out into our living room and hugged me. We were both absolutely unaware of the fear-filled nine months that lay ahead of us. We were just enjoying the idea of having a little baby to love and raise.

As my pregnancy went along, I picked an OB and suffered from morning sickness from six weeks on. One Saturday as I went about my business,

I noticed I was bleeding…not a lot, but enough…so I called my OB's office and immediately began to cry, thinking about what was to come, and that I was losing my baby. What had happened…and why? The doctor on call was a man, and he simply stated, "Well, if you're going to lose it, there is nothing I can do or anyone can do. Sit tight, and come in Monday."

Are you kidding me? MONDAY? It was Saturday morning. So we waited. The bleeding stopped, but by the time we went in on Monday I was as white as a sheet, fearing the worst. They said they saw a heartbeat, that the baby was fine, and that it was probably due to straining. They would see me at my 20-week ultrasound. Is this normal for most women, I wondered, not to be seen from week 6 to week 20? I had a nagging feeling about it, and for whatever reason, I decided that this practice and this doctor were NOT for me.

I switched to an all-women group of OBs and saw my new doctor that very same week. At this point, I was 13 weeks pregnant. She looked over my chart and said, "Well, I see you've had a LEEP procedure done." (I had had a LEEP six years earlier.) She suggested we watch my cervical length and do one ultrasound that day to know what my base length was. My thoughts were…HUH?

She explained that previous surgeries on your cervix can lead to a condition called incompetent cervix, something I'd never heard of. She was a very nice doctor, and I felt much more comfortable with her, so I didn't think another thing about it.

I had my first ultrasound, and my cervical length was 3 cm, not great. She said I could just be naturally short, and to come back in a couple of weeks for another ultrasound. I went about my life, and as my morning sickness lifted, I began to get excited. My mom bought a crib for the nursery, and I began to "glow." For the next appointment I had my husband join me. We went in, I had my ultrasound first, and then we saw the doctor.

The technician who did the ultrasound said, "Well, that's a little short. Let's see what the doctor says." She wouldn't elaborate, as they almost NEVER do, which is the worst thing, because as a mom you know when something is just not right, but it is policy that they relay the info to your doctor, and then the doctor explains it to you.

When we got into the room, the doctor said, "You're down to 2 cm. I want you to go home, lie down, and come back tomorrow. This could be a dynamic cervix, and I want to be sure before we move into more aggressive treatments." At this point I began to worry.

We went home, and the next day I told my husband to go on to work, that I'd call him after I left my appointment. I had gone to the doctor's straight from work, and this time it wasn't a question of how bad... it was BAD. My cervix had gone down to 1.6 cm overnight. I was allowed to call my husband and then was immediately admitted to the hospital.

He panicked and called my work, telling them I wouldn't be back for three weeks, that I was having a cerclage done, and that I would then be confined for a mandatory two weeks of bed rest. Neither of us really understood what a cerclage was, but one thing remains vivid in my mind from that day. As I sat in the exam room after absorbing all of this, I began to cry. Why me? Was I going to lose my baby?

The doctor came in to escort me out and noticed my tears. I'll never forget that she looked me dead in my eyes and said, "I'm not going to let anything happen to you, and I'll do my best not to let anything happen to your baby." I knew at that moment that she meant it. Switching doctors was the best decision I'd ever made. Had I stayed with the other doctor, well, all I can say is that it wouldn't have ended well.

So off to the hospital I went, and two days later I had what I now call my "magic shoelace" tied around and through my cervix. It was three days before Christmas, and the peri (high-risk OB) joked about using red and green stitching so I could show it to my family at Christmas. I stayed in the hospital overnight and then went home and began my journey.

The first two weeks of bed rest were nice. It was over the holidays, and everyone brought me goodies and catered to my every want and need. This was the only period in my whole pregnancy when I would ever say that bed rest was nice.

So, there I was. Now I had two OBs, one a high-risk specialist and one a regular doctor. The high-risk peri had worked in the army for years and was a gruff but BRILLIANT man who had helped develop the fetal heart monitor. I went in for a cervical-length check every week.

We had found out during my surgery that I had complete previa, so I was officially on bed rest when not at work, as well as pelvic rest. Now, most pregnant women are sex-driven creatures when they feel well, and I was no exception, except that I'd just been told that I could have NO sexual activity for the next five months. NONE.

Plus, the previa presents a real risk, which IC complicates. This is when your placenta covers your cervix. With IC, you're at risk for preterm labor, so add to that the previa, and both baby's and mom's lives are at risk. Great, what are the odds? Apparently, from what the doctors said, one in about 600 women get both. Sheesh. Go figure.

I continued to work with my feet up, being quite the spectacle at my office, as I was just inside the front door. Most people thought I was being lazy or had swollen feet. Talking about my cervix with strangers was something I wasn't quite up for, so I let them think what they wanted.

My cervix remained stable, with my McDonald cerclage at 3 cm for the remainder of my second trimester. At 28 weeks, however, when I went in for my weekly check, my placenta hadn't moved, and my cervix was only 2 cm. Off to full-on bed rest I went. I spent the next eight weeks on my couch with my dog. To most, it sounds heavenly, but let me tell you, it's anything but.

I was very fortunate; I never bled or had any major complications from that point on. With previa, they assured me I would almost certainly, at some point, bleed heavily, as I had a very "irritable" uterus and was on constant contraction meds. Nope, no bleeds.

We found out we were having a little boy, and although I thought I'd always wanted a little girl, let me tell you, I loved him long before he was here. So bed rest continued, until at 34 weeks they said, "Okay, if labor starts, you get in here ASAP, and you're having him." What, so early? Apparently after that point, it's better to get the baby out, so I prepared myself.

We finally allowed ourselves to finish the nursery, which we had put off, fearing I'd lose him and we'd have to deal with all of it. With previa, a C-section is mandatory, and though I didn't want one, I was scheduled for May 12, the day after Mother's Day. May 9 arrived, my last doctor's appointment. "Well, your placenta hasn't moved, so we'll see you Monday morning at 8 am." I couldn't believe it. The day was finally almost here.

Monday morning, I got to meet my little boy. I've never felt love like I did that day ever in my life. I was so incredibly grateful after all we'd been through. I couldn't believe it. I didn't sleep that night, but just held my little boy and smiled and loved him like I'd never loved another soul.

It's important for me to emphasize that the girls on the IC board got me through it all. I felt a bit out of place, as I hadn't had to lose two babies, which sadly I found was standard for so many doctors before they'd ever consider diagnosing you with IC. I hadn't even had to lose one baby, and for that I'm very blessed. For those who have, my heart breaks. That is a pain I cannot even imagine.

My OB is still one of my favorite people; I don't know many women who look forward to seeing their doctors when they go in for their annual paps, but mine gets cookies or brownies every time. I want nothing more than to see doctors becoming much more educated on this condition. I know most of us have written every daytime show, such as *Oprah*, with no response. Maybe this book will change that. I sure hope so. I tell anyone who will listen about what we went through. Then I show them a picture of Cohen Paul. Paul was my dad's name, and he passed away when I was 14. I know he was watching over us, because it was on his birthday that I got my cerclage and everything was caught. He was my angel who helped to get my son here, along with two amazing doctors, a husband who scrubbed bathrooms and cooked for me for months, and numerous friends and family...and of course my girls from the IC board. My son is nearly a year old now and is the joy of my life.

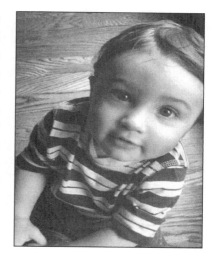

My Commentary:

There are many issues and themes you gals will run into throughout your pregnancies that are reflected in this story. Throughout the book, I talk about taking control of your care and having what I like to call a "consumer" rather than a "patient" approach.

Jamie's gut spoke to her, and she listened. Instinctively, we often know when something is off, but because of how we were raised, or our fear of speaking up, or even out of being polite, we don't listen. We worry about inconveniencing others or looking like a fool. Now is the time to knock that off. You have every right to switch doctors or get a second opinion, like Jamie, and you definitely have the right to question your doctor. Seriously, you can choose your doctor like you buy a car. Do your research, take a test drive, and pick one or two that work for you.

Never feel bad about asking questions and demanding answers. Sure, they may not have all the answers, but you should be able to have an open, frank, and comfortable discussion with your doctor. You shouldn't feel like you're on a conveyer belt or you're just a number at the deli counter. If you're not treated with respect, courtesy, or sensitivity, it's time to walk, girls.

Not all obstetricians are going to be knowledgeable about all our conditions, and some have the bedside manner of a Nazi commander, so I'm pleading with you; as much as it might be a pain, if you have any doubts about the doctor's experience with or knowledge of your particular condition (you don't want to be a science experiment, do you?) or the treatment you're getting that can't be resolved by good communication and discussion, or your visits leave you upset over the way you're treated...IT'S TIME TO SHOP AROUND.

Another important point this story touches on is that those of us with difficult pregnancies are just so grateful to eventually have healthy babies. We realize, maybe even more than others, in my opinion, just how special life really is and how precious our little ones are. So try not to worry about becoming a mom or how good a mom you'll be. You're already an awesome mom who's sacrificing so much to have your baby. The same goes for all the dads. You, too, have to sacrifice so much and do so much to support mom during this difficult, challenging time, so give yourselves a pat on the back.

A Rough Pregnancy Right From the Start

By Evette

Keywords: bed rest, bleeding, cerclage, infertility, miscarriage, PCOS, premature baby

I'm the proud mom of three. My first two were born between 34 and 36 weeks. I decided to have another baby and was told I have PCOS (polycystic ovary syndrome). Many women have it and don't even know it.

After fertility treatments, I miscarried. I decided to give up on the idea of having another baby. I finished school for billing/coding and took a trip to my native country of Jamaica. When I returned, out of nowhere, I was at the mall, and the scent of the food hit me, and I was sick. I told myself, "This is not right." I pondered the thought and stopped to get a pregnancy test. At home I took one, and it lit up so fast, I was shocked. Then another, the same thing.

I made a doctor's appointment, and they confirmed I was pregnant. I started to bleed. The girl said it could be from the checkup. So as the weeks went by, I found I started to bleed more if I stood. I went to the ER often. At one point my blood work showed my HCG level didn't change, and an ultrasound didn't show a sac. The tech said she didn't think I was pregnant anymore, to give it two days and repeat my HCG level. The test two days later showed no change. The nurse came out and shook her head and said, "I'm sorry, but you can go home and wait to bleed out. The level still hasn't changed."

I cried and thought, "No, this can't be happening." I went to look up HCG levels and found out all women have different levels, and some don't change. A website that really gave me hope was misdiagnosedmiscarriage.com. After reading some of the stories, I knew I had hope and I wasn't wrong about being pregnant.

As time went by, I found that if I stood to shower, wash my hair, or stood for about five minutes, I would bleed. I was in and out of the hospital. My regular doctor kept telling me he didn't see anything wrong. The high-risk doctor didn't know why and told me to stay off my feet. My regular doctor said it was okay to climb my stairs, that I was okay.

One day I was up, and I felt pressure in my uterus. I checked it and felt a bulge. I went to the ER again; at this point, I was 18 weeks. The ER exam showed I was 3 cm open. They told me I was in labor, and I would give birth in less than a week.

The doctor then asked me, "Do you want us to take the baby or give you a room to have it?" I chose to have a room. While I was waiting another doctor came and offered me a cerclage. If they are able to do the cerclage, then I have a better chance. If the baby made it 10 weeks, then I'd have a great chance of survival, but still I had the bleeding and no reason why.

I got P17 shots, as well as meds for the baby's lungs, hospital bed rest, and complete bed rest at home. Another strange thing was my uterus would contract and I would bleed clots of blood. Finally they kept me at the hospital and I asked the doctor why was I bleeding? They had no idea as to why this was happening. I cried because I felt so many doctors in one place and no one knew what was happening to me.

Well, on the day of the 28th week, 10 weeks from when I got my cerclage, my baby decided she was coming, ready or not. She was born crying on her own. The doctor said she was great and different at 28 weeks with a full head of hair, great lungs, weighing 2 lbs 9.6 oz. By 30 weeks, she was amazingly able to suck, breathe, and swallow. They were amazed.

A month after she was born, she developed NEC (necrotizing enterocolitis), and our world took a turn. The doctor called to say they needed to operate right away; she had given up. They called the clergy to baptize her, but in my heart I knew she wasn't going to die. After three surgeries and some intestine taken out, some six and a half months later, I took my baby home with a G-tube (a feeding tube that goes directly into the stomach) and Broviac lines. I became my own nurse. Today, my baby is four, very smart in school, and has no issues, thank god.

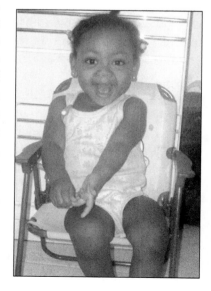

I pray you get great responses so that someone after reading your book realizes, don't always let a doctor's quick judgment let you have a lifetime of regrets. Trust your heart and instincts.

A Lesson in Letting Go

By Catherine Halpern

Keywords: bed rest, cardiomyopathy, cerclage, incompetent cervix, infertility, preeclampsia, premature baby

At the age of 40, after two years of infertility, I discovered I was pregnant. A blood test showed dangerously low progesterone levels, a risk for miscarriage, so I began treatments immediately. My blood pressure rose and my asthma got worse, both requiring medication, so I let go of my natural pregnancy.

At 22 weeks, I was diagnosed with an incompetent cervix, as my cervix opened when I stood up. My cervix was stitched, and I was placed on bed rest, my feet higher than my head. *[Trendelenburg position…yuck.]* My dedicated husband slept in this position with me. I was allowed bathroom and shower privileges but ate my meals lying down, and stairs were off limits. I remained in my bedroom, except for weekly doctor appointments, and I let go of my responsibilities at home. I went on disability from my job as a computer programmer and let go of the notion that I was irreplaceable at work.

The isolation and anxiety of bed rest were a challenge, although my relationship with my mother was transformed, as she came over five days a week to cook, do laundry, and help me pass the long hours. I hadn't spent this much time with my mom since I was a child, and even then I had shared her with three siblings.

After 11 weeks on bed rest, I developed preeclampsia, and my labor was induced. Jennifer was born seven weeks premature, weighing 3 lb 14 oz. She was healthy but tiny, and remained in the NICU. The sense of separation from driving away from the hospital without my daughter was a physical pain.

A day later, I was rushed to the hospital with dangerously high blood pressure and remained there for five days, with only a Polaroid picture of Jennifer and a T-shirt she had worn. When my husband needed a break from visiting two hospitals, a family member would visit Jennifer. They told me later that as each person held her, she looked deep into their eyes. I was diagnosed with cardiomyopathy, weakening of the heart muscle, and was given medication in the hope that my heart would repair itself. Breastfeeding was forbidden, so I let go of my dream of breastfeeding.

When I was released from the hospital, my husband drove me straight to Jennifer, and as I held her, she turned her head to my breast. We had been separated for five days, and I had never breastfed her, but she knew her mom. Jennifer came home at 15 days old, weighing 4 lbs 6 oz. I was so glad to have her with me.

One day, while I was holding her I started to cry, overwhelmed with fear that my heart wouldn't recover. Jennifer looked up at me and I felt my responsibility to her as though it was a physical thing. I had to be strong. This tiny person needed me. After that, my strength began to improve.

Against all odds, my story has a happy ending. Today Jennifer is a bright and creative 4th grader with a deep empathy for others. Her ambition is to be an author and illustrator. She's also a very talented viola player. Jennifer has no lasting effects from prematurity and my heart returned to normal within 6 months of her birth. She can light up a room with her smile and giggle. I appreciate my daughter every day, and I appreciate my health every day. I love being a mommy!

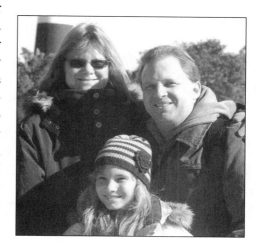

My Commentary:

This is such a heartfelt and beautiful story that packs so much emotion and feeling into relatively few words. Many of you will experience the let-down that Catherine felt when she was forced to leave her child behind in the hospital. Unfortunately, the many dips and turns of a high-risk pregnancy can quickly erode the dreams you had for your pregnancy and the birth of your baby.

Another point brought up is the potential for serious long-term effects from conditions related to pregnancy. (In her case, it was heart problems due to the preeclampsia.) For most women, the aches and pains of pregnancy disappear soon after birth (or a little later if a C-section is necessary). Many of you may also have to deal with the side effects from tocolytic drugs (i.e., contraction-stopping drugs), and even recovery time from the atrophy of your muscles, back problems, or bed sores following months of bed rest.

Often, women who have been on long periods of bed rest are surprised, after having their baby, at how difficult it is to then care for this child they worked so hard to bring into the world. They discover how hard it is to adjust and settle back into "normal" life, both emotionally and physically. After months of bed rest, they find themselves unable to walk up stairs without having to rest, they and are constantly tired and easily wiped out. Forget about caring for a newborn, taking on house duties, and enjoying a full, normal life again.

Remember, it can take time to rebuild your strength after months of bed rest. Just try to keep you chin up…it's completely normal. Frustration is natural, so express yourself if that helps you to cope.

A Story of Faith and a Blessing
By Aileen Abella
Keywords: bed rest, cerclage, pregnancy-induced hypertension, preterm labor

"I even came to thank God for the experience, because it allowed me to 'let go and let God in.'"

I'm a control freak, type A personality. Before getting pregnant, my husband and I set a series of goals, and having accomplished them, I thought that pregnancy would be a piece of cake. I was in good shape, living a healthy lifestyle, our finances in order. What could possibly go wrong? As it turned out, it seems like everything did.

I was experiencing a normal pregnancy until about 18 weeks gestation, when I started feeling heaviness in my uterus. Something didn't feel right. At the ER, an ultrasound detected that my cervix was less than 1 cm. The attending technician didn't really tell me what that meant, and so I followed up with my doctor on Monday.

I had an emergency cerclage put in on Tuesday and was placed on complete bed rest. I had a bout of preterm labor at 22 weeks, and then a few weeks later I developed pregnancy-induced hypertension (PIH). How much more bed rest could I do? I was put on phenobarbital and had several more short hospital stays over the next few weeks due to high blood pressure and an irritable uterus.

At 35 weeks, I was admitted with contractions, and my doctor said the stitch wasn't holding up. Nonetheless, they sent me home, but I was back a few days later. At 36 weeks, they removed the stitch…and nothing happened. I spent a few more days in the hospital and dilated to 4–5 cm without any contractions. My doctor said I was such an anomaly. He finally induced labor, and I had Chelsea, who weighed 5 lb 14 oz, and was 19½ inches long. She came out screaming, and I immediately knew the whole ordeal was indicative of her personality. :)

I will never forget how even the most well-meaning people can say some of the most insensitive things. To name a few: "You look fine; you're just milking the bed rest," "I would love to be home all day sleeping," "I knew somebody who had the SAME problem, and she didn't do bed rest," "I did aerobics until my eighth month of pregnancy; what's the big deal?" and "How much weight have you gained?" I felt so inadequate, so defective. It was a real emotional struggle.

My advice: get closer to God, figure out what His will for your life is and what purpose He has in this experience. It's also important to communicate effectively with your spouse. Call in all favors. Accept help from anyone who offers it, and don't isolate yourself. I was so annoyed by so many insensitive remarks that I shut out a lot of people who probably meant well. Keep yourself on a schedule (meals, shower, reading, TV, phone calls, Internet exploring). It helps the day go by faster and makes you feel like you actually have something to do. I decorated the nursery via online shopping, and I read a wealth of information on breastfeeding and child-rearing, which paid great dividends once my colicky baby with reflux was born.

My Commentary:

Most of us will need something to lean on to help us through this difficult time. It could be our faith, or specifically God, as for Aileen. It can be friends, family, your perseverance and strength, hope—maybe it's just daytime TV, movies or books, scrapbooking, knitting, or cross stitch, but really, it can be anything, whatever helps you to cope. Unless you've ever done time, as in bed rest, you will never understand just how difficult it is. Sure, the thought of it sounds nice—a break from life, a way to just sit back and relax, but that's not even close to what it's actually like. It's a time of fear, stress, isolation, depression, anxiety, maybe even anger, resentment, and second-guessing yourself and your desire to have a child. These are all normal feelings, and you shouldn't be afraid to express them to someone who'll be open to listening, non-judgmental, and reassuring.

As Aileen acknowledges, a high-risk pregnancy can quickly leave you feeling out of control. It affects the very core of your personality. Life quickly takes a sharp turn, and all your energy becomes totally focused on the business of having a healthy baby, even at the expense of everything you previously cared about. Maybe it's your relationships, how you present/take care of yourself (as in your looks), or your job. Things that used to drive and motivate you can now become nonexistent in your life. My advice is to try not to get completely wrapped up in being the victim in dealing with your pregnancy. You need to allow yourself to have some joy. Take some time "away" from it, even though you can't physically get away. Hang out with the girls and watch a chick flick. Pick up an old hobby or even learn a new one. Watch stupid movies you may not have dared watch before, just to get a laugh. Hey, even the dreadful Jerry Springer isn't off limits. Laugh at someone else who's making themselves look like an idiot if it makes you feel better.

Angels Lost but Never Forgotten

By Theresa

Keywords: bed rest, bleeding, losses, multiples, perfect pregnancy, PPROM, premature babies, preterm labor

My husband and I were married in October 1997. In January 1998, we started trying to conceive. It took only one month of trying, and on February 27, 1998, we found out we were pregnant. I was having some pain in my lower-right side, so the doctor sent me for an ultrasound to rule out an ectopic pregnancy. The ultrasound showed that I was carrying a 4-week-2-day-old embryo. Everything looked great. We were so happy.

On March 3rd, I began spotting. There wasn't much blood, just a little smear on my panties, so I called my doctor and he told me to take it easy and stay in bed to see what would happen. He said that if I was going to lose the baby, there wasn't much he could do to stop it this early on.

I continued to bleed, so three days later I had another ultrasound. This ultrasound didn't show what was causing the bleeding, but it did show that everything was still okay, so I was instructed to stay on bed rest until the bleeding stopped. The doctor felt the bleeding was from implantation, and although it took about a month, the bleeding did eventually stop. It was during my time on bed rest that it was discovered that I was carrying twins.

Except for the normal aches and pains, my pregnancy progressed nicely. On June 17th, I made an impromptu visit to Labor and Delivery because I thought I was having preterm contractions. I was 20 weeks 2 days along. Upon examination, I was told that my cervix was not dilated and I was not contracting, so I was sent home and told to relax.

On the morning of June 27th (a Saturday), I was having slight abdominal cramps and noticed a change in my vaginal discharge. I had been constipated for several days prior to that, so I assumed that was what was causing the cramping. After a few hours, I had a really loose bowel movement, and the cramping stopped. I started feeling better and didn't think any more of it, since the cramping had gone away. I went about my scheduled activities. On Sunday, I noticed that my discharge was still different, so I decided that I would call the doctor first thing Monday morning.

When I called the doctor, he told me to go right over to Labor and Delivery so he could see what, if anything, was going on. He asked me what my symptoms were, and even before he examined me, he said, "You should have called me Saturday morning. Next time, don't wait." Those words will stay with me for the rest of my life. I will always wonder what would have happened if I'd come in on the Saturday. Would my babies be alive today?

Upon examination, the doctor discovered that I was 2 to 3 cm dilated with a bulging membrane, and I was contracting every three minutes. I couldn't feel the contractions, even when I saw them on the monitor. My doctor called them "silent contractions," and said that a lot of women had them.

Since I had a bulging membrane and I was contracting, the doctor could not give me a cerclage. At this point, I was only 22 weeks along, and the babies were not viable if they were to be born. A neonatologist came in to speak to us about what to expect if our babies were born that day. The doctor also told us that the odds of carrying to viability would be slim. With the condition I was in, he didn't hold out much hope that I would be able to carry more than another day or two.

My husband and I discussed it, and we decided to try to do everything we could to bring our babies to the point of viability, at least 24 weeks. The doctor said our best chance would be to carry to at least 28 weeks.

An IV of magnesium sulfate was started, my bed was tilted so my head was lower than my feet to keep the pressure off my cervix, and I began receiving steroid shots to mature the babies' lungs in preparation for an early birth. Unfortunately, I had a bad reaction to the magnesium. I couldn't focus my eyes, I couldn't bend my joints, I had a severe headache, chest pains, and my whole body just ached. It felt like the worst case of the flu that I'd ever had. After two days, the contractions stopped and I was taken off the magnesium and put on Terbutaline to keep the contractions under control.

Five days later, the contractions started again, and I was put back on the magnesium. This time, it was only for $1\frac{1}{2}$ days. Since I had such a bad reaction to the magnesium, the doctor decided to try a Terbutaline pump, and I had a small catheter inserted in my leg through which the Terbutaline was administered. This drug made me extremely nauseous, and I couldn't keep any food down, but it was keeping the contractions under control, and that was all that mattered.

On July 7th, at 23 weeks 1 day, the doctor told me that the NICU at the hospital was full, and that if I were to deliver my babies there, they would not be able to care for them. I was told it would be safer to transfer my babies in utero, rather than wait until after they were born, so he suggested that I move to another hospital that was better equipped to care for my babies. On July 8th, I was transferred by ambulance.

When I arrived, my contractions were still under control, and there was no sign of infection. My membrane was still bulging, and I may have been a little bit more dilated. They continued with the Terbutaline pump and monitored me. On July 10th, I began leaking amniotic fluid. An ultrasound was ordered, and it showed that Eric's foot was resting in my cervix.

I'd had a catheter inserted for urination on the day I was admitted to the first hospital, and this was now taken out. In the early morning of July 11th, I had a sensation that I had to urinate, but when I tried to do so, nothing happened. I thought that this was happening because I had been catheterized for so long, and my body didn't know how to react without the catheter. I continued to have this feeling about every 45 minutes, and now realize that I was probably having contractions, but at the time I didn't know that.

At around 5am, I felt something in my vagina, and then my water broke. An ultrasound showed that Eric had stretched, and his foot had come through my cervix, rupturing both his and Joshua's sacs. The doctor told me that it was highly unusual for both sacs to rupture at the same time.

At this time, since I was only 23 weeks 6 days along, the doctor offered to perform an abortion to end things right away. In Pennsylvania, an abortion is only legal up to 24 weeks, and he wanted to give us that option while he still could, but after having spent the last two weeks in the hospital trying to save my babies, there was no way an abortion was an option for me now, so we declined. Even though the sacs had ruptured, we decided to try to keep the babies in as long as possible. The doctor told us every day we could keep them in would increase their chances of survival.

The following day, however, an ultrasound showed that Eric was halfway through my cervix, and there was nothing we could do to stop his delivery, so the doctor discussed our delivery options with us. He said we could do a C-section, but since I was only 24 weeks along, they would have to do a conventional cut rather than the bikini cut. It was his recommendation that I have a vaginal delivery, because he didn't think the babies would survive, and he didn't want to put me at risk with the conventional C-section. We agreed, and Eric was born at 4 pm, weighing 1 lb 4 oz. He was pink, active, and screaming, and received an 8 and 9 on the

APGAR scale. The neonatologist felt he had a good chance of survival, and they whisked him off to the NICU.

After Eric's birth, my cervix closed up and my contractions stopped, so the doctor gave me a Pitocin drip to bring on the contractions again so that Joshua could be born. Five hours later, I was lying in the birthing room, with only my husband and my mom with me because my contractions were not that strong, when suddenly I experienced a severe pain. I knew something was wrong, so my husband ran out in the hall to grab a nurse, but before they arrived I felt another sharp pain, and Joshua was born. I delivered him myself, with no nurse or doctor present.

Like Eric, Joshua was pink, active, screaming, and scored 8 and 9 on the APGAR scale. He weighed 1 lb 6 oz. The neonatologist felt Joshua also had a good chance of survival, and so he joined his brother in the NICU. The doctor said that at 24 weeks, we couldn't have delivered better babies to him, and so we had high hopes for their survival.

The main reason I'd ended up giving birth so early was because I'd been having contractions but couldn't feel them. The next day, the nurse who had been caring for me prior to my delivery said to me, "Now you know what contractions feel like." I thought this was a very insensitive, unthinking thing to say at that time, or at any time, for that matter. *[I have a word for people like that...bitch.]*

The next time I saw my babies, they had ventilator tubes in them and all kinds of needles and IVs. It was horrible seeing them like that, but we thought, if that's what it would take to save them, then that's what they had to do.

Ultrasounds of their brains showed that they had no brain hemorrhages, which was attributed to the fact that I had been on magnesium, which is known to prevent brain hemorrhages. This was a good thing.

When Eric and Joshua were seven days old, a nurse discovered white pimples in their mouths, and she suspected that they had a fungal yeast infection. Three days later, a blood culture confirmed that she was right. The doctor told us that this was the worst infection that they could have and started them on some horrible antibiotics to try to stop it. As time went on, the antibiotics did slow up the infection, but not before it had done terrible things to their tiny bodies.

When Eric was 14 days old he was doing well, so his nurse asked me if I wanted to hold him. I couldn't hold Joshua because he was too sick. I held Eric for 20 minutes that day, and while I was holding him, the nurse said all his vitals were perfect. That was the only time I held either of my babies until the day they died.

Three days later, Joshua went into cardiac arrest, and it took 45 minutes to get his heart pumping again. We didn't know what damage had been done, but shortly after, it was discovered that his kidneys were no longer functioning. The doctor said that at this age, babies could go a lot longer than adults without functioning kidneys, and he hoped that in a day or two his kidneys would start working again, but this never happened.

Four days later, Eric's ventilator blew a hole in his lung, and he couldn't breathe, so the doctor had to put a chest tube in him. There wasn't much time, so my baby had to undergo surgery without anesthesia.

The next day, the doctor came to talk to my husband and me. We were prepared for him to tell us that it was best for Joshua if we let him go, but not only did he tell us that we should let Joshua go, he also told us that it would be best for Eric, too. The infection had damaged Eric's lungs to the point where they would be unable to recover, and so after 23 days of inflicting pain and suffering on our little babies, we were now being told that it had all been for nothing, because they were going to die anyway. Imagine the guilt that my husband and I were feeling, knowing that we had done this to our babies.

We gathered the family together and spent the day washing and dressing our babies in pretty little outfits. Up until then, they'd only worn diapers. We read their favorite Dr. Seuss books to them and told them over and over again how beautiful Heaven was. We told them that it was okay that they were going, that we would miss them terribly, but we wanted them to be happy and pain-free, and that someday we would all be together again. The most important thing we told them was that we loved them.

They were given a shot of morphine in their IVs to calm them, and then all tubes and needles were removed. I held Joshua and my husband held Eric until they died. We wanted to die with them.

We called the funeral director and asked him to come and take our babies away. There was no way we were going to let them go to the hospital morgue. We waited until he came and made sure that he took them with him. Two days later, we had a small graveside ceremony with just the immediate family in attendance. Eric and Joshua were buried with my grandparents.

If I had it to do over again, I would have a full-blown mass and funeral for everyone to attend, because since no one outside of the immediate family ever saw Eric and Joshua, they don't think of them as real; they simply think of them as the results of a pregnancy gone bad. If they'd been at their funeral, they would think differently.

At my six-week postpartum consultation/checkup, we asked the doctor his opinion as to why things had gone bad and I'd delivered early, but he said he didn't know for sure. He didn't know if I'd started to contract first, causing the dilation, or if I'd dilated first, causing the contractions. If I'd dilated first, that was a sign I had an incompetent cervix. If I'd contracted first, that was a sign of preterm labor, attributed to carrying twins. There was no way of knowing which came first; however, it was his opinion that I most likely would be able to carry a singleton to term if I were to get pregnant again. He also recommended that we shouldn't wait too long to try to get pregnant again, since I was already 36 at the time.

My doctor told me that if I was to get pregnant again, he would watch me very closely and address any problems immediately should they arise. His course of treatment would be vaginal ultrasounds every two weeks, starting at 12 weeks. We waited until after my due date of November 1st and then began trying to conceive again. Once again, we conceived in the first month of trying. This time, I was pregnant with a singleton.

As discussed during my postpartum consultation, the doctor ordered vaginal ultrasounds starting at 12 weeks, and at 16 weeks an ultrasound detected cervical funneling, so I was confined to modified bed rest. I had to stay in bed for most of the day, but I was allowed to eat my meals at the table and shower every day. We have a two-story house, so I was allowed up and down the steps only once a day. My cervix was 4 cm, which indicated that I did not have an incompetent cervix, and the doctor felt that a cerclage was not warranted, since my cervix was so long.

At 26 weeks, my cervix suddenly shortened to 1 cm. By this time, I was too far along to receive a cerclage, so I was confined to total bed rest.

I ate my meals in a reclining position and was only allowed to shower once every three days as long as I wasn't up for more than 15 minutes. I was no longer permitted to go to my weekly doctor appointments, so my doctor arranged for a nurse to come to my house once a week to examine me. I remained in bed until I reached week 37.

I was required to have a C-section, as a result of uterine surgery I'd had two years earlier to remove a fibroid tumor, and I eventually delivered my daughter at 38 weeks 5 days. We named her Jessica Erin in honor of her older brothers, Eric and Joshua.

Although the doctor could not say for sure, he said that I'd probably lost my twin pregnancy due to my funneling cervix. I'd been with a different doctor with my twin pregnancy, and he hadn't been watching my cervix during that time, so I don't know if my cervix had been funneling at the time.

Had he been watching it, maybe my babies would be alive today. I asked my doctor why it wasn't standard practice to watch everyone's cervix like they'd done for my second pregnancy. His reply was that it's just not cost effective, and insurance doesn't pay for it unless you have a past history of cervical problems. It's sad to think that it took the death of two babies to save a third.

Two years after having Jessica, my husband and I decided to try for another child, because we wanted Jessica to grow up with a living sibling. We talked to my doctor, who warned us that, given my pregnancy history, I had a 99% chance of being on bed rest during this third pregnancy. We discussed it and determined it was worth the risk. We had a good support system of family and friends, so we moved forward with our plans. Once again, I became pregnant the first month of trying, and once again, it was a singleton.

Much to everyone's surprise, my third pregnancy was picture perfect. I had no problems, no bed rest was required, and I was able to work full-time right up to delivery. The doctors were simply amazed and had no explanation as to why this pregnancy was so different from the other two. At 39 weeks, I had another baby girl via planned C-section. We named her Abigail Rose.

Our girls are now 10 and 7 years old, and they both know all about their older brothers in Heaven. They regularly tell people (friends and strangers) about their brothers, and periodically we take out their memory boxes and photo albums and look through them. Eric and Joshua will always be a part of our family. We love them, and we will always miss them and what might have been.

My Commentary:

What can I say . . . even after having read this a dozen times, I still have to wipe away the tears. You just shouldn't have to experience what this family went through, and yet they did it and then went on to have healthy children, and they have come to terms with the loss of their precious sons. Even though Theresa went through this ordeal about 11 years prior to writing this account, the pain was still very real and very raw. The pain from losing your baby (or babies) will stay with you every day of your life. Yes, it gets more manageable, and we learn to cope, but it's not something you'll ever fully "recover" from.

Theresa addresses guilt and how we question ourselves, the "what-ifs." If only I'd gone to the doctor earlier. What if I hadn't done so much, walked around, had sex, etc.? There's terrible guilt that we can carry for many years, and sometimes even for our entire lives. I know I still carry mine on my shoulders; if only I'd called the doctor on Thursday, when I first noticed a change in my discharge.

Some of us, like Theresa, will be asked to consider abortion/terminating. When you're "pre-viable" or on the edge of "viability," many doctors will offer this option. It can seem like the most insensitive, rude, and appalling suggestion you've ever heard, but try to stay calm. Don't be rushed into making a decision without having all the information. My husband and I were completely insulted when, at 22 weeks, I was told that we could just end it right now and abort. I hadn't come this far to just give up and kill my baby.

After all the research I've done, I can now appreciate a little bit more where they're coming from when looking at the possibility of a very sick/disabled baby. This is an extremely personal decision for any family to make, and no one should ever judge anyone who has chosen or will choose to abort.

Theresa's story is a testimony to how strong people can be. Her story rips at my heart each time I read it, yet she made it through these terrible experiences to have two precious children. I can't imagine the choices she had to make and the guilt she experienced regarding her two little angels.

It's important to note that each pregnancy is different. IC, preterm labor, and other conditions that lead to preterm birth can show themselves in many different ways, or maybe even not at all. So keep your hopes up, and if you've had a previous loss or difficult pregnancy, know that you're not necessarily doomed again.

A Broken Heart Is Never Totally Repaired

By Chrissy

Keywords: bed rest, bleeding, cerclage, incompetent cervix, loss, multiples, premature babies, preterm labor

Back in 2001, I found out that I was pregnant with my first child. I was only 23 years old, so I was nervous, but also a bit excited. My husband and I had only been married for a year, but were ready to take on the adventure of having a baby. Everything was going great, and I was really hoping for a girl, but we went in for an ultrasound and found out it was a boy. I was slightly disappointed, but we went home and got the nursery all ready. The room was blue, painted with clouds, and it had Jimmy's name written in the clouds.

We went on a trip to Florida, where we went to some amusement parks and I rode on some of the rides but stayed off the big attractions, the more violent rides. We returned home and went about our lives as normal. So far, I was having what seemed to be a normal pregnancy.

I was working at a hotel, and on February 25th, at 20 weeks, I didn't feel well all morning, and I felt like I had to use the restroom all the time. I also had back pain but chalked it up to normal pregnancy back pain. I kept trying to go but just couldn't. I went to lunch, and when I returned, I tried to use the restroom again.

At that point, something went very wrong. I looked down and saw that part of the amniotic sac was bulging out. I just sat there, scared and not knowing what to do. I waited for someone else to come into the bathroom so I could ask them to get help, but nobody came, so eventually I had to get the sac back inside and call my husband, who rushed to collect me, but I just knew that it wasn't going to be okay.

We went straight to my OB's office, and I could tell from the look on his face that it was not good. I was taken out of the OB office in a wheelchair with tears in my eyes, and all I could see were the looks of sadness on people's faces. I knew I was going to lose my baby.

I was immediately taken over to the high-risk unit at the hospital, where they gave me many meds, and I was basically placed nearly upside down in the bed to keep weight off my cervix. I really don't remember much of that day. I remember they kept doing ultrasounds, and Jimmy kept kicking them, but for much of the time I was drifting in and out of consciousness.

When I finally woke up, they told me it was time to push. I couldn't believe this was actually happening. It was all over quickly; there was no crying, no excitement. It was one sad, quiet room, not like the excitement you see on TV. They asked me if I wanted to hold him, and I said no. My mom was in the room, and she held Jimmy first. Then the nurse came over and told me she felt it was best that I see him and hold him, so my husband held him, and then I held him.

I think I was scared of what he was going to look like, because I was only 20 weeks pregnant, but he was the most beautiful baby I had ever seen. At that moment, I did not see the bruising or how small he was. All I knew was that I wasn't going to be able to see him grow up. We spent about 10 minutes with him and then handed him over.

One of the hardest parts of the whole experience was being on the floor with all the new mothers. You could hear babies crying, and my milk came in. I had all the after-effects of giving birth, everything that went along with having a baby, just no baby to take home with me.

The hospital made a great memory box for me, with Jimmy's footprints and a gown, and they also took some pictures of him for me. I was wheeled out of the hospital with nothing but that box and went home with an empty heart to an empty nursery. We shut the door and hoped everything would go away. However, there was a funeral to attend, and people were stopping by, but I was in no shape mentally to see anyone. Thank goodness my parents took care of the burial arrangements, because we couldn't handle it. We went to the funeral, and that day we buried our son.

After that, it was almost like he didn't exist for anyone. I was told I had to come back to work immediately, because the company I worked for was going to switch over, and I wouldn't be paid my severance if I didn't come back. I'd only taken five days off work, and now I had to return. Many people thought I had a live baby and that everything was great. One vivid memory I have is of when a housekeeper looked at me and said, "You had your baby?" I just had to say no and walk away. The poor lady looked so confused, but I didn't know what to say.

Other people were downright rude about the entire situation, so I just did my job in order to get my severance and then left as soon as I could and never returned. I simply wasn't in the right frame of mind to have returned to work so soon, so I pretended that everything that had just happened was all a dream.

Another difficult time was when I had to go to my OB for my follow-up appointment. Sitting in that waiting room with pregnant women was not easy at all. I was so sad. I went in for my exam, and my OB explained that I had an incompetent cervix. He also explained that they'd made two attempts to place an emergency cerclage the night I was admitted to the hospital, but they'd been unsuccessful.

He was great, but I still just felt emptiness inside. He explained that I should try to get pregnant again after three months, but any subsequent pregnancies would require a cerclage to be placed at 12 weeks. I left there feeling nothing, looking at people in the waiting room with hatred, because that should have been me.

I went home and took some time out. In that time I thought, what did I do wrong? Maybe if I hadn't gone to Florida, maybe if I hadn't ridden on some of those rides, maybe if I hadn't drank that one Coke, maybe if I'd only known those were contractions I was having, and not back pain.

I'd done everything right—no seafood, no caffeine, no smoking, and no alcohol. WHY DID THIS HAPPEN TO US? Was it because I was upset that I was having a boy at first? Why?

We received information from the hospital about an infant-loss support group, so my husband and I went along to a meeting, but we only made it to the door before we turned and walked away. I just envisioned a bunch of sad people sitting in a room crying, and I didn't want to listen to their stories. We went back the next time, and this time we made it inside. I was right; it was a bunch of sad people, but they were all in the same place I was. I was so sad and depressed, and I felt so alone, but at least in this small room was a group of people who knew exactly how I was feeling.

We talked and cried a lot, and listening to other people's stories was somewhat helpful. I remember listening to people for whom it had been 5+ years since their loss, thinking, "I cannot believe they are not over their loss yet." We went to several more meetings and then stopped going.

I had to return all of the stuff I'd purchased. All of the bedding went back to Babies 'R Us, and they asked us why we were returning it. I kept the bibs and the first outfit I'd bought for him, because I just couldn't bring myself to return them. I just felt like I was throwing away everything that had to do with him.

I became obsessed with getting pregnant again. I felt like if I got pregnant again, this pain inside me would go away, that if I could just replace Jimmy with another baby, I would feel so much better. I think that, mentally, I just wasn't sure what to do.

I got another job but couldn't concentrate because I was depressed, even though I put on a happy face whenever I was around people. I don't think they ever knew that inside, I was dark, I was depressed, and I was crying myself to sleep every single night. My obsession with getting pregnant grew and grew.

It was around Father's Day that we found out we were pregnant again, but when I saw the positive pregnancy test, all the happiness I'd thought I would feel simply wasn't there. Instead, all I felt was fear. I called my OB, and we went in. I had an ultrasound to see how far along I was. I was about six weeks, and we saw a strong heartbeat.

Two weeks later, I was shopping at the mall with my little sister when I suddenly expelled a huge amount of blood. I called my husband and my mom, and we went to the OB, where he did the exam, gave me that sad look again, and sent me straight over to the hospital for an ultrasound. My husband and I went into the ultrasound room knowing it was going to be bad news. The tech just looked at me and said, "I see their heartbeats." "THEIR?" We replied in unison. "Yes," she said. "Didn't you know you're having twins?"

She then left the room to get the perinatologist, while we just sat and waited. The doctor arrived and told us it that looked like we were having twins, and that the bleeding had come from a "threatened miscarriage." I walked out of the room and held up two fingers to my mom, although sadly, I wasn't very excited, because all I knew was that two babies were now going to put a lot of extra weight on my cervix. We went back to the OB, who could not believe that I was actually still pregnant, given the amount of blood that I'd lost. I then went and quit my job.

I spent the next few weeks lying in bed, not excited, just waiting to mis-carry my babies. In my head, I simply couldn't connect with my preg-nancy. Eventually, I made it to $13\frac{1}{2}$ weeks, having bled off and on through the entire pregnancy. It was time for the cerclage, which went off without a hitch.

After that, I was terrified of putting any weight on my cervix and remained lying down for most of the time. Whenever I left the house, I used a wheelchair. When I went in for my OB exam at 24 weeks, I said, "If my babies are born now, they will be alive, right?" I think my OB must have thought I was crazy, and he told me I needed to wait longer. I still couldn't connect with my pregnancy, though.

We found out that they were identical girls, but I still wasn't excited, because every day I expected to lose them. As crazy as it sounds, I felt like it was bound to happen. I was having contractions, I couldn't stand up, and I knew in my mind that this time, I was going to have two of my chil-dren die. Throughout the pregnancy, we'd been going to a pregnancy-after-loss support group, which was helpful, but I still just felt like I was getting fat. I went to get monitored for contractions and was immediately admitted, because I was having them but couldn't feel them, and they were close together. I was drugged up yet again and hospitalized for a few days.

This was the first of a series of stays in the hospital, and I decided I didn't want a baby shower, because I didn't want to have to return the stuff to the store again. We didn't even have cribs or anything for the girls, and we had to paint over Jimmy's name in the nursery.

My mom finally decided to throw a baby shower for me when I was 33 weeks pregnant. I got a lot of stuff and managed to put on a happy face, even though I was still convinced I was going to lose them. Two days later, I was at the mall, went to the restroom, and lost my mucous plug, so off to the hospital we went, and I was admitted for the last time. I was hooked up to all the machines, and three days later I gave birth. When it came time for me to push, the reality that I was getting ready to have two live babies suddenly hit me, and I freaked out. I wasn't ready for it, and they were coming fast.

Emotionally, I don't know how I handled it. It was a lot of tears and a ton of pain. Allison was born at 9:00, and Zoe was born breech at 9:02. They were each 4 lb 13 oz, while Allison was 18 inches long and Zoe was 18½ inches. I couldn't believe that they were all right. They stayed in the NICU for 10 days, and then we brought them home.

My parents had bought cribs for them while I was in the hospital, but we didn't have anything, since I'd never really thought that they would survive, so on nurse shifts I went to the store and bought diapers and clothes and stuff like that.

Our girls are seven years old now, and we decided not to have anymore children. I feel like I was lucky to make it through their pregnancy, and I don't think I could handle going through another pregnancy. Even after eight years, I still cry for Jimmy and miss him every single day. Whenever I see a little boy of around his age, I wonder what he would have been like, but I also know that I wouldn't have my girls here with me if he was alive.

Losing Jimmy was the single most difficult thing that I have ever gone through or will ever go through in my life.

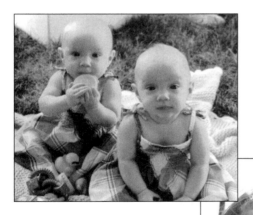

My Commentary:

What can I say? Chrissy's story says it all, and I can relate to so much of it, and I'm sure some of you can, too. Dealing with the loss of your baby will surely be the single hardest thing you will ever have to do. Words are unable to truly describe what it's like to lose your baby.

I never thought I would be whole again after the loss of my son. Like Chrissy, I thought that getting pregnant again would fix everything, but it doesn't. It's a normal reaction to believe that another baby will fix our heads and our hearts, but my advice is to talk about your loss and come to a place of acceptance, if possible, before you try for another baby; otherwise, another pregnancy just tends to bring out any unresolved issues and emotions, which are not so easy to deal with on top of a high-risk pregnancy.

Not connecting to your pregnancy following a loss is common. There were some people in my family who didn't even know I was pregnant again until I was almost seven months, because I didn't want to tell anyone for fear of having to explain to people again that my baby died. Going back to work and explaining to people that you weren't off on a short maternity leave, and having people assume that you had a healthy baby, is extremely difficult.

Elsewhere in this book I talk about the importance of connecting with your baby during your pregnancy, even though you're in fear of losing your baby. Seriously, this defense mechanism, refusing to connect, just doesn't work. If you lose the baby, it doesn't make it any easier or the pain any less real because you weren't connected. Enjoy every moment you have. There's a very good chance that this time around, you won't be leaving the hospital with empty arms.

An Angel and a Healthy Baby ... Beating IC

By Lindsey Nelson

Keywords: bed rest, cerclage, incompetent cervix, loss, PPROM

At first, I had a relatively normal pregnancy with my daughter, which was my first pregnancy, but when I went in for my 20-week ultrasound, that all changed very quickly. My husband and I were so excited that day, because we were going to see our baby and hear the heartbeat, and we would finally get to find out the sex of the baby. We found out we were having a girl, which my husband had known all along.

The ultrasound tech took all of the baby's measurements and then said she would be right back, and left the room. She was gone for a few minutes and then returned with another tech. After looking at the screen for quite some time, they then both left the room. My husband and I had no idea what was going on. They were gone for about 15 minutes, and then they both came back in, this time accompanied by a doctor.

He told me that I was starting to dilate and that he had already called my OB, who wanted me to go straight to the hospital. We went to the hospital, and I was taken to Labor and Delivery triage, where my OB met me and explained that I had an incompetent cervix, was dilated to about 2 cm, and had bulging membranes (the sac of fluid that the baby was in was starting to come out of my cervix). I was admitted to the high-risk perinatal floor and put on strict bed rest in Trendelenburg position. This was on a Thursday. I was evaluated by the maternal/fetal medicine specialists the next day, and they said I was a candidate for a rescue cerclage. My surgery was scheduled for Monday morning. I was kept in Trendelenburg the entire weekend and wasn't even allowed to get up to use the restroom. (Try peeing in a bedpan when you're lying upside down.) I was miserable, and I kept getting headaches and throwing up (probably from being upside down), but I was committed to doing whatever it took to get a healthy baby.

By the time Monday came around, we were very anxious and ready for the surgery. I was prepped and taken to the OR where the high-risk doctor was going to do my cerclage. When she got me all ready, however, she realized that I'd dilated further over the weekend (to about 4 cm), and now I had no cervix length left, so she was unable to put in a cerclage. I was devastated. She told me that this indicated fetal loss and wanted to induce me.

I was taken to recovery, and the high-risk doctor spoke with my OB, who convinced her not to induce, which was my preference; I wasn't ready for that. I couldn't understand why they hadn't done my surgery on Friday, when everything was still okay, and I still wonder about that to this day. Maybe my daughter would still be here.

I went back to the high-risk floor, where I stayed on strict bed rest in Trendelenburg for the rest of the week. The high-risk doctors still rounded on me every day, and I felt like they pitied me more than anything. I preferred my OB doctors, because they seemed so much more compassionate and understanding. Nine days after I was admitted to the hospital, I woke up and felt wet. I was checked, and they discovered that my water had broken, so my OB came in to discuss all the options with me. I wanted to wait until my daughter had a better chance of survival, but being only 21 weeks at the time, it was very unlikely that I would make it another three weeks.

We decided to go ahead with the induction and went to Labor and Delivery. I had a pretty quick delivery, and my beautiful daughter, Anna, was stillborn, weighing only 12.5 ounces and measuring just 10 inches long. I guess we made the right decision, because when my placenta was delivered, there was a hole about the size of a quarter where infection had set in. Later, pathology results showed that the umbilical cord also had a severe infection (chorioamnionitis), even though I had been on antibiotics for days.

That was the hardest thing I have ever had to do, going through labor knowing my daughter was not going to make it. Everything happened so quickly. Within 12 hours of discovering that my water had broken, I'd gone into labor, delivered my daughter, and returned home.

I probably went home a little too quickly, but I really didn't want to be on the postpartum floor with all of these happy women who had their babies with them, so my doctor said that if I wanted to go home, he would expedite the process. To make matters worse, my body didn't realize that I didn't have a baby to feed, and so my milk came in a few days later, which was extremely painful.

Our daughter had been supposed to bring us happiness. My husband and I had lost his mom and my brother in the months before I got pregnant, so we were so excited about bringing a new life into this world, but now I felt completely lost. The grief, coupled with postpartum hormones, left me slightly depressed, I think. There were days when I just didn't want to get out of bed, and I was having a really hard time sleeping, so I was prescribed sleeping pills. I was afraid to go out in public, because I had a really hard time seeing other pregnant women. I wanted to be happy for my friends who were pregnant, but I just couldn't. I should have still been pregnant myself.

I found that most people don't know what to say to you, and I heard many hurtful things, such as, "You're young; you can have more children." I didn't want more children. I wanted my daughter, Anna. I realized later that people weren't trying to be hurtful; they just didn't know what to say or how to act. A lot of prayer and supportive friends and family eventually got me through. It really helped me to be able to talk to other people who knew what I was going through. It also helped to look at my daughter's things. I'd made a scrapbook of the pictures we had taken with her, and I had a little mold of her hands and feet. I even had a necklace made with her footprints engraved on it (which I still wear almost every day).

I got pregnant again six months later and had the choice of going to the high-risk doctors or sticking with my OB. My OB said that he understood if I felt it was just too hard to keep coming to them, but I felt exactly the opposite. I felt comfortable with them and didn't want to have to start over with a new doctor. They were confident that they could handle my incompetent cervix, and I had a cerclage put in at 14 weeks.

I was already starting to dilate when my OB put my cerclage in, so as a precaution I went on bed rest at 18 weeks. Everyone kept telling me they couldn't imagine having to be on bed rest for so long, but I think having experienced the loss of my daughter really helped me keep things in perspective. I was willing to do whatever it took to get my baby here healthy and full term.

It was hard at times, because we didn't have any family in the area to help out, but my husband was very supportive, and my family came up about every other weekend. We had frequent doctor's visits and ultrasounds to check my cervix, and after 4½ months on bed rest, I was finally allowed to get out a little bit. My cerclage was taken out at 36 weeks and 5 days, and 12 hours later my water broke, and I delivered a healthy 7 lb 12 oz baby boy, who brings us so much joy.

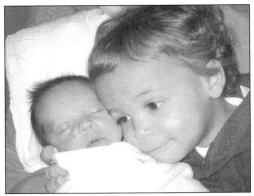

We recently had the two-year anniversary of Anna's birth/death, and it's still hard some days, but I know that she is in a better place, and I will get to see her again one day.

In this picture are Lindsey's boys, Noah (born after her loss) and baby Andrew (born at 33.5 weeks).

A Difficult Pregnancy Far From Home

By Anonymous

Keywords: bed rest, IUGR, preterm labor

I had difficulty maintaining a pregnancy with my first baby (a son) but managed to go to 41 weeks. My second full-term pregnancy was plagued with problems from the start, and a move 10,000 miles around the world in connection with my husband's naval career didn't help things.

Shortly after our arrival in Japan, our home was burglarized while my husband was at sea. I was 26 weeks at the time and under a great deal of stress, so I dismissed the signs of preterm labor. About two weeks after the burglary, I went into unmistakable labor and had to get my three-year-old to a daycare provider in order to get myself to the hospital.

This was no easy feat. We lived out on the economy, not on the base. I drove myself the 9 kilometers, through eight tunnels, in heavy traffic, to the base. My husband was preparing to leave for three months that morning, and I didn't want to "mess up" his day by worrying him, but when they could not determine the cause of the preterm labor, nor stop it, the decision was made to fly us to Okinawa, where I would remain until I delivered or reached full term. I was 28 weeks pregnant at the time and would not see my three-year-old son for another 12 weeks. My husband accompanied me on the helicopter ride to Yokota AFB and then on the Red Cross jet to Okinawa. I was barely aware of what was happening. We did learn just before we took off that the baby was a girl, so we named her Meara and prepared for what could be the worst trip of our lives.

I spent 10 weeks in the Army Hospital on Okinawa, alone. My husband took our son to Boston to live with my parents while he attended to his duties aboard the ship. This was in 1995, and there were no computers for us to use, and so snail mail was my only means of communication.

It was determined that my daughter was suffering from IUGR and had a blocked renal collecting tube, resulting in too little fluid, so I was monitored very closely and had regular sonograms to determine her growth. I took Procardia and basically stayed still and quiet for 10 weeks.

I was incredibly lonely, but every "pity party" initiated another round of contractions, so I had to just endure it for Meara's safety. When I reached 38 weeks, I was given the go-ahead to move into a duplex across the street from the hospital for two weeks. The consensus was that if she was born at that point, she would be fine. I continued my bed rest, but with slightly more room to move around.

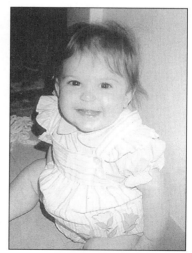

At 40 weeks, I flew back to Yokosuka and waited for Meara to arrive. My mom brought our son back to Japan, and my husband returned from his deployment. My mom stayed a week with us, and we were certain she would arrive during that time, but she didn't. My mother-in-law arrived, and the next morning, I knew I was in labor.

Meara arrived that afternoon, after just 20 minutes of intense labor and four pushes. She was a healthy 7 lbs, with a good set of lungs owing to the steroid shots I'd had earlier. Her first year was a challenge in terms of health concerns, but she grew and thrived, and today Meara is a freshman in high school and an accomplished Irish step dancer, as well as a budding marine biologist.

Nine Months of Bed Rest ... and Back for More

By Lisa

Keywords: bed rest, bleeding, cerclage, incompetent cervix, loss, preterm labor

July 4, 1998, 20 weeks pregnant

In the midst of a major kitchen renovation, I decided to vacuum the dust. Later, I felt cramping and had some spotting. I rang my doctor, who said to go to L&D for an exam. I did that and was sent home with instructions to take it easy and to keep off my feet, which I did, but the light spotting continued, so I returned to the hospital on July 6 to get checked again. Once again, I was discharged and sent home with the same instructions. I celebrated my 28th birthday with my feet up, and that evening, I had severe cramping, diarrhea, and bleeding. We rushed to the hospital, and I was feeling numb, like an out-of-body experience, thinking, "I'm going to lose this baby."

I was told that the membranes were protruding, and that I had two choices: either let nature take its course or have my membranes pushed back in, which included the chance of infection, risking both the baby's and my life. I decided to let nature take its course—a decision I still struggle with—to let go of my first child, a little girl we named Sarah. What if I'd made the other choice that day? I still think about it over and over.

This was the first true loss my husband and I had ever experienced. It was such a heavy, indescribable feeling that no one can ever fully understand. You're given blank stares of helplessness from family, friends, and coworkers who don't know what to do or say to help heal your pain.

Incompetent cervix, "IC," was the diagnosis, and we were told that this experience was how you learned that you had this condition, and how I was lucky, because I could help to prevent it during my next pregnancy with a cerclage and bed rest.

Getting pregnant again became the main goal now, but it wasn't a fun time. It was very nerve-wracking, with all the fear of not having a normal pregnancy. Seven months after our loss, we discovered that we were pregnant again, so I proceeded to hold my legs tight, move gingerly and carefully, and limit my activities.

Then, at eight weeks, I started bleeding, not spotting. "I cannot lose another baby," I thought, so we went to the OB and found that it was due to a tear in the placenta. I was told to go home and stay in bed, and that there were no guarantees.

This was when my complete bed rest started. I was in a state of paralyzing fear, with blood pooling, and having absolutely no control over my body. The bleeding eventually subsided after five days, and I stayed on complete bed rest and had a cerclage placed at 12 weeks.

My bed-rest experience

My husband and family furnished my bedroom with all the necessities — a dorm-sized refrigerator, a microwave, a toaster oven, and a TV/VCR — and he would stock the fridge with my breakfast and snacks every morning before leaving for work. My mom came for lunch every day, and I would heat up leftovers for my dinner. I spent hours sleeping, reading, watching TV, teaching myself to crochet, needlepoint... anything to help the time pass.

The worst part of bed rest is the loneliness, quietness, and the loss of contact with the world. I felt like everyone's lives continued on without me being a part of them. Visits were infrequent, and phone calls were few and far between. I think I had more conversations with my nurse from the home-monitoring company than I did with my friends. Looking back, I know I did a poor job communicating my needs. I needed my friends to be there more, either by visiting or calling.

My husband felt the stress too, because he needed to take care of me and the household (food shopping, cleaning, household chores), in addition to working his job. He also had the stress of job hunting, because he needed to find a better job to supplement his income, since I was no longer working, so there was the financial stress on top of the emotional stress of taking care of me and the baby.

I looked forward to my OB appointments every two weeks. I would shower, get dressed in nice maternity clothes, and go out into the world for an hour. I would hear the heartbeat or see a sonogram, and the fears would subside.

At 24 weeks, I went into preterm labor and had to be hospitalized. I was put on the dreaded magnesium treatment and hung upside down. After one week, I was discharged with a terbutaline pump to control the contractions, and I eventually delivered my first live child, Nicholas, at 37 weeks, a day after my cerclage was removed.

Returning to everyday life after being on bed rest was a difficult transition. My muscles were weak, and my endurance was poor, and it took a while to get strong enough to be able to go up the stairs without getting winded. Just being able to go out on a regular basis was a bit weird, almost like the world had changed in the nine months I was confined to a bedroom.

I went on to have two more boys, was on modified bed rest with both of them, took Brethine to control preterm labor, and hired a wonderful woman for five hours a day to help out with childcare, food shopping, laundry, and any other activities that I couldn't manage.

The things I would recommend to those who are, or will be, on bed rest are:

1. Communicate; let family and friends know what you need and want, including visits and phone calls.

2. Try to be financially prepared, if possible, to alleviate some of the stress.

3. Go online for support. (I did not have this, but I do feel it would have helped.)

4. Keep a routine—i.e., time to sleep, TV time, reading time, visit time. This does help the days go by quicker.

5. Talk about your feelings or write in a journal (even all the nasty, bitter feelings).

6. Let your church, community, or coworkers know if you need any help with errands or chores, to alleviate your spouse's stress.

Feelings today

I love and adore my three sons, now aged 10, 8, and 6. They bring me so much joy, and sometimes aggravation, too. My little girl in heaven is also a part of my life. We have her footprints on a magnet in the kitchen, my sons ask about her occasionally, and we go to the cemetery to plant flowers.

It's difficult when people say, "Are you going to try for a daughter?" How does one answer that question? It depends on the mood I'm in that day and how much personal information I feel like sharing. Another situation that really upsets me is when the granddaughter question is raised with my parents. My angel is never mentioned.

Seeing women carry pregnancies with no complications is also difficult. Do I wish negative things on people? No, but it's hard to watch even close relatives—i.e., my sister or sister-in-law, have healthy, active pregnancies with no complications. I just tell myself that my experiences have definitely made me a stronger person and more appreciative of my children.

Three Tough Pregnancies and Three Wonderful Babies

By Beth

Keywords: bed rest, premature baby

My first child was born at 29 weeks after a near-perfect six-month pregnancy. We were told that he probably wouldn't survive the first 12 hours, and to prepare ourselves for that. Even after the specialists told us this, I wasn't allowed to see him. I can only imagine the grief I would've felt had anything happened to him before I'd had the chance to see him. They told us if (and it was a big "if") he survived, we would have a long road of brain damage to deal with, as he was born without a heartbeat and wasn't breathing, and they had no idea how long he'd been down.

Today, he is an amazing six-year-old with seemingly no ill effects from his preterm birth. The first year and a half were awful, trying to find specialists and dealing with all of his preemie delays. A friend once told me that when you have a preemie, you hope and pray for this fire in their belly to allow them to "fight the fight" in the NICU. Unfortunately, you can't leave that fire at the NICU doors. My boy had a fire in his belly like no other I have ever seen. I mean, I'm headstrong, and he's a lot like me, but his "preemie fire" was like nothing we've ever seen. It's frustrating at times, but I know that he's destined for greatness, and one day we will be thankful for his strength and determination. We spent more than three months in the NICU, and our hospital did not have any type of support group, so I felt very alone. My husband and I dealt with our son's prematurity very differently, and while the stress of the situation may have brought us closer, our vastly different coping skills were painful at times. I felt very alone and uncomfortable in our home and was only comfortable at my son's bedside, even though my world had been shattered. I was depressed and felt like I'd been cheated out of the full-term birth that we'd both dreamed of.

My second pregnancy was not without stress. I was admitted to Labor and Delivery at 26 weeks after they found my cervix to be 50% effaced, and I was put on modified bed rest for 11 weeks. I was told to prepare for another preemie and that I would never see my due date. I eventually delivered at 39 weeks 6 days, had an amazing birth experience (VBAC), and felt that the polar opposite birth experiences somehow made us stronger.

Both of my children had proven the medical field wrong. What's funny is that our preemie now has a personality similar to his birth. He does something on a whim, without a whole lot of thought. He sort of bulldozes his way through things and, surprisingly, he comes out okay. Our second son arrived right before his due date, and that's how his personality is: he really thinks about things before he does them.

Our third child was born following a similar pregnancy story to our second. At 29 weeks, it was determined that I was 80% effaced. Up until that point, I was feeling great but sort of waiting for the other shoe to drop, and I wasn't at all surprised when I was put on bed rest again. I had been hoping for the best but preparing for the worst. I was released from bed rest on 4th of July (MY very own Independence Day!) and was very reluctant to do anything, as I was 36 weeks and really wanted to make it to full term. I continued to take it easy and decided that as I approached 38 weeks, I would do a little bit each day. During the 37th week, my husband and I took the boys to Babies 'R Us, and it was then that I realized how much I'd missed out on while I was on bed rest. (I called it 'house arrest.')

I'd forgotten how much people like to ooh and ahh over pregnant women, and I got all the attention. People were commenting on how good-looking our boys were, asking what we were having (we didn't know the gender), asking if we were hoping for a boy or a girl, etc. It felt good to not only be out of the house, but to get so much attention.

On the day I hit full term, I was having very regular contractions. Around 5 pm, we decided to head on in to the hospital, but the traffic was awful and what should normally have been a 35-minute ride to the hospital took an hour. My contractions had gotten significantly worse in the car, and I felt myself starting to push. I was really worried that I was going to have the baby in the car.

We eventually arrived at the hospital, and my parents met us at the emergency-room doors. Seven minutes after we arrived at Labor and Delivery, our daughter was born. She was full term and in quite a hurry to get here. It was another amazing VBAC experience, although I don't recommend only being in the hospital for seven minutes. That was a little rushed.

Knowing that this was our last baby, I had a very emotional few weeks after she was born. It took about a week for me to come down from my high of my labor and birth, and the shock that we now had a little girl. (I'd been sure that we only made boys.) I mourned the end of my pregnancy, the fast labor (which went so fast I never really had a chance to "enjoy" it), and all of the boy clothes that I'd saved. Even though we'd wanted three children, and we now had them, it was still hard knowing that I would never experience pregnancy or childbirth again.

I am a mom of three now; I often have to remind myself of that in my head. I'm thrilled to know that my sons will experience having a sister, and I'm looking forward to the future and watching these little people grow up into adults, while also enjoying these moments of time that go by way too quickly. We learn amazing things from these little beings.

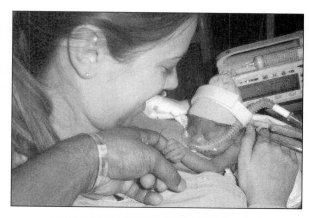

My Commentary:

For her last two pregnancies, aside from bed rest, Beth was also on 17P (a.k.a. progesterone). Based on her history of a preterm birth, and the

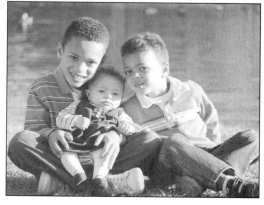

fact that she was effaced by 29 weeks with her next two babies, there's a good chance that this helped her to carry her babies to term.

Beth's boy reminds us that doctors don't really know for sure. She was told that he wouldn't survive, and that IF he did survive, he would have major brain damage from the lack of oxygen. He not only survived, but is thriving and a "normal" six-year-old.

Another issue addressed by Beth is the rift that can form, or grow, between you and your spouse/significant other during times of stress. A complicated pregnancy, the loss of your baby, or a preemie can put enormous strain on any relationship.

Even those of us who've dealt with far less than ideal pregnancies still enjoy being pregnant. Knowing that this phase of our life is over can be tough, while others say, "Thank goodness that's over and done with." Some of you will grieve the end of the childbearing journey, even in light of everything you've gone through. For some, this will be by choice, while for others, the decision will be forced upon you due to various circumstances, including the outcome of a previous pregnancy, your age, and/or fertility issues.

I want to give Beth a round of applause for following her dreams of a natural birth and not forgetting that, even in the midst of complicated pregnancies. There's a chapter elsewhere devoted to the idea of a natural (or "naturalish") birth, even following a rough pregnancy, and I hope that those of you who may have considered this for even a split second reconsider it, research the possibility, and speak with your doctors. Don't give up on your dream to have the kind of birth you desire.

A Very Early Rupture and a Leap of Faith

By Telisia Marie Montano and Martin Anthony Valdez, Jr.
Keywords: bed rest, bleeding, diabetes, miscarriage, PPROM, premature baby

Well, there is nowhere to start but from the beginning:

My boyfriend and I had gotten pregnant almost three years ago. I made the mistake of announcing it to everyone right away. Unfortunately, I had a miscarriage about three days after I found out. I was sad for awhile, but after struggling with type 1 diabetes since the age of 13, I had a spark of hope. I had been trying to get pregnant with no luck for a couple of years, and this brought a new sense of relief within me.

After finding out I was pregnant this time around, I was ecstatic. Although my diabetes wasn't quite where I wanted it to be as far as control, it sparked me to try and get it under the best control possible. Everything was great. This time around, I held off on telling people just to give it awhile. I found out at about two-and-a-half months. With diabetes, my periods were always irregular, so to miss a couple was not abnormal for me.

After about the three-month mark, I began to tell family and friends. I was again ecstatic! My boyfriend was so happy, as his sister was pregnant too. We talked about them growing up together, being about the same age. We thought about names and decided I picked if it was a girl, and he picked if it was a boy.

Appointments were all going well; my baby had a strong heartbeat, and from ultrasound pictures, a big head like the dad, of course. (Actually, I found out their heads are about a third the size of their body at that age…I still say it's the dad.) They asked if I wanted to know what it was, so I found out it was a girl. (I PICK THE NAME…YES!) It was so neat to see her little body forming and hear her heart beating.

One night I started bleeding a little bit. I had my mom take me to the hospital ER the following morning, where they examined me and gave me an ultrasound. I was told my cervix was still closed and that some women have their periods during pregnancy; I might just be one of those women. I felt a little relief. I continued to bleed for about the next four days and then it stopped. Whew.

Late one night, about midnight [she was exactly 15 weeks], I woke up to a feeling of gushing fluid. I knew I wasn't peeing, and it felt a little more like when you leak during your period…only heavier. WAY heavier. I had that feeling during my last miscarriage, but never to that extent during my periods. I got up to check, and lo and behold, my underwear was covered in blood. I cried. Not again, God, please not again. This time I WAS already attached. My boyfriend lived a state away, and I was living with my mom at the time. So I put on clean underwear and a pad, and decided I would wait. I had an OB/GYN appointment at 9 am the next morning anyway. The next morning it happened again, and my concern really grew.

I told my OB what happened, and they gave me an ultrasound. PPROM. I was told I was going to have a miscarriage probably within the next day or so, was written a prescription for painkillers, and was told to see him again in a week. I was devastated. I went home and cried, with my mom comforting me as much as possible.

The day went by. Then the next. Then the week, and I went back to the doctor. After another ultrasound, I was told my baby still had a strong heartbeat, but there was very little fluid, and it wasn't growing. Again, I was told to be expecting a miscarriage and to come back in a week. I went home and prayed. My family prayed and waited until the next week. The next week was about the same—strong heartbeat, no growth, and little fluid. Only the doctor had expected a miscarriage by now.

All I knew was my baby was alive. If my baby was fighting to live, I wasn't giving up hope just yet. I prayed and cried and prayed some more. I drew on whatever faith I had in me that God's plan for my baby was greater than any doctor's, or even my own.

I have to break into the story here to talk about my faith and what I was taught to believe. My parents raised me to have faith in God at all times. I begged him to give my baby a chance at life. I refused to let it go. Not yet. I refused to give up. God just help my baby to grow. Please, Please, PLEASE…I am begging not only for myself, but for the life of my child. I continued to pray. The next week I went back, and my baby had grown. Little fluid, strong heart, and GROWTH. I cried. God had heard me. So to this day, I continue to pray.

I went back week after week, and the same story kept on. They would find little patches of fluid here and there. Growth, and now the growth of a penis. What? Yes, I am having a boy. My son.

I was referred to a neonatal doctor, who kicked me back a few notches. He told me yes, my baby was alive, but that he would have cardiovascular growth issues, lung development failure, amnio banding, and more likely than not, be stillborn. "Don't have too much hope," I was told. Really? Thanks for that, Dr. Harris. I was told if I was to have an abortion, now was the time.

So I researched it on the Internet. I read exactly how abortions are done. I am not in any way judging anyone who has chosen to have an abortion. But, for me, it wasn't going to happen, not that way. I would let God take my son, but I wouldn't make that choice. After all, he was growing, and his heart was beating, and now I could feel him moving. Nope. Not for me.

I researched babies that lived through PPROM. Many were ill. Many lived in the hospital for months, many had physical problems. BUT THEY LIVED. I still hold on to that hope for my son.

Needless to say, I had myself referred to a different neonatal doctor. I was told at 24 weeks I would be hospitalized for the remainder of my pregnancy and put on bed rest. Two days shy of 24 weeks I was having abdominal pain, and was admitted to Labor and Delivery right away. It stopped, and I was eventually moved down to the OB unit. I went in on 11/22/10, so I was there for Thanksgiving, my birthday (27th), his birthday (29th), and was now six days away from Christmas.

I am exactly 27 weeks and four days today, and I have prayed every day to hit 28 weeks, and then 32 weeks, and if possible 34 weeks. I take it day by day right now, but still have belief that my son will survive this.

It's not easy, and some days I do get scared and worried, but I am human. I allow myself to feel these feelings, cry, worry, and do what I have to do to relieve them and then move on. I just don't lose hope.

I still leak amniotic fluid daily; my placenta never resealed. My fluid measures at a 3.2, considered to be a low amount, and my son weighs about two pounds. He's breech, or "transverse" so I'll have to get a C-section. I've had shots of steroids to aid lung development, shots to prevent contractions, IV iron to prevent blood transfusions and blood loss during birth, fluids pumped in me in every IV location possible, not to mention high and low blood sugars galore. But he's still surviving. His heartbeat remains strong, he moves like crazy, and he is producing fluids on his own. He's practicing breathing, gets the hiccups, and hates to be strapped down and monitored. He's alive, my little guy, and every day with him is a blessing.

I toured the NICU unit where they take preemie babies after birth. It was hard to see such tiny babies with tubes and IVs. However, I think God has a purpose for each one of those darling children, as he does for my son. There are still risks and unknowns. The staff here at this hospital is vey supportive. They let me know what could be but encourage me to continue to have faith. They have a very knowledgeable, highly trained team of doctors fighting alongside me and my son, which is reassuring.

To any mother out there who struggles with fear, worry, and uncertainty...don't lose hope.

My Commentary:

After rupturing at 15 weeks, she carried her baby, against every odd, to an amazing 28 weeks and 5 days. He was born weighing 2 pounds, 12 ounces. She wrote this story from her hospital bed and when I read this, I could feel each and every emotion she went through. She writes, *"They put so many things in my head about what was going to happen to my baby. That was the hardest part, but his little heart kept beating. I said no matter the outcome I would love my son, with whatever problems and or issues he had; his mom would be there for him. I felt so guilty at times that I was going to cheat my son out of a normal life, out of a healthy future, and did I really make the right choice? Was it me being too selfish to let him go? I wanted him soooo very much to live."* Then *"he's beautiful . . . he's in the NICU now..."* (January 2011)

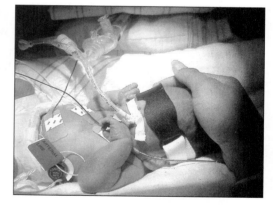

Liyah's Song

By Kimaiya

Keywords: bed rest, HELLP, loss, preeclampsia

Where do I start? It's been almost seven years and it still seems like yesterday that this "song" was forever engraved in my mind and heart. I told myself that I would keep this to myself; it's much easier that way, or so I thought, but I've been inspired, and I'm gonna share my story. As sad as it may seem to some, it has a happy ending, a blessing that came my way. A miracle that appeared itself, or should I say herself, on December 30th, 2009. You see, the saying "time heals all wounds" holds true, and sometimes it takes witnessing the struggle of another person and the way they overcome to inspire you, and yes, I've been inspired. So here it goes, "Liyah's Song."

"Ms. Taylor, you have a disease known as preeclampsia, and we have to put you on strict bed rest until your delivery." "Pre what? You mean I'm going be in this hospital until February 14th? It's only October 20th! What about my baby? Is she going be okay?" I think. My head hurts, and I think I need to get my eyes checked because my vision has been a bit blurry these past few weeks. So you see, doc, I can't possibly stay in this hospital for four months; can't you just monitor me from home? Foolish little girl, I didn't realize the danger we were in. I'm only 21; this seems like something a middle-age-woman should be going through. Five days later I would soon find out the meaning of preeclampsia and HELLP syndrome. I would witness them firsthand and live to sing this song.

October 24, 2004, was not a normal day for me. I'm pregnant, on bed rest, my head is hurting, well, pounding. I've spoken with my doctor, who informs me that she is going to do everything she can to keep the pregnancy as long as possible, but my blood pressure and the protein that's spilling in my urine may prevent that from happening. I'm only 26 weeks pregnant, so of course, the next step is to introduce me to the neonatologist, who, "in the event of an early delivery," will care for my baby. I'm not really sure how I feel about the things he's telling me about the process of the NICU and the dangers of having a baby this early. I'm more concerned with the pain in my upper abdomen that I mistook for indigestion and the needle that my nurse is holding, preparing to give me steroid shots to help mature my baby's lungs. Oh yes, there's definitely going to be an early delivery—Lord help me!

It's 12 am, October 25, and I can't sleep. My nurse is coming in every 15 minutes to check my blood pressure and reporting the findings to my doctor. My head feels like someone is cracking my skull with a hammer, and I can't seem to focus on anything. "Should have had that eye exam before leaving Tampa" is what I'm thinking.

My nurse comes in and informs me that I'm going to be moved to Labor and Delivery because my blood pressure is very high, and delivery is basically inevitable. "Ma'am, can you wait a second? I need to call my mom. She's going to be worried when she comes in the morning and I'm not here." I'm whisked away to Labor and Delivery. I'm not sure if I blacked out for a second or minutes, but my parents are suddenly in front of me, smiling, obviously trying to hide the worry they must be feeling right now.

I don't remember much of what happened from about 1:00 am to 7:00 am, but I do remember my dad rubbing my head and holding the basin as I vomited violently. The result of the nurse putting what I later learned was magnesium sulfate in my IV to try and bring my blood pressure down. I remember my mom saying, "Calm down and try to rest, Maiya." Easy for you to say; you don't have a hammer at your skull right now mommy. My mom tells me this went on throughout the night, with my blood pressure getting up to 210/over something.

She tells me that she and my dad took turns sleeping on the little couch, while the other stood guard over my bed. I finally was able to rest a bit, after getting a dose of Phenergan to control the nausea and vomiting. The breaking point, she tells me, was when the doctor came in and told them that the bloodwork done through the night revealed my liver enzymes were elevated; my liver, kidneys, and every other organ in my body were about to shut down. I, along with my unborn baby, would, unfortunately die. They had to make the decision—deliver MY baby to save my life. Sounds harsh, but this disease is only cured by delivery of the baby, so Aliyah Le'Shun Sheffield was about to make her grand entrance into the world.

My mom sat near my head during the surgery and tells me that I slept throughout the entire thing. As I'm being taken to my room, I'm wheeled through the NICU. There she is. "Focus Maiya. Where are my glasses? I need to see my baby." I'm not in any pain, but I can't seem to move my body. I manage to move my arm up to her isolette and touch her foot, which is no bigger than my thumb. I later learn that she weighs 14 ounces. That's the size of a cordless phone.

The next few days are filled with pain medication, blood pressure medication, and more ultrasounds. My incision is full of fluid, and someone mentions something about going back to surgery. No way! I just wanna see my baby. I have to get better so I can take care of my baby. Somebody please take me to see my baby, better yet, I'll just get out of this bed and walk over there myself. I'm a SURVIVOR. I walked out of St. Mary's Hospital with my belongings and a prescription for Procardia (a blood pressure medication) a week and a half after delivering my 14 oz baby and a near-death experience. Aliyah, on the other hand, had a long way to go.

Being born so early due to preeclampsia and HELLP syndrome caused

Liyah to be very premature; her lungs and all her other organs were just not strong enough, but I wasn't blessed with a wimp. She fought, oh boy did she fight. Most new moms take their babies home and spend the next few weeks recovering: sleepless nights, frequent feedings, etc. I, on the other hand, spent the next seven weeks making trips back and forth to the hospital, sitting at her bedside for hours at a time, singing her songs, reading her stories from her first Bible, praying and telling her she's never going to believe how far God brought her. Laughing at the silly doctors and nurses that were telling me that she may not make it. What did they know? She's doing so well, tolerating breast milk that I faithfully pumped every two hours and brought up to hospital. No one could make me believe that I would never bring her home.

On December 13th, 2004, Liyah surrendered to an illness known as NEC (necrotizing enterocolitis), which is the death of intestinal tissue, primarily affecting premature infants and sick newborns. I often blamed myself, "If I hadn't been such a weirdo, having preeclampsia, she would have never been born early, never developed NEC." During the weeks following Liyah's birth and death, I never really had a chance to think about and dwell on the actual disease, I just knew that I hated the name. I hated the doctor in Tampa who missed all the signs and symptoms that I was displaying at each visit. I hated the fact that I waited so long to come back home to see another doctor. I hated being in the NICU and hearing the doctors and nurses discuss Liyah's condition and then mention mine, as if to say, "It's her fault." (My thinking at the time.)

I hated the sight of those stupid blood-pressure pills, which I threw in the trash the minute I came home from Liyah's funeral. Liyah is gone; what reason did I have to live? BUT GOD…

Have you ever heard a song, maybe even a verse of a song, and no matter how long ago you heard it or how hard you try to put it out of your memory, it's always there? You wake up humming the lyrics, you find yourself repeating the words, it's always on your mind; well, that's my Liyah, like a song.

I'm always mentioning her name—cautious, up until a few months ago, not to say too much, though, out of fear of someone asking too many questions. I had a fear of being looked at as a freak, I mean, most people like myself have never heard of preeclampsia, let alone dealt with it, so it seems a bit strange for a young woman in perfect health to have experienced something so life-changing. I have so much more to say, there's so much more to my story, but that would take days or maybe even weeks and months to get it all out. One day I'll get around to it—oh yes, I would love to share with the world my struggle and walk that began on December 13th, 2004.

It has not been easy; I'm sure there's someone out there who needs to know the power of prayer, the meaning of family and unconditional love. Someone needs to know that there is a light at the end of the tunnel and a rainbow after every storm. In the meantime, I'll just continue to share Tayler, my miracle baby. The one that wasn't discovered for $10\frac{1}{2}$ weeks. The little girl that came seven weeks early, due to another round of preeclampsia, my RAINBOW after my STORM. I've also been inspired to join a wonderful cause, to be a voice for other mothers and infants affected by preeclampsia, eclampsia, and HELLP syndrome, both those alive and those who have passed on. I'm inspired, and I plan on doing my part. I'm going to continue to sing "Liyah's Song," and my prayer is that this small bit of my story will inspire you to join the cause and sing along with me.

Story is courtesy of the Preeclampsia Foundation. For more stories or information or to donate to the cause, please visit www.preeclampsia.org.

The Story of a Woman Full of Strength and Determination—Erin's Story
By Kelly Whitehead

As I walk into your hospital room, I become you at that moment.
My senses react. I'm sorry, but I can't help myself.
I cry for you ... you are only 25 weeks and
you shouldn't be here ... again, no less.
Your body has failed you ... again.
I cry because I understand what it's like for
your own body to turn against you.
I understand the fear and sadness that is
swimming around in your mind.
Your dreams of a low-stress natural birth, a celebration,
and a big plump baby are shattered,
a million miles away from that dark hospital room.
You are only 25 weeks.
And I know what the future can hold for
such a tiny, precious being.

But you, unlike me, are so calm and assured.
Not a mess or an emotional wreck.
How can that be?
I am so impressed by your strength and faith.
I need to pull it together, and fast.
I am so sorry for you having to be in that bed, hooked up to
tubes and monitors, unsure of what the future holds.
Not you, though.
You are happy and grateful that your baby is
still alive and well…kicking and moving.
Grateful for every moment he stays inside.

26 weeks, and I am frozen in time.
Filled with fear and scared. Really, really scared.
I can't get over how small this little guy is.
I look at his fingernails, making a teardrop look big.
His tiny penis, no bigger than my pinkie nail.
His miniscule arms and legs flail about.
His immature lungs strain in an attempt to make noise.
Pissed at the world to be out in the cold before he is ready.
Words cannot accurately describe the
effect of seeing a baby so small.
He is strong, and he is starting his existence with a fight.
More so, a battle for his very life.
The shock of his tiny body is much too real.
The memories of my own son, who died before
he had the chance to fight, slam into my brain,
as well as thoughts of your angel son.

Not this little guy, though.
The washcloth-sized blanket,
which can be wrapped around his body,
will be a source of stories for him when he is grown.
Through the shock and the tears
of those in the room where he lies,
tears we try to hide mom from seeing.
Hours after being taken from the womb of his mother…
there is hope.
Lots of hope and laughter at his bright future.

His mom, who has yet to glance upon or
touch her precious son,
is two floors below.
Recovering from and digesting the past week's events.
She hopes, and has faith, that he will be prevail.
Still grateful that at least he is alive.
And triumph over his battle he does.
A true miracle of life!

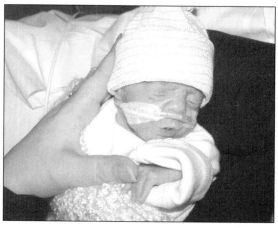

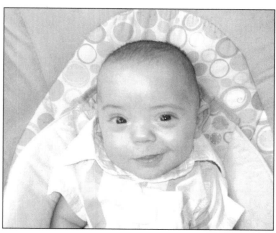

Baby James. Born on January 15, 2010, at 26
weeks, weighing 1 lb 9 oz. He celebrated his
first birthday as a "normal" one-year-old.

Key Abbreviations

BMI	Body mass index
BV	Bacterial Vaginosis
CL	Cervical length
FDA	Food and Drug Administration
FFN	Fetal fibronectin
IC	Incompetent Cervix
IUGR	Intrauterine growth restriction
OB	Obstetrician
PTB	Preterm birth
PPROM	Preterm premature rupture of membranes
PROM	Premature rupture of membranes
PTL	Preterm labor
ROM	Rupture of membranes
SPTB	Spontaneous preterm birth
STL	Second trimester loss
TAC	Transabdominal cerclage
TVC	Transvaginal cerclage

Index

"Lean On Me"
pregnancy and birth coaching services

A note from author Kelly Whitehead...

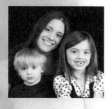

- *Like the idea of having your own personal one-on-one high-risk pregnancy advisor?*
- *Someone to turn to for answers, reassurance and a friendly voice of experience?*
- *Someone who can help develop a birth plan that fits you and your circumstances?*

You're nervous and stressed about your pregnancy. You suspect it may be high-risk, but don't know where to turn to for information and support. Your doctor is great, but 10-minute office visits just aren't enough time to cover your concerns and calm your nerves. You want someone you can call on for more dedicated attention....

Someone like me, Kelly Whitehead....

- Who's been where you are, multiple times, and knows exactly what you're going through...
- Who's recognized as an "expert resource" on the subject of high-risk pregnancy
- Who can guide you through what to expect during your high-risk pregnancy, and, along the way, offer insights, advice, encouragement, tips, etc.
- Who you can vent to, commiserate with, and lean on throughout this experience
- Who understands all the ins and outs of maximizing the doctor/patient relationship
- Who can discuss your birth-plan options (there are a lot more than you may realize!), and help you develop the one best suited to you...
- Who's trained as a doula (labor assistant) and has performed that role for many families

Disclaimer: I am not a doctor. I do not dispense medical advice. On all issues requiring a professional medical opinion, I will refer you to your doctor.

*Due to work and family demands, I am accepting only a limited number of "Lean on Me" coaching clients.

Pregnancy can be one of the most joyous and stressful periods of your life. But, you don't have to go through it alone. When it gets too overwhelming, lean on me.* For full details (rates, terms, and availability of services) of the "Lean on Me" program, please visit:

www.hrpwhyme.com/leanonme

Quick Order Form

High-Risk Pregnancy—Why Me?
Understanding and Managing a Potential Preterm Pregnancy
A Medical and Emotional Guide

Email Orders: orders@hrpwhyme.com

Website Orders: www.hrpwhyme.com (credit card or PayPal accepted)

Mail Orders (Checks or Credit Cards):
Evolve Publishing, Attention: Orders, PO Box 276, McAfee, NJ 07428-0276

Name:_____

Address:_____

City:_____ State:_____ Zip:_____

Telephone Number:_____ Email _____

Credit Card Info:
Type: _____Visa _____ MasterCard

Name on Card:_____

Card Number:_____ Exp. Date:_____

Security Code:_____ [3 digit code (front)]

Billing Zip Code (if different from above):_____

# of Books/Total Cost:
    1 book ($26.95) + $2.82 shipping= $29.77
    2 books ($53.90) + $3.23 shipping= $57.13

International orders: email for shipping rates

For bulk orders of more than 2 books, or for those interested in reselling, see website www.hrpwhyme.com or email orders@hrpwhyme.com for discounts/terms available.

Sales Tax:
Please add 7% sales tax (or $1.89 per book) to orders shipping to New Jersey addresses. (Sorry… the government has to get their share of the pie!)

Westminster Public Library
3705 W. 112th Ave.
Westminster, CO 80031
www.westminsterlibrary.org